A Bold Profession

Women in Africa and the Diaspora

STANLIE M. JAMES AND AILI MARI TRIPP

Founding Editors

A BOLD PROFESSION

African Nurses in Rural Apartheid South Africa

Leslie Anne Hadfield

THE UNIVERSITY OF WISCONSIN PRESS

The University of Wisconsin Press
728 State Street, Suite 443
Madison, Wisconsin 53706
uwpress.wisc.edu

Gray's Inn House, 127 Clerkenwell Road
London ECIR 5DB, United Kingdom
eurospanbookstore.com

Copyright © 2021
The Board of Regents of the University of Wisconsin System
All rights reserved. Except in the case of brief quotations embedded in critical articles
and reviews, no part of this publication may be reproduced, stored in a retrieval system,
transmitted in any format or by any means—digital, electronic, mechanical,
photocopying, recording, or otherwise—or conveyed via the internet or a website
without written permission of the University of Wisconsin Press. Rights inquiries
should be directed to rights@uwpress.wisc.edu.

Printed in the United States of America
This book may be available in a digital edition.

Library of Congress Cataloging-in-Publication Data

Names: Hadfield, Leslie Anne, author.
Title: A bold profession : African nurses in rural apartheid South Africa /
Leslie Anne Hadfield.
Other titles: Women in Africa and the diaspora.
Description: Madison, Wisconsin : The University of Wisconsin Press, [2021] |
Series: Women in Africa and the diaspora | Includes bibliographical
references and index.
Identifiers: LCCN 2020035411 | ISBN 9780299331207 (cloth)
Subjects: LCSH: Women nurses—South Africa—History—20th century. |
Nurses, Black—South Africa—History—20th century. |
Rural nurses—South Africa—History—20th century. |
Nursing—South Africa—History—20th century.
Classification: LCC RT14.S6 H33 2021 | DDC 610.73/430968—dc23
LC record available at https://lccn.loc.gov/2020035411

ISBN 9780299331245 (paperback)

*To health care workers everywhere
who give their lives
to their people.*

Contents

	List of Illustrations	ix
	Acknowledgments	xi
	Introduction	3
1	Medical Systems and the Rise of African Nursing	20
2	The Politics of Ciskei Homeland Health Care	49
3	Remembering Clinic Work	74
4	Engaging Xhosa Beliefs and Practices	112
5	Negotiating Marriage and Family Relations	144
	Conclusion	173
	Notes	185
	Bibliography	239
	Index	255

Illustrations

MAP 1	South African apartheid homelands	xiii
MAP 2	Consolidated Ciskei	xiv
MAP 3	Ciskei health districts: hospitals and clinics	xv
FIGURE 1	Ander's Mission ·	42
FIGURE 2	"One of our rivals—with his 'dispensary'"	45
FIGURE 3	Ciskeian Nursing Association emblem	71
FIGURE 4	Qibirha clinic	78
FIGURE 5	District clinic building sketches	82
FIGURE 6	Gxulu clinic	85
FIGURE 7	"No tarred roads here!"	89
FIGURE 8	Sister V. V. Matthews attending to antenatal patients	103
FIGURE 9	*Imvo Zabantsundu* classifieds	118
FIGURE 10	*Imvo Zabantsundu* advertisement	119
FIGURE 11	A leading herbalist	134
FIGURE 12	Group of *amagqirha*	135

Acknowledgments

This project started with an interview I had with Nontsikelelo Biko and her neighbor Zotshi Mcako in December 2008. I had asked Mam Biko if I could interview her to gain a sense of what it was like to work as a nurse in the area around King William's Town as I completed research for my first book, *Liberation and Development: Black Consciousness Community Programs in South Africa* (2016). She invited her neighbor and longtime Ginsberg clinic nurse Mam Zotshi to meet with me as well at her house in Ginsberg. At the end of the interview, they told me that if I wanted to interview more nurses, they could introduce me to members of the King William's Town Retired Nurses' Association, which they had just formed. Many more meetings, introductions, interviews, and research trips later, I have Mam Biko and Mam Zotshi to thank for putting me on this path and for their continued support and care throughout the whole journey. *Ndibamba ngazibini mama bam.*

Many others have contributed significantly along the way. I cannot adequately thank each one here but acknowledge with gratitude the role of certain individuals in particular. First and foremost, I want to thank all those who graciously gave of themselves by granting me an interview. Each one has a valuable story, pieces of which have been captured in the historical record where I hope more will learn from them. Some also helped with referrals, visits to historic sites, and donations of written material. Some passed away before the book was completed. Along with Mam Biko and Mam Zotshi, the late Buyiswa Tunyiswa Vakalisa (Mam Vaks) acted as a research partner, introducing me to retired nurses' associations in Middledrift (Xesi) and Alice, traveling with me to villages and towns unfamiliar to me to conduct interviews, and supporting my efforts to gain feedback. She loved history. I hope she is pleased with this final product.

It was Fundiswa Mnyaiza who introduced me to Mam Vaks on a Saturday morning run around Xesi. This is just one example of how much Fundiswa and her whole household supported me and furthered my research over the years. I could not have done it without them, not least because they repeatedly provided me with a home in King. Fundiswa, Siyabu, Wathitha, Sama, I hope you all know how much you mean to me. Lungisa Jack was part of the Mnyaiza household for a time. Lungie deserves special thanks for acting as a research assistant at the Cory Library, traveling to Rabula and Gxulu, sifting through dusty old files at the old Ann Shaw clinic, and—though we would rather have not needed to—giving me firsthand experience helping someone seek health care in the Eastern Cape. And as always, the Sihlalo and Pumla Booi family continued to support me in many ways, but I especially appreciated my discussions with Dr. Sino Booi and former nurse Pum Pum as I worked on this project.

Archival and academic institutions also provided valuable assistance and insights. This research was almost entirely funded by Brigham Young University, through grants, awards, and leaves from the Women's Research Initiative, the College of Family Home and Social Sciences, the Kennedy Center for International Studies, and my own Department of History. I would also like to thank individuals and archives such as Koleka Jadezweni and colleagues at the Eastern Cape Archives and Records Service in King William's Town, Cornelius Thomas at the Cory Library at Rhodes University, Ammi Ryke at the Unisa Library Archives, Stephanie Victor at the Amathole Museum, Pratima Chitnis and Eunice Seekoe with health sciences at the University of Fort Hare, Luvuyo Wotshela at Fort Hare's National Heritage and Cultural Studies Center, and Glynis Smith at East London's *Daily Dispatch*. Mwelela Cele first helped at the Killie Campbell Africana Library, then as a friend and archivist at the Steve Biko Center in Ginsberg. The Center and its staff continue to lend their support to my research pursuits, including hosting the dialogue I held with retired nurses. Thanks go to Sifiso Nldovu as well for his continued advice and help. Research assistants and friends helped me balance my teaching and research while still advancing the project. Hannah Matheson, Scott Catt, and Charissa Pincock did the first interview transcriptions, and Krissy Scott helped with indexing. Justina Grubb became the "MVP," transcribing the bulk of the interviews and maternity registers and sharing her public health perspective. Chase Phillips and Garrett Nagaishi helped with Ciskei records on microfiche. (Chase was also my running buddy in King in 2013.) Last but not least, Hlumela Sondlo and Lindani Ntenteni came through in a pinch with hours of translation work on newspaper articles. *Ndiyabulela kwakhona Mama.* I am also grateful to anonymous reviewers and friends who gave feedback on drafts and Dennis Lloyd for all his good work with the publication process.

Finally, people who provide moral and intellectual support and just make life better all help complete a work such as this. I have thanked many of you already. I also believe in a higher power whose hand has been in this work and in creating this support network. I am grateful for all this and say thank you to all my dear family, friends, and colleagues in South Africa, Utah, and beyond.

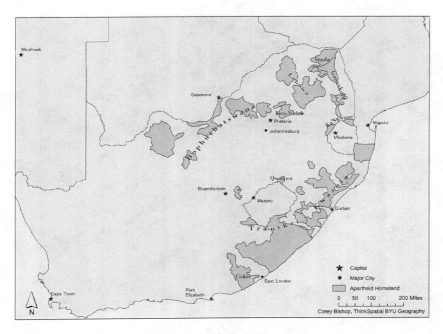

Map 1. South African apartheid homelands

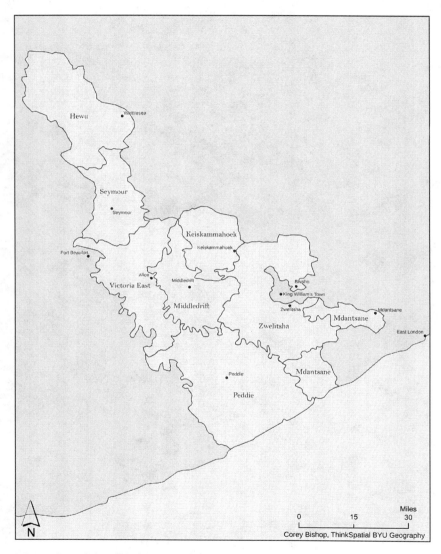

Map 2. Consolidated Ciskei

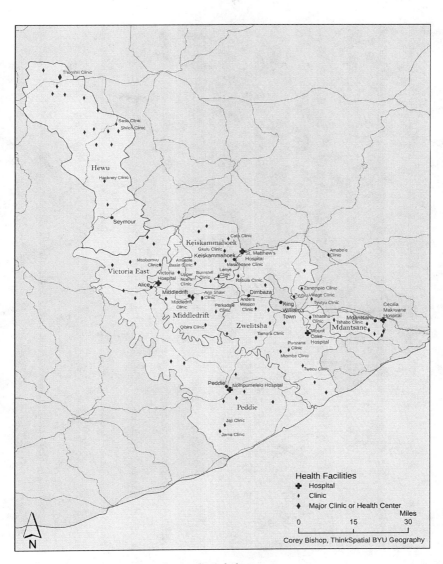

Map 3. Ciskei health districts: hospitals and clinics

A BOLD PROFESSION

Introduction

It's a bold profession. Dealing with people's lives is something very, very important.

—BUYISWA V. VAKALISA

And if you are *kwezaa* rural clinics, you are all by yourself there. You have got to be sure of yourself. You have got to know exactly what to do and what you are doing. Nobody is going to help you, that's the thing.

—THEMBISA E. NKONKI

The successes? As I say, . . . the side I liked most was maternity. Ever since I did that maternity, I never had a death. . . . Even if it's a twin delivery, I never had a death. That was my success.

—LINDA E. NGORO

I would think I would tell them that nursing is not a job. It's a calling. Because we have to endure so much. And when you are a nurse, . . . it must be within you.

—PHOLISA N. MAJIZA

BY THE MID-TWENTIETH CENTURY, Black female African nurses such as Vakalisa, Nkonki, Ngoro, and Majiza had become the backbone of rural health care systems in South Africa. Less concentrated in numbers, nurses working in the largely rural apartheid homelands nevertheless at times made up half the African nurses employed in South Africa throughout the 1970s.[1] As the majority of health practitioners in rural mission hospitals and a growing number of clinic outposts, nurses occupied a crucial position in both the health care system and in the communities where they worked. Their stories illuminate significant forces at work at the intersection of politics, health care, and gender in regions with some of today's most difficult health care challenges. They show how politics and a gendered profession shaped the context within which these nurses worked, yet they also demonstrate how the nurses acted—autonomously and with great success at times—to deliver

Western biomedical care and to influence notions of health and healing in rural communities. As the apartheid government adopted a more diffused comprehensive health care approach in the homelands, the Ciskei region of the Eastern Cape relied more and more on Black female clinic nurses to reach remote rural villages. Working intimately with rural communities, these nurses succeeded in delivering biomedical care because of their training, commitment, and approach to working with, rather than against, Xhosa practices and beliefs. They gave their lives to this demanding work while attempting to fulfill their family responsibilities at a time when all family members confronted changing roles for women.

In ways that have not been explored previously, these nurses' lived experiences reveal significant elements of three major aspects of South African history: the impact of politics on health care, exchanges between medical practices and beliefs, and the intersections of the careers and family lives of professional African women. First, in a place with a large public health system, various forms of government molded the system over time. While the political basis for apartheid homelands was flawed, desires to ensure a healthy Black population with limited resources meant that the apartheid government imposed a streamlined, comprehensive public health care system in the homelands. These systems relied on nurses acting as committed officials and skilled practitioners to sustain and extend them. Following this model, the Ciskei in particular succeeded in increasing the number and quality of its facilities, reaching many communities with comprehensive care and curbing some diseases. Improvements did not mean that the region met the ideal. Apartheid and Ciskeian politics made the impact limited and uneven. Yet politics also had its limitations. Nurses acted within the larger system with some autonomy to prevent, cure, and deliver. Second, the nurses' lived experiences show how Africans from the same ethnic group understood, used, and contested various medical systems while interacting with each other. Many Ciskei nurses worked with Xhosa beliefs, motivating patients to take treatments from both systems, while also using health education to change what they viewed as detrimental practices. Their approach helps explain how both biomedical and Xhosa systems adapted and persisted at the same time, even if nurses sought to change one more than the other. Third, taking into account the full lives of these women, this history provides a fuller understanding of the gendered considerations affecting their work and the hidden struggles and successes of twentieth-century professional African women. With their demanding careers that rarely accommodated family concerns, nurses often struggled to balance their work with their family responsibilities. This included negotiating gender roles in marriage as they moved into a relatively new role for women. Their stories demonstrate that changes in marriage expectations came unevenly, and the ability of a nurse to succeed in nurturing both her community and her family was largely dependent on the family support she had. The family lives of nurses in turn influenced the delivery of health care to some degree by affecting staffing and the quality of care individual nurses offered.

At a time when South African public health care struggles to maintain adequate resources and public nurses have a reputation for disrespecting patients, the positive aspects of this history may be surprising—even more so when some realize they occurred during apartheid. Historians are becoming more open to exploring the complexities of apartheid history that go beyond strong anti-apartheid political judgments, in part because of how those complexities can explain and inform current challenges. Other nations confront similar difficulties in ensuring their people gain access to quality health care, an issue brought to the fore by rapidly spreading global pandemics. Some debate instituting national health insurance and the role of so-called traditional medical practitioners, while others struggle to provide basic, well-equipped health care in urban and rural areas. The COVID-19 pandemic particularly highlighted in South Africa the importance of well-trained, compensated, and supported health workers who can deliver primary care in communities.[2] The complex history of rural South African nurses, as largely informed by those who worked on the ground, deserves closer scrutiny, as it offers insights into dealing with these challenges, including ways to provide health care to rural communities and to support and draw upon skilled women.

South African Nursing and Apartheid Homeland History

South Africa experienced intense political and social change during the 1960s through the 1980s. The Afrikaner Nationalist Party intensified racial segregation after its electoral victory in 1948 and increasingly implemented plans to engineer society for the benefit of white South Africans in the 1960s. Racial segregation shaped many aspects of society, including economic and educational opportunities and the provision of health care. This left Black populations gravely disadvantaged, evidenced by significantly higher infant mortality rates, higher rates of disease, shorter life expectancies, and astonishing discrepancies in doctor-to-population ratios: in 1972, 1:400 for white people, 1:900 for Indians, 1:6,200 for Coloured people, and 1:44,400 for Africans.[3] In the 1960s the apartheid state also increasingly suppressed Black opposition. The state declared opposition groups such as the African National Congress (ANC) and the Pan Africanist Congress illegal and jailed their leaders, forced them underground, or drove them into exile. At the same time, Black economic and educational opportunities expanded to include more and more people in a growing Black middle class, even those working in segregated professions. The apartheid state capitalized on this as it sought to implement "grand apartheid"—a scheme to separate and contain the different ethnic groups in South Africa by turning regions designated for specific groups into independent countries, referred to as "homelands."[4] This required a class of Black professionals and a civil work force—including many nurses—which the apartheid state hoped to lure into accepting the new system. Although the international community never accepted apartheid homelands as legitimate, Black politicians in these regions saw grand apartheid as an opportunity to gain power and resources and, in part, to elevate their people. They persisted in building their supposed independent countries even as popular resistance to apartheid intensified in the mid-1970s and 1980s and anti-apartheid forces infiltrated some of their structures. For example, the Transkei was the first to gain independence in 1976, the same year students in Soweto led uprisings against apartheid education and the year before apartheid security forces detained and killed Black Consciousness leader Steve Biko. The Ciskei gained independence in 1981, just a few years before the founding of the United Democratic Front in 1983 and before South Africa declared states of emergency in the mid-1980s. Apartheid homelands would struggle to obtain political stability until their official dissolution after the first fully democratic elections in South Africa in 1994. Yet over their years of existence, they reflected and caused many of the social and political changes South Africans experienced.[5]

Health care and nursing history in South Africa is wrapped up in this apartheid history. While others have examined the national and racial politics of the nursing profession or outlined homeland health care, most have yet to examine critical aspects of rural homeland health care and the significant work and lives of Black African nurses who worked in those regions. Shula Marks's *Divided Sisterhood* established a baseline for South African nursing history. Her examination of the racial and class divisions within the profession brought Black nurses into its history and exposed the racial discrimination that affected hospitals and national nursing organizations.[6] Yet with her focus on the high politics and development of the profession, certain topics such as patient perceptions, rural district nursing, and the impact nursing careers had on women's personal lives lay outside her purview. Even after scholars and former nurses themselves made further contributions, the critical work and lives of nurses who shaped health and health care on the ground in rural homeland regions is largely missing. Scholars have explored nursing education and delineated milestones in the development of the profession, from the perspective of both the white-dominated professional associations and Black nurses.[7] A number of authors have foregrounded the perspective of African nurses through oral histories,

Introduction

7

autobiographies, and biographies, including some district nursing work.[8] However, these works have focused on urban hospitals, presented life histories without a broader contextualized analysis, and almost entirely ignored nurses' family and marriage considerations. Exceptionally, Anne Digby outlined the overall approach of homeland health care and Elizabeth Hull examined the aspirations and relationships of nurses who worked at a former mission hospital in KwaZulu-Natal; but generally, authors have left out the large number of nurses who worked in homelands.[9] Moreover, a focus on hospitals has excluded important clinical work. Scholars have demonstrated that hospital records and employees make for a focused archive from which to build rich histories; yet nurses' rural clinic work reached a sizable population of South Africans as well.[10] As the first site of contact for many people accessing biomedicine, clinic nurses have a significant place in South African health care history.

The history of nurses working in rural homeland clinics opens a unique lens into the history of health care in South Africa, exchanges between medical systems, and the work and lives of professional African women. Combined with recent works by Simonne Horwitz on the Baragwanath Hospital in Soweto and Hull on the Bethesda Hospital in KwaZulu-Natal, this book helps create a fuller picture of the history of spaces dominated by Black nurses.[11] Yet homeland rural clinic nursing involved different working conditions, patient and community relations, and racial and gender dynamics. For example, in a system largely led by Black Africans, these nurses did not confront racial tensions in their day-to-day work as much as those working in the rest of South Africa. Since doctors visited clinics only a few times a month, the nurses also did not have as many interactions with male, mostly white, doctors.[12] Instead, the nurses I interviewed dealt more with cultural notions about what ailments they could treat as women. This history thus brings to the fore the different levels of autonomy African female nurses had in engaging and shaping different medical practices and beliefs as well as leveraging their skill and limited resources. This includes the delicate work of interacting with communities and patients and the interplay between nurses' careers and their family lives.

Concentrating on the Ciskei to understand rural homeland nursing is instructive and appropriate. Like other apartheid homelands, the Ciskei emphasized comprehensive and preventive health care and increased the number of professionals in order to staff more clinics. Although it had more financial resources than many of the others, the Ciskei still faced similar challenges of implementation, with a lack of doctors, financial deficits, and a comparable infant mortality rate.[13] It is also the region that produced the first female African nurses. A small group of Xhosa women trained as medical aides at the Native Public Hospital (later Grey Hospital) in King William's Town in the

8 Introduction

1850s, and Cecilia Makiwane became the first registered African nurse in 1908 after training at the Victoria Hospital in Alice. These two places became some of the major focal points of the region. Historically, the Ciskei referred to the area between the Kei and Fish Rivers occupied by the Xhosa. This area was indeed at one point the heart of a Xhosa chieftainship (the Ngqika), but various groups of what are now collectively referred to as the Xhosa lived farther west of the Fish River and farther east of the Kei. It was in the more western regions that the Xhosa first encountered Afrikaner farmers and cattle herders migrating east, then battled the British for control over their land. King William's Town later served as a center of the British colonial government that reshaped and divided Xhosa chiefdoms into administrative districts. Beginning in the 1960s, the apartheid government prepared the territory for self-government as an independent nation. It reorganized the local government authority and instituted various stages of bureaucratic control. In the 1970s the South African Department of Health began to implement comprehensive health care in the homelands. By 1975 the government had consolidated the land of the Ciskei territory and established a Department of Health and Welfare that continued to emphasize comprehensive health care after Ciskeian official independence in 1981. Thus the Ciskei serves as a representative example of homeland and rural health care in an area with a long history of African nursing.

Details of Ciskei health care history not found elsewhere provide important context to rethinking nursing and apartheid history. A previous neglect of this rural homeland history may be partly explained by the fact that in the past, writing histories that took apartheid homeland institutions seriously was politically unthinkable. Activists, scholars, and the international community recognized homelands as highly problematic apartheid projects. Eventually granting independence to ten apartheid homelands meant the apartheid government could contain Black Africans to 13 percent of the country's land while still benefiting from Black labor. This released the South African government from providing social services to those areas and led to the relocation of thousands of people. Many people in the Ciskei already suffered from the effects of migrant labor and a decrease in agricultural sustainability. Forced relocations to the Ciskei made these conditions worse. Rural poverty and corrupt leaders were clear evidence of apartheid homeland failures. For example, scholars of the Ciskei Les Switzer, Jeff Peires, and Luvuyo Wotshela examined the homeland's underdevelopment, corruption, and political and territorial reorganization that sparked resistance.[14] Peires forcefully wrote of widespread election abuses, clientelist networks, and ethnic politics that led to the "implosion" of the Ciskei and Transkei, claiming that the two regions "never achieved even the first prerequisite of government control, namely legitimacy."[15] Switzer discussed

Introduction 9

the implications homeland policies had for the health of the region. Understandably, impoverished people in the Ciskei suffered ill-health, especially those who ended up in relocation camps.[16] Estimates of the infant mortality rate for Africans in the Republic of South Africa in the 1960s and 1970s ranged from 140 to 180 deaths per 1,000 births, with a much worse rate for the Ciskei in the early 1980s at an estimated 250 per 1,000 births.[17] Authors decried the poor infrastructure of the health care system, the lack of personnel and supplies, and poor ambulance services.[18] Switzer wrote that the Ciskei had half the minimum number of beds per Africans set by South Africa's Department of Health and a ratio of 1 doctor to every 8,707 people.[19] It is no wonder that liberation movements condemned homelands as "a ploy to give apartheid credibility," and activists and scholars worked to expose the charade.[20] Wotshela has documented the intense local movements that challenged the Ciskei state's power from the beginning, showing that it met resistance from many sides almost constantly.[21]

Greater distance from apartheid has opened up the possibility of recognizing the more complex legacy of the homelands. In what scholars such as Daniel Magaziner, Catherine Burns, and others have characterized as "post-antiapartheid" scholarship, Meghan Healy-Clancy described historians as focusing less on the spectacular and more on the politics of everyday lives.[22] Recent scholarship on apartheid homelands has taken this turn. William Beinart argued in 2012 that it was time to go "beyond homelands," that it was time "to think about this phase in a longer perspective and, equally important, to discuss the history of these rural areas partly through analytical lenses that are not necessarily dominated by a critique of 'homeland' policy."[23] Beinart went on to discuss what we might learn from studying homeland links to other local and national dynamics, the cultural space even poor rural areas enjoyed, and homeland class formation. For him, looking at homeland history in a longer historical trajectory opened up possibilities for understanding legacies of popular resistance, patterns of government funding, and agricultural and environmental practices. Steffen Jensen and Olaf Zenker similarly argued in 2015 that homeland history greatly illuminates issues of land tenure and reform. They asserted that the loose ends of apartheid more particularly manifest themselves in former homelands, where the "dilemmas of post-apartheid South Africa are particularly acute," adding even more importance to examining homeland history.[24] Articles in the special journal issues wherein Beinart, Jensen, and Zenker's work appeared along with subsequent work shows that looking at the continuities and changes in the provision of social services across the temporal divides of apartheid can be instructive.[25] For example, while few retired nurses I interviewed spoke about HIV/AIDS as the epidemic did not fully manifest itself in the region until the 1990s, the nurses' work in communities prior to that laid a foundation for addressing that challenge in those communities. Indeed, the homelands were more than just corrupt politicians and their cronies or poor dehumanized people. There is much more to explore in the history of the people who lived through the homeland eras and the various processes that played out in different regions. Temporal distance allows us to see the intricacies of those places more clearly and to more seriously consider the important systems and everyday aspects of life in these regions.

Of course, those who lived through the homelands and currently reside in former homeland regions have little choice but to live with that historical complexity. It no longer surprises me to hear someone staying in the King William's Town area who opposed apartheid also point to achievements of L. L. Sebe, the former president of the Ciskei. People often hold up Bhisho as an example—the former Ciskeian capital and now administrative center of the Eastern Cape, with its (small) block of high-rise government buildings. Nurses I interviewed likewise acknowledged the problematic basis of the homelands while at the same time appreciating what the system gave them and the people they served. At a meeting I held with retired nurses wherein I presented this research, one nurse commented that she "had to say the homeland system on its own was bad" because of the segregation it enforced; yet it also gave them room to achieve as Black nurses. She continued: "But great strides were made because now, here we were in a position to have our officials now, independent and progressive, I can say."[26] A nurse who became the matron overseeing disaster management at the hospital in Mthatha held a similar sentiment. Lulu Msutu Zuma had been involved with the ANC Youth League as a student at the Lovedale Mission Hospital in the late 1950s. She made it clear that she did not approve of the homelands ("We are some of the people who didn't want to hear a thing about those governments. We wanted the real thing [democracy]."). At the same time, she counted her time as a matron as the highlight of her career. Under apartheid segregation in the Republic of South Africa, she had ideas to contribute, but racial discrimination meant that her suggestions and those of her Black colleagues remained ignored. In the Transkei, on the other hand, she could plan and do things. People believed in her and she had resources. "If there's a place that gave me a chance to display my capabilities and skills it was Transkei," she said.[27] Thus, while it may seem that the homeland system did succeed in co-opting Black nurses, not all of them had the wool pulled over their eyes. As Hull has argued, when analyzing homeland health care we need to see the limits of apartheid state power and recognize that, within the layers of the system, nurses exercised a degree of autonomy in the way they carried out their work and the way they understood and molded their place in the system.[28]

Introduction

Largely focused on the delivery of health care experienced by these retired nurses in an apartheid homeland, this history requires us to accept this complexity. It requires us to recognize that nurses who worked in the "independent" Ciskei were not immediately confronted with racial tensions in their everyday life, even if apartheid formed the backdrop to the system within which they worked. It asks us to acknowledge that while the Ciskei state had a problematic foundation and became unsustainable, the paradoxical, simultaneous expansion of clinics, subclinics, and mobile clinics meant that many homelands ended up with "more favorable ratios—in having fewer people to clinics—than did three out of four South African provinces."[29] As Horwitz and Jacob Dlamini demonstrate, improvements were at times made to some institutions during apartheid, and people have expressed fond memories of apartheid times. Delving deeper into the explanations behind these developments and nostalgia for apartheid times reveals the complex forces at work in both the past and the present and offers more meaningful lessons for the future.[30] In the case of Ciskei rural nursing history, delving deeper uncovers the failures and achievements of the health care system in the past as well as the dynamics of encounters between medical systems and the work and struggles of key women.

Medical Encounters

The relatively recent work of scholars has challenged us to shift the way we understand African medical systems in relation to other systems. Patient pluralism in seeking healing from various sources has long garnered the attention of anthropologists and historians.[31] Rather than focusing on the clashes between the two, historians have more recently emphasized the exchanges and mutual evolution between biomedicine and African medical systems in the past. The Comaroffs characterized encounters between the Tswana and Christian missionaries in the nineteenth century as a dialectical conversation that changed everyone involved.[32] Scholars such as Anne Digby and Helen Sweet, Barbara Mann Wall, Karen Flint, Ruth Prince and Rebecca Marsland, David Baranov, and David Gordon have taken a similar approach in examining exchange rather than competition.[33] Their work has demonstrated that Africans have not simply been passive recipients of coercive colonial medical campaigns or European visions of health and health care but have sought out and engaged biomedicine in various ways. Furthermore, Flint and Gordon have reminded us that the history of the relationship between different biomedicine practitioners and African practitioners took different turns depending on the contours of the broader context.[34] Overall, these perspectives have more fully portrayed Africans, as Wall has argued, not as "passive recipients of a foreign culture" but people with their own objectives who have at times helped create hybrid practices, as Nancy Rose Hunt has also demonstrated.[35]

Scholars have also more fully· acknowledged the cultural, political, and social construction of biomedicine, African influences on biomedicine, and the similarities between African and Western biomedicine. Baranov in particular challenged the concept of African medicine as devoid of science and biomedical elements, arguing for the use of the term "African biomedicine" to more accurately describe the beliefs and practices that have evolved into today's systems across the continent.[36] I use the terms "biomedicine" and "Xhosa medicine" to describe the two main medical systems in the region that I focus on. In doing so, I do not imply that Xhosa medicine has no biomedical elements or that either system has remained static over time. I also recognize that "Xhosa" is a broad identity that can include various groups. These two terms best define the systems in the time and the place on which this history focuses and best illuminate how the two interacted in that context. As Baranov wrote, the disease etiology of the two systems was the primary distinguishing factor between the two. Whereas African healing systems have recognized multiple causes of ill-health ("with a broad spectrum of overlapping forces that intersect the natural, supernatural, and social worlds"), European or Western biomedicine developed a belief that ill-health was strictly caused by natural forces.[37] This difference has led some to define African systems as pluralistic in contrast to a Western biomedical approach focused on one cause of disease. The fact that African medical systems have also long been open to incorporating effective elements of other medical systems has deterred others like Digby from using "traditional" to describe African systems.[38] To reflect the pluralistic and dynamic nature of the healing practices and beliefs of people who lived in the Ciskei region outlined above, I use the term "Xhosa medical systems." Even if Xhosa practitioners added more biomedical elements to a system that already believed in natural causes, the basic worldview and practices of the system persisted, including recognizing multiple causes of ill-health. I use biomedicine mostly without a qualifier for the sake of brevity but also because the basic worldview of the system remained the same even as the practitioners who shaped it changed from European to African or Xhosa.[39]

Since African nurses have often occupied the middle ground between different systems and have dominated the nursing profession on the continent since the late twentieth century, the perspectives of African nurses are especially important to understanding the exchanges between African health practitioners and medical systems. Digby, Sweet, Wall, and Hunt have explored the role of African nurses as cultural brokers who translated biomedicine linguistically and culturally. Wall particularly emphasized the agency of nurses

Introduction   13

who "influenced [biomedicine's] cultural translation" as they acted as "partners, colleagues, or resistors."[40] Yet there is still a need for further investiga-
tion into the work of African nurses in rural communities, where nurses had
close relationships with the people they served and encountered African practitioners and beliefs more than those working in urban centers. Although African medical practitioners work in urban as well as rural areas, people in rural
areas often have just as much or more access to African medicine as they do to
biomedicine. This was true of many places in the Ciskei in the 1960s through
the 1970s. Furthermore, examining the interactions African nurses have had
with African medical practitioners and beliefs allows us to see the complexities
of the exchanges between medical systems within African communities on a
deeper level than when we focus just on the encounters between Africans
and Europeans. While scholars have written about the training of African
traditional birth attendants and village health workers (VHWs), few have, like
Hunt, focused on how biomedically trained African nurses understood, used,
and contested medical beliefs and practices originating from within their own
communities.[41] In the Ciskei, nurses exercised their agency as African practitioners in contesting, sharing, and negotiating Xhosa beliefs. Their approach
to encouraging rather than discouraging their patients ultimately contributed
to the continued coexistence and adaptation of both systems, even as Xhosa
systems may have incorporated more biomedicine than vice versa.

Professional African Women

Skilled and economically empowered professional African women have been
influential historical actors. While historians have investigated the history of
female African economic and political roles, late twentieth-century professional
women have received less attention. Professional women have been included
in a few volumes addressing a range of issues, such as Gudrun Ludwar-Ene
and Mechtild Reh's *Gender and Identity in Africa*; Jean Allman, Susan Geiger,
and Nakanyike Musisi's *Women in Colonial Histories*; and more recent surveys
by Iris Berger and Kathleen Sheldon.[42] A few others have centered their analysis on professional women and their relation to democracy and development
(such as Ifi Amadiume), education and respectability (such as Corrie Decker),
and their entry into certain professions, such as nursing.[43] Yet these works are
few, and the number and influence of professional African women is large.
In the late twentieth century, the number of women entering professions significantly increased with greater education and economic opportunities and
African independence. Nurses have constituted one of the largest groups of
professional African women. As was true for the rest of the continent, nursing and teaching were for some time the only professions widely accepted as

appropriate for African women in South Africa. Moreover, nursing made high demands on a woman's time and resources. As the number of professional African nurses grew in the mid to late twentieth century, more women from diverse socioeconomic backgrounds joined the profession. This meant that more women faced the shifting marriage and family relations that came with entering a professional class than the educated elite of earlier times.[44] The experiences of nurses in the late twentieth century is particularly revealing when exploring how professional women grappled with the demands of work and family life. However, the literature on nurses rarely intersects with the history of marriage and motherhood.[45] Moreover, the history of marriage and motherhood in South Africa has been dominated by histories of the educated African elite of the early twentieth century on the one hand and the struggles of low-wage-earning women and political activists during apartheid on the other. This has left out the important family life of professional Black nurses.[46] Nurses who worked in the Ciskei in the 1960s through 1980s shared many struggles in balancing their professional work and domestic work. Their experiences give us valuable insights into how professional women dealt with the tension between the demands of work and family life while caught in the process of changing gender roles in families and marriages.

Sources and Methodology

To construct this history, I drew upon a myriad of archival sources and original oral history interviews with retired nurses. To understand the larger context, I consulted hospital and government records held in archives in King William's Town, Grahamstown, Cape Town, Johannesburg, and Pretoria. This included the records of three prominent mission hospitals in the region up until government takeover in the mid-1970s: Victoria Hospital at the Lovedale mission in Alice, Mount Coke at the Mount Coke mission station south of King William's Town, and St. Matthew's near Keiskammahoek.[47] To obtain general statistics and track changes over time in the self-governing Ciskei, I consulted Ciskei government records available on microfilm and at the Documentation Center for African Studies at the University of South Africa (UNISA). The annual reports of the Ciskei Department of Health at UNISA proved extremely valuable in providing a picture of the system's aggregate numbers, challenges, and plans. The Ciskei legislative debate transcripts also offered insights into Ciskei politics and health-care-related deliberations. Relying on Ciskeian and mission hospital records is problematic, however. Biomedical and mission biases in the records amounted to the dismissal of Xhosa beliefs and practices at times, while at others, exotic or sensational descriptions of Xhosa systems obscured daily, common practices. Aggregate numbers from just a few short

Introduction 15

years of the Ciskei's brief lifetime also masked local variations, and others had a political agenda to bolster the Ciskei. Furthermore, many Ciskei records were discarded or filed away in various new government offices when it was dissolved in the early 1990s. Current Eastern Cape provincial health offices and facilities focus on maintaining medical records only five years deep. In search of more nuanced and deeper perspectives, I hunted for more local records. With the permission of the Eastern Cape Department of Health, I visited hospitals and a few select clinics; however, searching in clinic closets and through old hospital files only uncovered a few reports and registers. I also consulted contemporary studies and read two local newspapers, the East London *Daily Dispatch* and *Imvo Zabantsundu*, the Xhosa-language paper published in King William's Town. These papers had their own political biases and bent toward the sensational.[48] Along with the other written records, they also required critical analysis. Still, they added valuable different perspectives that helped provide a fuller picture of the context within which Ciskei nurses worked.

Among all these records there are only small glimpses of what the nurses who worked in the Ciskei experienced. For example, Mount Coke Hospital staff files offer information on salaries and proof of employment, but other reports rarely highlight individual nurses or discuss their experiences. This applies to government reports, although some Ciskei Nursing Council publications include biographies of some prominent nurses. Moreover, because of the interest of scholars, record keepers, and researchers in the past, there is very little written evidence of the family life of nurses or how they engaged Xhosa medical practices and beliefs. To understand what Ciskei rural health care looked like on the ground and what it meant personally to those most important to carrying it out, it was necessary to draw on oral history.

Between 2011 and 2013, I conducted interviews with sixty-seven Black female retired nurses who had worked in rural clinics and hospitals throughout the Ciskei region during the 1960s through the 1980s. The sixty-seven I interviewed were a small number of those who worked in the Ciskei (in 1991 alone the Ciskeian Nursing Council counted 3,668 on its register).[49] Even if they do not constitute a valid statistical sample, taken together, their interviews are historically characteristic of the various experiences of African women working in the region during this time. Surviving historical sources do not always allow for statistical accuracy. However, as Joe Lunn discussed in his history of Senegalese World War I veterans, "collective trends are readily discernable" when several different interviewees explicitly attest to them and other actions and sources corroborate them.[50] Such was the case with the interviews I conducted. Trends in responses became overwhelmingly clear as I reached the end of the interviewing process. Nevertheless, I attempted to gain a geographically representative sample of women who worked in rural clinics. For instance, I made sure that I interviewed women with extensive experience in all major districts or hospital catchment areas, with more interviews of those who worked in the larger districts that had more rural clinics.[51] I recruited interviewees through three retired nurses' associations based in King William's Town (the Nightingales), Middledrift, and Alice through other interviewees and through my own friends living in the area.[52] This meant that I interviewed women who had worked in a range of locations and had different training and career trajectories. Almost all the women were Xhosa and had significant ties to rural areas in the former Ciskei (either through their work or family), but they came from different socioeconomic backgrounds. For example, of the fifty-two who talked about their parents' occupations, at least 60 percent said their parents had little education or relied on menial labor or agriculture to make a living.

The process that generated these memories consisted of a combination of my own questioning and the more natural remembering of those I interviewed. I approached the interviews as a history of the woman's career as it related to her broader life history. As feminist historians have argued, to fully understand women's history or allow women to shape the construction of history, we must listen to how women interpret the past in the context of their own full lives, where aspects of everyday life are given considerable consideration.[53] Because I wanted to add a broader analysis of nurses' experiences to anecdotal accounts already existing, I did not conduct full life histories.[54] Yet I worked to conduct the interviews with predominantly open-ended invitations to the women to share with me what they found most important and to include the personal or private aspects of their lives. Feminist history work along with work on the importance of emotion in oral histories influenced me to pay attention to issues relating to a woman's experience, emotion, and meaning.[55] At times I asked about the mundane, at other times I asked about the more outstanding aspects—their challenges, successes, fears, joys, and motivations. Contemporary conditions also provided points of comparison to the past. I was cognizant of the political context within which we spoke, as well as the cross-cultural, racial, linguistic, and class dynamics of the interviews. I am a younger, white American woman who was mostly a stranger. I had to be sensitive to my position as I asked women about cultural practices previously disdained by white societies or about the details of their intimate relationships. Being an ignorant outsider can help one gain information from interviewees, even information an informant knows the outsider could not disclose to anyone close to her; but it can also restrict an interviewee from sharing private information. Also, since most interviewees belonged to one of three retired nurses' associations that

Introduction

celebrated their careers, they may have been more inclined to focus on the positive aspects of nursing in the Ciskei at the expense of more negative aspects. At the time I interviewed the women, nurses in public hospitals had a reputation for treating patients rudely or neglecting patients in favor of striking for better working conditions. The public health care system in the Eastern Cape was often under fire from the media for misuse of funds and failures to deliver on its promises. Some former Ciskei nurses felt slighted by the ANC-led government when they did not receive pensions. In fact, the King William's Town Retired Nurses' Association was founded in part to take care of nurses who felt forgotten by society. This context gave interviewees an urge to reaffirm the standards and respectability of their profession and praise the Ciskei's health care system and former corrupt homeland leaders as "excellent," "wonderful, wonderful, wonderful," and "number one."[56]

With these dynamics in mind, I employed various strategies to probe interviewees and analyze the meaning behind their expressions and the way they remembered the past. These strategies, along with the number of interviews I conducted and the archival evidence I found, combined to help correct for nostalgia and flesh out a more accurate history. For example, I signaled to the nurses that I saw Xhosa medical practices as possibly effective by asking leading questions about the merits of Xhosa medicine. When a woman was reluctant to speak about her own marriage relationship, I asked what she had heard about other nurses. Interviewee personalities, interests, and memories also shape what comes out of interviews, but I asked questions about emotions and motivations to offer the women different avenues of expression. I asked why others would quit and what kept them in the profession. Furthermore, my shared female gender, my younger age, my ability to conduct an interview in Xhosa, and the connections I had with trusted women who referred me to interviewees helped some feel comfortable speaking with me. Nostalgia also is not just an obstacle. The way people remember the past is also telling. For example, comments about how important it was to view nursing as a noble calling as they did in the past were directed more to young nurses at times than they were to me. These comments revealed not only how these nurses felt about the current direction of the profession but also how they had constructed their own professional identity in the past. Remarks about inadequate salaries, the negative effects of their work on their children, and aspects of their work they did not like also demonstrated that the women were willing to talk about the not-so-glamorous aspects of nursing as well. Moreover, complaints about Ciskei politicians interfering with work showed that not all of them harbored loyalty to the Ciskei. Overall, the questions I posed, the memories and interpretations the nurses shared, and analyses of the interviews help

18 Introduction

us understand what was most significant to these women about their careers as lived in the past and as shaped by the present context.

Finally, to gain the most accurate understanding and show respect and gratitude to interviewees, I also sought to involve them in the interpretation process. I gave each woman a copy of her interview almost immediately afterward (mostly in audio format). A few women listened to the interview and later offered further comments. Although I obtained informed consent from each interviewee, I also met with three women to ask for their approval of what I wrote about them. My main effort to gain feedback, however, came when I was drafting the book manuscript. I invited all whom I had interviewed and the three local retired nurses' associations to come to a meeting in Ginsberg (next to King William's Town), where I presented my book and invited their comments and questions. About thirty-five women attended. During this two-hour session, some who had not previously been interviewed added their own experiences and those I had interviewed reminded me of aspects they felt were important to include. I clarified questions I had and sought their feedback on where I should include certain topics. We also discussed the complexities of Ciskeian history and nurses' history. After talking about nurses' challenges in marriage, for instance, one participant remarked that it was good to discuss the negative and the positive of nursing. More than one later commented that our meeting felt like a "debriefing session"—a meeting where they could address previously unspoken issues and make sense of what happened to them in the past. The way this session influenced the history that follows, along with other sources, is highlighted in each chapter.

Chapters

The first two chapters provide important background and contextual information. Chapter 1 presents historical background on Xhosa medicine and the growth of Western biomedicine and African nursing in the Ciskei from the time of British colonialism through the 1950s. The first female Xhosa nurses were trained in the colonial hospital in King William's Town, but mission hospitals took the lead in training African nurses and delivering biomedicine in the rural Ciskei after the turn of the century. The chapter discusses the growth of these hospitals and the training of African nurses throughout this time, while also highlighting biomedicine practitioners' engagement with Xhosa medicine and practitioners. Chapter 2 then outlines the impact of apartheid homeland restructuring on the development of the Ciskei health care system, starting with a new state commitment to extending district services through rural clinics in the 1960s, then charting the adjustments, successes, and challenges of the system through the 1980s. It underlines the growth in comprehensive community

Introduction

19

health care and the Ciskei's problematic political and financial basis and argues that nurses exercised their own agency within the Ciskei system, with a degree of autonomy not necessarily aligned with Ciskei politics.

The next three chapters examine the nurses' experiences, drawing largely on the oral history interviews conducted. Chapter 3 explores what nurses experienced delivering health care from rural clinics as they remembered it years later. As it analyzes memories of the daily grind and dramatic incidents, it highlights the challenges and successes these nurses faced in executing Ciskei health care plans. Nurses handled a myriad of cases, ranging from minor ailments, chronic diseases, and tuberculosis to childhood malnutrition and high-risk maternity cases—all with a lack of personnel and infrastructure. This made for heavy responsibilities that required skill and stamina. Nurses also learned to cultivate good relationships with their patients and their community leaders. The chapter concludes by discussing how the nurses' training and commitment significantly contributed to their success in delivering health care under these circumstances. Chapter 4 focuses on how nurses negotiated, shared, and contested Xhosa medical practices and beliefs. It examines the position of the nurses in relation to the two medical systems and then outlines the different approaches they took to working with rather than against patient beliefs. The chapter also highlights the gendered limitations placed on women working as nurses in rural Xhosa communities. Chapter 5 investigates how nurses' careers intersected with their family lives. It explores how the women balanced home and family responsibilities with their work in a system that did not generally accommodate family concerns. It also examines changing marriage expectations and the impact nurses' careers had on their marriages. While some found that their careers exacerbated or caused marital tensions, others had supporting husbands and extended family members who helped them balance their families and their professional work. It ends with suggestions about how family considerations may have affected staffing and the quality of care individual nurses offered.

The book concludes with a brief description of the end of the Ciskei, the challenges of transitioning the health care system into the postapartheid era, and an analysis of the nurses' dissatisfaction with the nursing profession in the democratic era. It also presents messages the nurses I interviewed had for present-day nurses and the current health care system. Ultimately, these nurses played a leading role in providing critical health services and influencing health and healing in their communities. This examination of their life experiences changes South African history by providing a more analytical and detailed understanding of a critical aspect of South African health care, deepening the history of exchanges between different medical systems and revealing the intersecting dynamics of a group of influential professional African women.

CHAPTER ONE

Medical Systems and the Rise of African Nursing

In January 1908, Cecilia Makiwane became the first registered African professional nurse on the African continent. Makiwane and her sisters were some of the first young women from the Xhosa Christian elite in the Ciskei region to attend the Lovedale Girls' School and the Lovedale Missionary Institute in the town of Alice. Makiwane's father, Reverend Elijah Makiwane, was a teacher and the second Black minister to be trained by the Presbyterian Church in South Africa. Her mother, Margaret Majiza, taught at the Lovedale Girls' School until her death at an early age in 1883. Reverend Makiwane subsequently ensured his daughters received a good education. Cecilia earned a teacher's certificate before training at the Lovedale mission's Victoria Hospital and qualifying as a registered nurse. Her oldest sister, Daisy, was the first African woman to pass the matriculation exam in mathematics. Another sister, Thandiswa Florence, taught at Lovedale before studying music in England.[1]

It is no wonder that the first registered African nurse came from the Lovedale mission. The institute provided the education necessary for young African women to continue on to further training and education, and the hospital was at the forefront of the mission hospital movement in South Africa. With Cecilia Makiwane's achievement as its chronological center, this chapter explores the history of the African women who came before and after Makiwane in the nursing profession as they fit in the Ciskei context. African female nurses became important actors in delivering biomedicine in the region throughout an ebb and flow of state- versus mission-driven medical systems. The views of certain hospital superintendents as well as the impact of British-Xhosa conflicts paved the way for the training of female African or Xhosa nurses as the British established their colonial government in the Eastern Cape in the mid to late nineteenth century. Around the turn of the century, mission hospitals

Medical Systems and the Rise of African Nursing

such as Victoria took the lead in training African nurses, as missions became highly invested in providing health care intertwined with Christianity to rural African populations. Mission hospitals continued to train African nurses into the 1940s and 1950s, a time when African nursing in the Ciskei became linked to the national history of nursing in South Africa, more tied to the state, and influenced by broader politics.

This all unfolded against the backdrop of Xhosa medical practices and beliefs already in the region. In the Ciskei, interactions between Xhosa medicine and Western biomedical institutions began with British encroachment in the region and shifted throughout the rise in African nursing. Although some biomedical doctors were more open to certain Xhosa practices in earlier years, colonial officials and mission doctors and nurses subsequently sought to counteract Xhosa beliefs and practices. Xhosa and Western biomedical understandings of the causes of ill-health differed fundamentally, with the Xhosa believing in multiple causes of ill-health and Western biomedicine offering increasingly rigid explanations focused on natural causes. African nurses, especially those trained in mission hospitals, undoubtedly adopted a similar approach to European doctors and nurses to some degree; however, evidence suggests that Xhosa practitioners of both healing systems left more room for accommodation and adaptation than Europeans throughout.

Xhosa Healing Practices and Beliefs

Europeans brought Western biomedicine into a region with its own established medical system. It is difficult for historians to accurately describe Xhosa medical systems as they existed in the late eighteenth and early nineteenth centuries. Historical records written by colonial officials, missionaries, settlers, and anthropologists are problematic, with their biases and limited understandings. As Europeans attempted to understand African medical systems (to categorize or contain them), they emphasized certain characteristics over others and, as Karen Flint has demonstrated, some aspects changed during the encounter with Europeans.[2] Anne Digby has similarly argued that "traditional African societies were transformed in the very process of being observed, so that the customs and practices of their world before the arrival of the Europeans remains obscure."[3] This is in part because Xhosa medicine has never been static or uniform. Like other Nguni medical systems, healing depended largely on individuals with specialized skills who were open to incorporating any effective approaches and therapies that increased their abilities to help people. As a pluralistic medical system, it could accept various explanations and effective treatments, even if for simple pragmatic reasons.[4] These characteristics led Digby to use the term "indigenous" to describe Xhosa healing systems rather than "traditional" to more fully reflect the dynamic nature of the systems.[5] Despite the challenges of painting an accurate picture of Xhosa healing history, it is still necessary and even possible to describe the basic worldview and practices held by the Xhosa when Europeans moved into the region and started training African nurses. The biomedical and European bias in the archive can be revealing and countered with critical reading. I also privilege sources that foreground a Xhosa perspective, such as the writings of Xhosa scholars, historians emphasizing the validity of Xhosa worldviews, and an anthropologist trained in Xhosa medicine. These sources require skeptical analysis with their largely Christian commentary and temporal distance from early Xhosa history. However, employing these strategies, it is possible to create a sense of the basic philosophies and practices that have persisted over time, even as techniques and materials have changed.[6]

Similar to the Zulu as described by Flint, it is evident that the Xhosa believed ill-health came from three main causes: natural forces linked to one's environment and physical state, spiritual forces, and social forces.[7] Scholars have been fascinated with describing those aspects of Xhosa medicine that are more exotic from a Western biomedicine perspective (the "supernatural" forces and the diviner's work). Yet Flint demonstrated that while Zulu healing systems maintained basic beliefs about the link between the spiritual realm and social relationships and one's health, Zulus held other beliefs about the impact of the environment on health, the spread of infection and disease, and the need for proper sanitation and personal hygiene. For example, Zulu public health initiatives included community planning that avoided malarial areas and tsetse fly zones and the architectural use of cow dung and certain woods to ward off insects. Frequent bathing and application of grease and red ochre protected people against vermin. They used quarantine measures when faced with communicable diseases. Zulus also considered fevers, the common cold, and coughs as caused by natural forces.[8] Evidence presented by scholars suggests that the Xhosa held similar beliefs about the link between one's environment and one's health. Measures taken to prevent the spread of disease among livestock, for example, would indicate an understanding of the infectious nature of certain diseases even if the Xhosa did not believe in a germ theory. For example, Peires wrote that in 1856, when lung sickness threatened the Xhosa cattle herds, some secluded their healthy cattle in mountainous areas, others quarantined "strange and colonial cattle" within their borders and refused to accept new cattle, while others burned the grass around the perimeter of their pastures.[9] The Xhosa also had an understanding of the natural functions of the body and its fluids, even though they did not perform invasive surgeries. For example, women who assisted other women in childbirth (birth attendants) were known to have

Medical Systems and the Rise of African Nursing

expertise in this natural process, even if it was at times influenced by spiritual forces. Alfred Bitini Xuma, a Xhosa medical doctor and president of the African National Congress in the early twentieth century, asserted that the Xhosa viewed slight sicknesses, gastrointestinal ailments caused by eating certain foods, infectious diseases, and accidents as all having natural causes.[10] David Baranov argued that this aspect of African health systems makes them an antecedent of biomedicine.[11]

Beyond the natural influences on one's health, the Xhosa also held the view that the unseen, spiritual realm had a direct relationship with the seen, temporal realm. Thus ill-health or misfortune indicated something was amiss in the relationship between the two. It could also mean that a person in the temporal realm was using medicines to harm another. Peires wrote that, for the Xhosa, "health and fertility were accepted as the natural condition of things, and any deficiency was attributed to dereliction of duty or the influence of malevolent persons."[12] While Peires's use of the word "any" might not be accurate, it is true that the Xhosa did see many incidents of ill-health as caused by forces beyond natural ones or consequences of something wrong in one's relationships with kin or community. The Xhosa believed in some spirits that were linked to nature, such as the people of the river (*abantu bomlambo*) who could cause physical and mental illness or initiate diviners. In describing Xhosa medical systems, scholars have also emphasized the centrality of one's relationship with one's ancestors for maintaining health.[13] David Gordon categorized Xhosa medicine as one of the systems characterized as "cults of affliction," which saw sickness as "an attempt at communication by ancestral spirits."[14] Anthropologist and trained *igqirha* (diviner) Manton Hirst stressed that Xhosa society was characterized by a patrilineal ordering of people, with senior males in Xhosa clans or male homestead heads presiding over family rituals. These senior males acted as representatives of, and to, ancestors. Once they passed on, they became ancestors themselves who could influence people's lives by either giving or withholding protection, healing, increasing one's resources, or in extreme cases, inflicting harm.[15] A person's ill-health could be caused by an offense to the ancestors, who might be punishing the living directly or leaving an individual or an entire group vulnerable to harmful elements and malicious people. Misfortune and ill-health could also be caused by envious people seeking to injure someone through the use of destructive medicines. A person may employ someone with skills to poison or harm another. People believed to have an "innate psychic power to cause illness and misfortune" were known as witches (*igqwirha* for females, *umthakathi* for males).[16]

Two examples clearly illustrate common Xhosa explanations for the occurrence of ill-health and misfortune caused by spiritual or social forces. Although these two examples may not necessarily reflect the exact beliefs and concerns of people of two hundred years ago, they do demonstrate basic Xhosa beliefs. The first is the *impundulu*, or the lightning bird. Xhosa Christian minister and scholar John Henderson Soga described it in 1932 as a harmful bird that caused or came from lightning.[17] Hirst and Philip and Iona Mayer described *impundulu* as the "familiar" of witches—an animal or other being that carries out the evil designs of a witch. A witch may send *impundulu* or may be asked to send one on behalf of another person. The *impundulu* was believed to feed off human flesh and blood and could act quickly (especially since it could fly). It may also have attracted other dangerous beings by depositing a strong-smelling substance in a person's skin. People attacked by *impundulu* were believed to suffer more acute illnesses and display symptoms of wasting away, often accompanied by a cough. In the early to mid-twentieth century, Xhosa people often explained the symptoms of tuberculosis, or TB, as the effects of being "kicked" by the bird. Mayer and Mayer quote an informant as describing the "work of *impundulu*" as causing someone to rapidly lose weight, cough "incessantly, particularly at night," and to sometimes cough up blood.[18]

A less dramatic cause for ill-health or misfortune was the neglect of ancestral duties or rituals. Ancestors expected their living descendants to follow the moral code of the community and family as well as perform rituals to qualify for ancestral protection. For example, two rituals immediately important upon a person's death are *ukukhapa*, the killing of an ox to accompany the deceased to the land of the spirits, and then *ukubuyisa*, a ritual performed usually one year later to welcome the deceased back to the family's homestead as a lineage ancestor. It was not uncommon for people who found themselves suffering from a reoccurring illness to be told that their ancestors were either trying to send a message or had withdrawn protection because certain rituals such as these had not been performed. For example, Hirst shared a case of a diviner's potential initiate who apparently suffered from what might be diagnosed as depression. A diviner interpreted a reoccurring dream of the initiate as a message from her ancestors that she and her family had long neglected certain rituals that were supposed to be performed after a certain person's death.[19]

The consequences of ancestral neglect or moral impurities could apply on a larger scale to communities and chiefdoms. As Xuma put it, "The concept includes and involves within its scope the individual, the family, the Chief, the tribe, their crops, animals, and other possessions, success or failure and well-being of those concerned."[20] Heads of families and chiefs or kings performed communal ceremonies to secure protection against harmful powers of nature, to ensure a successful harvest, or to show gratitude to benevolent ancestors. They could only expect protection from the ancestors against their group's

Medical Systems and the Rise of African Nursing

enemies if they had done all they could to appeal to their ancestors. Otherwise, they would be left vulnerable to the destructive powers and substances of those who sought to harm them. In the case of the Xhosa Cattle Killing of the mid-1850s, the Xhosa were told that if they purged themselves of impure cattle and crops, people from the spiritual realm would bring new, healthy cattle and help them drive out the British.[21]

The causes of ill-health determined the treatment or remedy. Minor ailments such as coughs, common colds, or fevers could be cured by home or folk remedies. These included herbal teas known to ordinary people and easily attainable in the immediate environment. One of the herbal remedies widely used in the twentieth century was *umhlonyane*, a tea made out of leaves from the herb *artemisia afra* (or wild wormwood) to ease coughs and common colds. Anyone who knew *umhlonyane* could pick the leaves and make the tea. Other imbalances in bodily fluids or functions or pollutants might be treated by bleeding and purging. This type of treatment would require more skill. For the more serious or complicated illnesses, people turned to a medical practitioner with specialized knowledge.

The Xhosa had two main categories of health care practitioners. *Amaxhwele* (sing. *ixhwele*) acted as herbalists or chemists—experts in working with plant materials to create healing agents or medicines (although they also utilized some animal materials).[22] *Amaxhwele* were known for their vast knowledge of plants and the local landscape, although some could also obtain expertise in treating certain illnesses or creating particular protective medicines. Gordon wrote that the first stage of the Xhosa's "therapeutic quest" in the mid-nineteenth century was to visit an herbalist for a natural treatment.[23] Soga described herbalists as able to administer basic treatments to relieve stomach pains and headaches, reset dislocations, and perform blood-letting and cupping procedures.[24] While they may have possessed some additional spiritual power, *amaxhwele* did not usually divine information about ill-health, nor did they have ritual expertise or authority. They generally learned their craft from other *amaxhwele*. Because of this, the role of *ixhwele* was often passed down from one family member to another. Scholars agree that it has been a predominantly male role, although women could be *amaxhwele* as well.

The other main category of Xhosa healers were diviners or *amagqirha* (sing. *igqirha*). Soga described them as mediators who advocated for the cause of the family and could deal with crop failures and natural calamities as well as illness.[25] Digby called *amagqirha* jacks of all trades.[26] They had the ability to explain and intervene in various aspects of life—roles reflected in the variety of older terms once used for various *amagqirha* (e.g., *itola*, the war doctor; *igqira lemvula*, the rain maker; *igqirha lokumbulula*, the revealer of charms;

and *amagqirha aqubulayo,* extractors of infection).[27] The homogenization of these different terms to *amagqirha* (or the Zulu *isangoma*) reflected the reduction of the roles of *amagqirha* during British colonialization.[28] Perhaps most importantly, *amagqirha* had the training and spiritual connection to diagnose or divine the cause of ill-health and misfortune and then determine the best treatment or remedy. Their connection to the ancestors and spiritual realm also meant they could prophecy, discover harmful substances and lost objects, and interpret dreams. They could mix up protective medicines for those about to embark on a long journey or go to war. They knew herbs, but they did not have the kind of knowledge *amaxhwele* had. Thus, they would at times work closely with *amaxhwele* to provide treatment. Before British colonialism, *amagqirha* also played an important role in Xhosa politics. The heads of families, chiefdoms, and kingdoms were both political and religious leaders. They carried out and supervised communal ceremonies and judicial cases; however, these leaders were usually not *amagqirha* themselves. Thus they needed to work closely with *amagqirha* to secure a person or group's power against enemies, protect the community or chiefdom, and discover the cause of illness and misfortune. Soga called them "national high priests" because they had the expertise and authority to direct rituals. *Amagqirha* were particularly important in dealing with witchcraft. In fact, an old term for witchcraft specialists is *isanuse* or *igqirha elinukayo,* terms linked to the way that they "smelled out" witches or other causes of afflictions.[29]

Amagqirha usually began their training or apprenticeship with an established *igqirha* after a series of dreams or inexplicable afflictions revealed to be a message from the ancestors that the person must become *igqirha.* This process of calling by the ancestors is still known as *ukuthwasa.* It is viewed as proof of the person's special ability to communicate with the ancestors and may start in one's childhood. Once the prospective *igqirha* recognized the call, she or he then would choose *igqirha* to train her or him to become a full-fledged diviner (this process also often involved some sort of revelation on the part of the initiate or the *igqirha* who would do the training). The trainer was paid to apprentice the initiate for a period that could last up to a few years. The initiate was taught about rituals and medicines and to cultivate his or her "psychic sensitivity and intuition."[30] A final ritual ceremony where the initiate proved his or her power marked the initiate's graduation, after which the new *igqirha* would wear certain regalia common to a full-fledged *igqirha,* including white beads.[31] In the twentieth century, an initiate often started wearing white beads but then, once fully initiated, wore a hat and girdle made from the skins of small wild animals. She or he would also carry sticks, spears, or a hippo hide switch.[32]

Medical Systems and the Rise of African Nursing

Anthropologists writing about *amagqirha* in the twentieth century presented them as predominantly female (with one giving a ratio of two females to every one male).[33] Some explained this gendered aspect as linked to the peripheral position of women in Xhosa society and the perceived nature of women as more sensitive, empathetic, and emotional (characteristics apparently making them more able to understand an ill person and receive spiritual messages).[34] Hirst argued that while some *amagqirha* may have occupied a marginal position in society as individuals, the explanation that more *amagqirha* were women because they were peripheral to society does not match the historical essential role of *amagqirha* within Xhosa society.[35] Flint's work on the changing gender ratios of Zulu healers over time also suggests that the gender ratio could have shifted with British colonialism in the Eastern Cape as it did in the Natal colony.[36] In any case, it is clear that both men and women could become *amagqirha* throughout time.

The main means of divination for the Xhosa included *igqirha* receiving what W. D. Hammond-Tooke called a psychic prompting by "tuning in" to the ancestors.[37] Historically, this divining process was usually initiated by a small group of family members or friends of an afflicted person (what others have called a "therapy group") who took the sufferer to *igqirha* to divine the cause of illness or misfortune.[38] Without being told why the group of people came to consult her or him, *igqirha* would attempt to describe the ailments or problems to the group. As *igqirha* "mouthed the divinations," the people in the group would beat a drum and say if they agreed. The people responded to *igqirha*'s statements with different volumes of clapping and stating, "*Siyavuma!*" (we agree), or "*Asiva*" (we do not hear if they disagreed). If *igqirha* could tell the people hidden information they already knew to be true, they could trust in his or her abilities. Gordon characterized this process as "an attempt at a consensus between the voices of the ancestors spoken through the *igqirha* on the one hand and the therapy group on the other."[39] *Amagqirha* may have also required sacrifices and feasts or have taken a singing approach, dancing and chanting with a small group of *amagqirha* to alter their state of mind and prepare them to receive messages from the ancestors. If the therapy group was satisfied with the divination, *igqirha* would be paid. If they were not satisfied, they could search for another *igqirha*. If the cause was identified, *igqirha* offered a remedy—usually involving medicines and/or ritual performances and the services of an *ixhwele*. Treatment could require another payment. Soga and Hirst described similar processes conducted in various decades of the twentieth century.[40]

Amayeza, or medicines, were the central materials for healing, protection, attracting a potential lover, and inflicting harm. Hirst distinguished *amayeza* from charms, or *amakhubalo*, by the way each was used: charms may be used for washing but are never ingested. Most *amayeza* still consist of ingredients from plant materials, though again, some animal materials are also used. Baranov has argued that Africans employed scientific methods to learn the effectiveness of these therapies—they used empirical observation and trial-and-error testing to create recipes for "tried and trusted" medicines for particular ailments (such as stomachaches, pubic lice, bile, acne, coughs, colds, and asthmas).[41] Medicines could be dissolved in water and drunk, rubbed in incisions, smoked, or used to steam or wash a body. Medicines were also used to induce vomiting or other purging to remove harmful elements in the body. Others would counteract natural poisons. For example, certain plants were known to cure snake bites and spider bites. Peires claimed that anthrax and tapeworms were the most common human illnesses prior to British colonialism and that the Xhosa knew that "the aloe killed tapeworms, and the starlike *cluytia* cured anthrax in men and cattle."[42] When used for protection, medicines could be swallowed, carried, worn, rubbed into the skin, or placed in a home or homestead. Peires mentioned that nineteenth-century Xhosa travelers may have protected themselves with the herb *inyongwane* (*dicoma anomola*), which would cause a person to vomit poisoned food the moment the food was ingested. He also described how the blue-flowered plumbago and pelargonium were believed to ward off lightning and to stop wounds.[43] Hirst wrote that when a person was "inflicted" by *impundulu*, a common protective treatment included "scarification, cupping, bloodletting and the rubbing of protective medicines into incisions made in the skin."[44] When used to harm someone, medicines were often concocted using some object from the victim's body or house to direct a harmful being to the victim. Alternatively, harmful medicines would be placed on the victim's person or in their home to attract evil elements. Medicines used to attract the love of a certain individual may have been used in a similar way.

Xhosa healing beliefs and practices were not completely opposite of Western biomedicine in the mid-nineteenth century when Western biomedical institutions were established in the Ciskei. Europeans held similar ideas about herbal remedies, natural pollutants, and the importance of keeping bodily functions and fluids in balance. Yet the basic worldviews of health and ill-health began to differ significantly in the late nineteenth century. While the Xhosa looked to a plurality of forces linked to one's health, biomedicine on the other hand was evolving to focus almost entirely on natural causes and define itself as scientific, with studies of anatomy supported by human dissection. African practitioners had employed empirical observation and experimentation found in Western science, yet the preeminence of science as defined by Europeans at

Medical Systems and the Rise of African Nursing

the time became a distinguishing element for those who promoted biomedicine in contrast to what they viewed as backward African systems. Studies supported the underlying belief that human bodies functioned according to a normal physiology. Ill-health came when normal functions were interrupted or damaged by malfunctions, imbalances, or external factors. Specialists who understood the human body were seen as having the expertise to heal it. Physicians and surgeons were the main types of healers in the mid-nineteenth century. Physicians were the product of rigorous schooling, the holders of specialized knowledge obtained in universities. They were the only practitioners allowed to be called "Doctor." Unlike the Xhosa, who expected *amagqirha* to divine the cause of illness, biomedicine patients explained their problem to a physician, or doctor, who would then investigate with his or her various tools and perform tests, prescribe medicines, and conduct procedures as necessary. By this time, surgeons also went through academic training and had gained more professional prestige. Unlike physicians, surgeons focused on developing the practical skills to perform invasive surgeries and corrective procedures. Biomedicine also had specialists in preparing medicines or drugs from various herbs and compounds that could be ingested or applied externally—apothecaries or, later, pharmacists; however, they held a less prestigious position and played a much smaller role in biomedicine in European colonies in Africa. Nurses—practitioners trained to assist doctors and provide basic first aid and general care—would become more integral in the latter part of the century, with Florence Nightingale working to formalize nurses' training in England in the 1860s and Henrietta Stockdale establishing a nursing school in Kimberley, South Africa, in the 1880s.

While the study of anatomy and empirical observation came to define Western medicine at this time, it was not until the late nineteenth century that many of the causes of diseases were fully understood. This led John Rankin to describe biomedicine in the first half of the nineteenth century as lacking consensus and certainty. There were those who believed in constitutionalism, the theory that an individual's natural makeup, age, and way of life determined his or her health. Others looked more to the influence of a person's environment to explain disease, while others adhered to miasmatic theories.[45] This was also the time of "heroic medicine," where physicians used aggressive treatments like bleeding, purging, and potent medicines. Rankin has argued that although it brought effective vaccinations against infectious diseases, biomedicine at this time was not necessarily superior to African medicine, nor was it applied uniformly. Still, in the minds of the British, biomedicine exemplified the achievements and superiority of European civilization.[46] Indeed, the link to European colonialism is an important aspect of biomedicine's history in

Medical Systems and the Rise of African Nursing

Africa. Those who established the first hospital for African patients in the Ciskei and trained the first female African nurses did so with a similar colonial mindset.

British Colonial and Mission Hospital Nursing

Over the course of almost one hundred years, the British encroached upon the Xhosa, beginning with conflicts over land use and ownership in the late eighteenth century, erupting in various violent conflicts now known as the Frontier Wars or Wars of Dispossession, and culminating in the final war and further annexation of Xhosa territory into the British Cape Colony in 1878–79. Throughout this time, many European actors moved into the land of the Xhosa—Christian missionaries, the British military and colonial government, and German and British settlers. Colonial officials and later missionaries came to see biomedicine as a vital part of achieving their goal of civilizing and Christianizing the Xhosa. The establishment of hospitals for African patients and the training of African or Xhosa nurses came as a result of these ambitions, the work of British colonial doctor John Patrick Fitzgerald, and the circumstances caused by British-Xhosa conflicts.

After a destructive war in 1834–35 that included the killing of Xhosa Gcaleka King Hintsa, the British declared much of what became the Ciskei as part of the Cape Colony (first known as the Province of Queen Adelaide). A decade later, the British declared the region its own colony, known as British Kaffraria from 1847 to 1865. King William's Town served as the capital. In 1854, after two further wars that depleted Xhosa resources, Sir George Grey became the governor of British Kaffraria. Taking a different approach from his military predecessors, Grey started to implement a more uniform system of administration and embarked on a mission to civilize the Xhosa. As part of this mission, Grey emphasized the importance of establishing a public hospital. He hoped such a hospital would pull people away from Xhosa healers and what he and the colonial government saw as superstitious beliefs. Grey was aware of the influence *amagqirha* had in shoring up the power of Xhosa chiefs and particularly saw their role in sniffing out witches and "confiscating property" as detrimental.[47] He believed that if the superiority of European medicine could be displayed, it would undercut the spiritual and political power of *amagqirha*. He thus established the first so-called Native Public Hospital in King William's Town in 1856.

Grey recruited John Patrick Fitzgerald as the district health surgeon for what he hoped would become a central hospital with a number of branches in the surrounding area. Fitzgerald had worked in New Zealand when Grey had served as governor there and shared Grey's enthusiasm for the colony's civilizing

Medical Systems and the Rise of African Nursing

mission.[48] However, Fitzgerald apparently did not share Grey's "deviousness and egotism." According to Peires, Fitzgerald became known for treating Africans as equals and restoring the sight of the blind. The small hospital initially consisted of six huts, but the number of people seeking medical attention there grew quickly. Fitzgerald began to see fifty patients a day and saw six thousand within his first ten months.[49] To help him manage the workload, he recruited Xhosa men to work as interpreters and medical aides with elementary medical education. The first Xhosa women to work at the hospital apparently did the laundry.[50]

The Xhosa Cattle Killing of 1856–57 drastically changed the relationship between the Xhosa and the colonial government and opened the way for the training of Xhosa nurses. At the beginning of 1856, the Xhosa, still suffering from a recent loss against the British, were hit by a lung disease among their cattle. Word soon began to spread that people from the spiritual realm had appeared to a young girl named Nongqawuse to tell her that the Xhosa's cattle were impure because of the use of witchcraft by the people. Echoing similar prophecies from previous wars, Nongqawuse's message was that if the people cleansed themselves of witchcraft and destroyed their defiled cattle and crops, Xhosa ancestors would return, bring new cattle, and drive the British out of their lands. As Peires wrote, when understood from a Xhosa worldview, the cattle-killing movement was a "logical and rational response . . . by a nation driven to desperation."[51] Although not everyone had faith in the message, Nongqawuse's prophecies did attract many believers. In the end, this led to devastation. An estimated 400,000 heads of cattle were destroyed, 40,000 people died, and 150,000 people were displaced.[52] Grey's responses exacerbated the situation. He mercilessly used the movement as a way to force the Xhosa into the colony. He offered relief for starving people in exchange for labor, sent chiefs to Robben Island on convictions of plotting against the colonial government, attacked the Gcaleka King Sarhili, and carved out Xhosa land for British settlement.

In the wake of the Cattle Killing, starving people flooded the Native Public Hospital in King William's Town. This pushed Fitzgerald to seek the help of Xhosa female nurses from the nearby Brownlee mission. Anna, one of the four women sent, had worked as a domestic servant of the mission. At the hospital, Anna and the other three women had roles beyond just taking care of the laundry, however. Fitzgerald trained them to serve as medical aides. Their successful work, in addition to Fitzgerald's attitude toward the Xhosa and the influence of Florence Nightingale on him, led Fitzgerald to believe that training African female nurses was possible and desirable. In 1859 the Native Public Hospital was converted into a permanent hospital structure and renamed

Grey Hospital.[53] Fitzgerald staffed this new hospital with a number of Xhosa men and women. His eventual goals were to train African male doctors and female nurses. He first trained male orderlies, aides, and attendants. In an attempt to train Xhosa male doctors, he recruited William Daniels and Govane Koboka, graduates from the Lovedale mission near the town of Alice. Racial prejudice and the lack of Western-style education frustrated Fitzgerald's ambitions. Daniels and Koboka abandoned their courses because of funding difficulties and "questions of [the] suitability" of training African doctors.[54] On the other hand, Fitzgerald had success in training Xhosa female nurses, though the lack of education for young women and racial discrimination prevented the nurses from being fully certified. He recruited European women with nursing experience to do the training, such as a soldier's widow named Ellen Parsons. In 1866, the year after British Kaffraria was reincorporated into the British Cape Colony, Grey Hospital had two European orderlies, two Xhosa orderlies, one European nurse, one Xhosa nurse, and temporary Xhosa nursing maids. Although the Xhosa nurses and nursing maids trained at Grey had not qualified in the British system, they reportedly subsequently used their skills in many hospitals.[55]

In this initial development of nursing history in the Ciskei, European notions of gender and nursing influenced the training of Xhosa female nurses more than broader racial ideology or Xhosa notions about gender and healing. By the late nineteenth century, the nursing profession in Europe was firmly considered a woman's profession, even though men had and would be involved in nursing (especially in predominantly male sectors such as war fronts and mining compounds).[56] Many scholars have analyzed how the development of the profession with Florence Nightingale was based on notions of femininity, that women were particularly suited for the care of sick people. Whereas men were seen as being more scientifically minded, natural leaders, and thus suited for the position of physician, women, especially in European Christian societies, were seen as nurturing, devoted, and passive but not capable of scientific understanding and decision-making.[57] The Xhosa men and women who went to train at Grey Hospital in this period had also associated with Christian missions and thus would have been influenced to some degree by the gender roles preached there. Marks successfully demonstrated that the gendered nature of nursing in South Africa has a complex history, since ideas about race initially meant that Europeans preferred African men in domestic and hospital service.[58] However, in the Ciskei, European notions of gender had a bigger influence in determining that female Xhosa nurses would be trained at Grey early on.

Similar to the early interactions of Europeans and Africans in KwaZulu-Natal, it appears that in the early years of Grey Hospital, "the great contest

Medical Systems and the Rise of African Nursing

between science and superstition which Grey had envisaged never occurred."[59] While the Xhosa were drawn to Fitzgerald because of his services, particularly in ophthalmic surgery, his hopes that his "kind charity" and medical treatment would win the loyalty of the Xhosa more likely only won himself personal loyalties and a reputation as a powerful, foreign *igqirha*.[60] On the Xhosa side, there tended to be an adaptation of new medicine rather than a displacement—as Peires wrote, they could "swallow Fitzgerald's medicine without in any way giving up their beliefs in the powers of the Xhosa doctors."[61] Gordon highlighted how the encounters between Western biomedicine and Xhosa healing began as more of a process of exchange than a contest, also arguing that "Africans could accept the beneficial aspects of this colonial medicine without conceding their central ideas about the nature of healing." Gordon continued to assert that "colonial medicine was also transformed as Fitzgerald began to accept and incorporate different African medical practices." Although he did not provide details, Gordon cited meetings between Fitzgerald and Xhosa doctors, such as a man named Gota, wherein they exchanged therapies. Gordon also described interpreters and aides as cultural brokers.[62] Even if Europeans like Grey had more disdain for Xhosa beliefs, the Xhosa were more eclectic, and practitioners such as Fitzgerald learned to adapt as well.[63]

Gordon argued that the period of colonial government support at Grey Hospital began to wane after the departure of Grey in 1861 and the reincorporation of British Kaffraria back into the Cape Colony in 1866. He also viewed the end of Fitzgerald's career in 1891 as signaling the end of a more collaborative era.[64] Indeed, the late nineteenth century saw some significant changes in medical systems in the region and their relationships with each other. Although the colonial government did not provide stronger support for Grey Hospital, by whittling away at Xhosa political power in general it undermined the status of *amagqirha* in Xhosa society. By the mid-1880s, the British had annexed all Xhosa territory into the Cape Colony. As the chiefs lost power and authority under the British, *amagqirha* began losing their public role: "the expectation that they would control public conditions of health" through communal rites, dealing with natural calamities, or rooting out witches. Under British colonialism, they could no longer be "national high priests," but their work became more localized and individual.[65] The professionalization of biomedicine within South Africa further marginalized *amagqirha* in the broader society. The same year Fitzgerald retired, the Cape Medical Act of 1891 established the registration of biomedical-related professionals in the colony, leaving out diviners such as *amagqirha*. Only the Natal Colony had a professional association for the less-threatening herbalists at this time. In 1895 the Witchcraft Suppression Act was passed, making offenses related to the practice of witchcraft illegal, providing further legal means to suppress the practices of *amagqirha*. Heading into the twentieth century then, the role of *amagqirha* had been reduced and proscribed by British colonialism.[66]

The turn of the century also marked a rise of a new hospital movement with a nongovernmental impetus. In the years following the establishment of the hospital in King William's Town, revolutionary developments occurred in biomedicine that shaped it into the more technical, effective, and universally oriented medicine of the twentieth century. The introduction of antisepsis and asepsis in the late 1860s drastically reduced the number of deaths and infections in hospitals, leading to hospitals gaining acceptance in Europe as the central place for healing. Physicians became "powerful and respected representatives" of biomedicine, and nurses became essential to the work of hospitals, clinics, and community outreach.[67] In addition to offering curative care, hospitals trained nurses and doctors, dispensed medications, and housed the technology to perform invasive procedures. The development of the germ theory in the 1870s also drastically improved the effectiveness of biomedicine. The isolation of microorganisms led to the development of "magic bullet" treatments—chemical compounds or medicines that could isolate a harmful microbe inside the body and destroy it—as well as new vaccinations and sanitation and hygiene practices.[68] As it adopted these new theories, biological medical science was universalized by its practitioners, even if it was in reality applied differently to Africans.[69] Scholars like Baranov, Steven Feierman, John Janzen, and Megan Vaughan remind us that biomedicine has been socially constructed and is multilayered; yet those practicing it often operated within a worldview that believed Western science and medicine constituted independent universal truths.[70] As it became more and more scientifically and materially focused, biomedical practitioners left little room for recognizing the influence of a person's social relations or spiritual forces on her or his health. This trend would continue well into the late twentieth century, when biomedicine became even more linked to high-technology devices to detect and treat illnesses, ranging from the stethoscope, thermometers, and microscopes to X-ray machines and CAT scans. As Baranov put it, "The human body itself is laid before biomedicine as a soulless, multifunctional machine whose detailed internal structures require precise probing via a sophisticated complement of capital-intensive biotechnology."[71]

The hospital movement in Europe greatly influenced Christian missions in Southern Africa. Missions soon took the lead in establishing hospitals and training African nurses in the Ciskei. Christian missionaries in Southern Africa had a long tradition of combining medical care with their evangelization efforts. Other scholars have explored the origins and complexities of medical missions

Medical Systems and the Rise of African Nursing

in depth, highlighting the range of their motivations from the religious and spiritual to the humanitarian and utilitarian.[72] Similar to earlier colonial officials, in addition to providing charitable physical relief, many missionaries believed that demonstrating the superiority of Western culture in such a powerfully personal way could discredit *amagqirha* and win converts to Christianity and Western civilization. As the Comaroffs put it, they believed they would save souls by "tending the flesh."[73] The establishment of mission hospitals in the late nineteenth and early twentieth centuries took the relationship between Western biomedicine and missionary work to a different level. Hospitals had the potential for a much greater impact than the missionary doctors who had worked in earlier times. As biomedicine became more effective, technical, and sterile, missionaries and health practitioners believed it exemplified the best of Christian civilization. Often situated in remote rural regions, the hospitals could take Christianity intertwined with biomedicine to the margins of the civilized world and act as an example of cleanliness and order.[74] Christian medical officers and nurses would primarily relieve suffering but, in the meantime, hoped to "eradicate and replace" African beliefs with faith in biomedicine and a Christian God.[75]

One of the first mission hospitals built was the Victoria Hospital of the Lovedale mission of the Free Church of Scotland. The Glasgow Missionary Society founded the mission station in 1824, near the town of Alice, along the Tyumie River. Seventeen years later, it established the Lovedale Missionary Institution for the higher education of Africans, which promoted the education of young women, such as the Makiwane sisters. With the completion of the Victoria Hospital in 1898, the mission was at the forefront of the mission hospital movement in the Eastern Cape and positioned itself to train the first registered African nurses. Dr. Neil Macvicar, a pioneering superintendent, arrived at Victoria Hospital in 1902 and shortly afterward introduced an official three-year training course in general nursing for African women.[76] Although he was more "scientifically minded," Macvicar was a strong proponent of the special characteristics of mission hospitals.[77] The Lovedale Missionary Institute and others advocating for the training of African women as nurses also believed that missions could make the most effective change in African societies by targeting women, especially those giving and receiving maternal and child care.[78] Two women "handpicked from the daughters of the Christian African elite in the Eastern Cape," Cecilia Makiwane and Mina Colani, began their training in Macvicar's program, under the tutelage of Matron Mary Balmer.[79] The Lovedale mission provided the ideal trainee in Makiwane (and supposedly in Colani as well, although little is written about her). With its emphasis on the education of young women, the mission had opened a way for Makiwane to gain the necessary academic abilities to begin nursing training. She was also from a prominent African Christian family, and the Victoria Hospital wanted nurses who could do "Christ-like work" in African communities.[80]

The two women finished their training at Victoria Hospital, then worked in Butterworth for further preparation before taking the Colonial Medical Council examination. The Cape Medical Act of 1891 did not place any racial restrictions on this professional certification, opening the way for Black nurses to enter the profession. Makiwane passed the exam in general nursing at the end of 1907 and became the first Black professional nurse to be registered in South Africa and the African continent in 1908. Makiwane's success proved that African women could become fully qualified nurses. However, her training was not without its difficulties. Balmer enforced strict discipline on her trainees, and the disrespectful way white male patients treated Makiwane and Colani (including sexual harassment) contributed to tensions between the hospital staff and donors over whether or not the hospital should even admit white patients.[81] Still, upon her registration, Makiwane returned to Victoria Hospital, where she worked for a number of years and was known for her dedication to her duties.

Few trainees followed Makiwane's example in the ensuing decade. Marks highlighted a number of stumbling blocks for the training of African women in nursing in the early twentieth century. Although the first nurses came from the educated, Christian elite, these communities still saw certain nurses' tasks as "unseemly for young unmarried women." Women were also largely still expected to contribute to agricultural production and to build a life around marriage, yet hospitals at the time did not train or employ married women.[82] Nevertheless, Makiwane paved the way for the growth of African nursing in the region and throughout South Africa.[83] Victoria Hospital graduates began to gain a reputation for their skill and service to the communities throughout the Eastern Cape. Almost all came from mission-educated families. Graduates who immediately followed Makiwane included Agnes Kakaza (1914) and Violet Donga (1919). Donga worked at the St. Matthew's Mission Hospital and later returned to Victoria Hospital, where she eventually took charge of three wards. After completing midwifery training in Cape Town, where she was one of the first African women to receive formal training in midwifery, Donga also took charge of Victoria Hospital's maternity work.[84] Thandiwe Jacobs became the first district nurse to serve in Cradock and Duncan Village in East London. Jacobs reportedly inspired Dora Nginza to train as a nurse.[85] Nginza was one of the first district nurses in New Brighton (near Port Elizabeth), appointed there as the solo nurse in 1919 before she was joined by two others trained at Victoria Hospital. She gained notoriety for her work there among a population of more than six thousand as well as for her position as the wife of a headman or chief.[86] Mount Coke and St. Matthew's hospitals soon established training as well. Eight miles (fourteen kilometers) south of King William's Town, Mount Coke Mission Hospital was opened in 1933 in an effort to revive the Methodist mission. The St. Matthew's Mission Hospital was established in 1923 by the Anglican mission just over thirty miles (fifty-two kilometers) northwest of King William's Town and sixty-five kilometers northeast of Victoria Hospital.

Little in the secondary sources about these early Ciskei nurses indicates how they interacted with Xhosa practitioners and Xhosa beliefs about health and healing. Much of the literature about them is simply laudatory. Comments by those celebratory authors about the role nurses played in combatting witchcraft and superstition and how "western and Christian norms and values" prepared the ground for professional nursing may reflect the same sentiments of these early nurses, especially if the nurses who came from Christian, mission-educated families felt a missionary zeal for their work.[87] However, these statements reveal more about the authors of those statements than the views of the nurses at the time. If evidence from later times are any indication, the beliefs and actions of African nurses were more complex and varied, as demonstrated further below.

Tensions and Engagement in Early Twentieth-Century African Nursing Expansion

African nursing from the early twentieth century into the 1950s expanded exponentially, with each decade seeing a new development along with changes in South African health care and politics. The South African war, the establishment of the Union of South Africa, and the 1918 influenza epidemic all brought with them a demand for an expanding nursing workforce. Nurses formed the South African Trained Nurses Association in 1914 to gain more control over the profession as it grew. Marks demonstrated how gendered and racialized concerns about white women nursing Black men added weight to calls to train African nurses.[88] Increased Black urbanization, more educational opportunities and hospital use by Africans, and a greater desire by the state to have a healthy Black population also contributed to the demand for more African nurses. Nursing became a more desired and more acceptable profession for African women as the demand for female African nurses in public services grew. The first half of the twentieth century was also a time of tension between different medical systems and greater racial tensions. The centers for training African nurses moved from the few mission hospitals, like Victoria Hospital, to include others of both mission and government origin in different regions of the country. Throughout, training programs maintained a strict regimen, with Christian, civilizing mission overtones that many African nurses internalized and others challenged. The rise in Afrikaner nationalism in the 1930s and the Nationalist Party victory of 1948 resulted in the institution of apartheid. This heightened racial separation led to practices that threatened to block Black advancement, with white female nurses gaining more control over the profession. Trends in nursing in the Ciskei region reflected much of what was happening in the rest of the country as the nursing profession and health care in general became more uniform.

In predominantly rural areas such as the Ciskei, government officials, missions, and hospital staff advocated for African district nurses to help alleviate overflowing hospitals that lacked funding. Mission hospitals in the Ciskei were small, with limited staff, yet they catered to large rural populations. Throughout the 1930s and into the 1950s, patient attendance grew dramatically. Biomedical treatments for certain diseases such as TB, venereal diseases, typhoid, or enteric fever, cases of malnutrition, gastroenteritis, acute respiratory diseases (e.g., pneumonia, bronchitis, whooping cough), and childbirth and surgery attracted more people.[89] In 1941 Victoria Hospital reported that it had 275 beds for Africans, and the outpatient department saw 4,000–5,000 cases annually. Outstation clinics saw another 3,000 annually, making a total of 7,000–8,000, double that of a decade earlier.[90] Within a three-year period in the mid-1940s, Mount Coke's daily average attendance went from 49.6 to 73.4, and its outpatient numbers rose by almost 2,000, from 5,575 to 7,121.[91] The hospital could barely manage the number of maternity cases as the number of Xhosa women seeking to give birth in the hospital rapidly increased.[92] In 1955 the hospital board reported over four times more births given at the hospital than a decade earlier, with a total of 419, and commented that the hospital had to implement shorter lying-in times to open up space for more cases.[93] From 1935 to 1946, St. Matthew's Hospital reported a 270 percent increase in the number of inpatients. The number of outpatients had doubled. In March 1954 the superintendent reported double the number of patients over the previous three years, and in 1955 the number of outpatients had risen to just over 9,000, more than four times the number nine years earlier.[94] The hospital reported that it "became so congested that it was impossible to carry on the work effectively."[95]

Funding for mission hospitals was almost always tight. Many of the rural patients could not afford to pay fees, and the mission hospitals consistently reported a financial deficit in their end-of-year reports. The hospitals thus relied heavily on subsidies from the government and donations from various civic and religious sources. St. Matthew's Hospital even closed for six weeks in 1935 because of the lack of funds. In an urgent appeal to the Department of Public

Health for immediate financial relief in 1945, it reported that the hospital had cut back operations by a third to reduce costs.[96] By 1958 Mount Coke had grown so much that the state provided 85 percent of its expenditures, and the Cape Provincial Administration had taken over the Lovedale Hospital completely.[97] The South African state took responsibility for rendering health services free of charge for the general population and for curbing and preventing the spread of infectious diseases. Various forms of TB were the biggest cause of worry. Randall Packard has examined why TB grew predominantly among Black urban and rural areas in South Africa during this time.[98] The Ciskei was similarly affected by migrant workers who brought the disease to their rural homes from urban areas where they worked and lived in poor conditions. This led to the opening of new TB wards in the hospitals. Lovedale even built a separate TB hospital, the Macvicar Hospital, opened in 1940 (referred to as the Lovedale Hospitals when lumped together with Victoria Hospital). Recognizing that mission hospitals provided the care the state did not, the national government's Department of Health, the provincial administrations, and the Native Affairs Department (working with regional and local councils) all took some responsibility for financing aspects of mission hospital and clinic work. The provincial administration was responsible for general hospital services, the central government provided specialist services, and local authorities were charged with preventing the spread of infectious diseases and providing mother and child welfare services.[99]

As the hospitals grew, hospital staff and government officials wanted to extend health care services to the people in scattered villages. They desired to reach more people with both preventive and curative care and alleviate the number of patients coming to the hospitals. In the late 1930s and early 1940s, there was a push to establish more clinics and district nursing services to bring health care closer to people in the Ciskei as well as South Africa in general.[100] District nursing services had begun in Kimberley and in the Western Cape around the turn of the century, in urban areas and primarily among white populations. Midwives played a particularly important role in district services in those early years, taking their midwifery bags with them to people's homes at all hours of the day and night. In the mid-1930s, people concerned about African rural health advocated for more nurses to work in rural communities— nurses who came from the same communities and could relate closely to the people. The government, civic organizations, and mission hospitals held conferences on rural nursing in 1934 and 1935 to discuss the need for, and implementation of, district nursing.[101] With the Nursing Amendment Act of 1935, the government passed a regulation that allowed state funding of district nurses employed through mission hospitals in order to extend district nursing to areas

40 Medical Systems and the Rise of African Nursing

that did not have government hospitals.[102] Subsequently, the Ciskei region moved to establish Xhosa district nurses in addition to the few already working from mission hospitals. A social health care movement and the National Health Services Commission (or Gluckman Commission) of the 1940s, discussed further in the next chapter, added motivation for community-centered health care.[103] In most cases, a system developed whereby the central government's Department of Health paid one portion of the nurse's salary, the Native Affairs Department paid another portion, and a final portion might come from other sources, either the Ciskei General Council, local community, hospital, or charitable donations.[104] Local authorities and hospitals were responsible for applying for new clinics to be built and ensuring continued support for the clinics in the local communities.

Despite the challenges of obtaining resources, rural clinics and district nursing grew substantially from the late 1930s into the 1940s. Records indicate that government officials made long-term plans to build a network of clinics. The idea was to eventually have a district nurse in every location, although the funding was certainly not available and securing fully qualified nurses willing to relocate to rural clinics could be difficult. Each clinic also needed to be supervised by a medical officer—either a district surgeon or doctors based in mission hospitals.[105] Other challenges included having buildings in good repair and with enough space for both a nurse and her clinic work. Some situations required the nurse to find accommodation within the community, while other clinics started with three different rondavels donated by the village— one serving as the main clinic, one as a dispensary, and one as the nurses' accommodation. Plans for clinic buildings became regularized as time went on, with a standard rectangular building, but then ambulances or other motor vehicles also became important to rural district work and required constant upkeep. Still, within a decade the number of clinics rose from a small handful to over a dozen (if the East London and Lady Frere areas are included). Among the clinics built during this time, three public clinics were established at Lovedale, King William's Town, and Middledrift in 1938–39. In 1948 a public health center was opened in Zwelitsha as well as a clinic at Hackney in Wittlesea where district surgeons visited weekly.[106] In other areas, the mission hospitals ran the clinics, with grants from the government (e.g., in 1945 the chief Native Affairs commissioner granted money to erect six clinics in Ciskei).[107] These hospitals had already sought to extend their services to villages but had more resources to do so at this time with government support.[108]

In a memo to the National Health Services Commission in 1943, a committee of various entities reporting on health care in the region pointed to Mount Coke's clinic system as a model to follow.[109] Starting in 1939, it had established

Medical Systems and the Rise of African Nursing

clinics, believing "the solution of many of the health problems of the Native people can only be found in large scale District work, aimed at combating disease at its source—the people's home."[110] By the mid-1950s, Mount Coke had five extension clinics: Tamara, Tshabo (established 1947/48), Ander's Mission (1941), Mtombe, and Twecu (1953), ranging from fourteen to twenty-seven miles (twenty-three to forty-three kilometers) away from Mount Coke.[111] Each clinic had one African nurse fully trained in general nursing and midwifery who ran the clinic and administered the bulk of the services. Covering such a wide area meant that nurses would often walk miles or ride horses to make home visits. The ideal was for a doctor to visit each clinic once a week, but that did not always happen, especially as the number of people attending the hospital itself grew. In 1956 the hospital reported that the doctors attended 5,636 district services patients during the year, of a total 13,232 attended to at either the clinics or in-home visits.[112] This number continued to grow. The year 1959 saw a 35 percent increase in the number of patients attended to through the clinic work, up 6,992 people from the previous year's 18,133, compared with 2,248 inpatients and 17,434 outpatients attended to at the hospital in the same year.[113] These numbers show that by the end of the 1950s, African nurses working in these clinics were shouldering a large portion of the health care work in the Mount Coke area and acting as an important point of contact for a great number of people seeking biomedical care. Nurse Queenie Dikwayo deserves special mention at this point. Stationed twenty-four miles (thirty-eight kilometers) away from Mount Coke at the Ander's Mission clinic for six years as the sole fully qualified nurse, Dikwayo died at the clinic in 1947. The hospital report commented that she had "proved a most conscientious and reliable nurse of the Christian character."[114] The records do not indicate the cause of her death but give the impression that this nurse gave her life to the clinic where she undoubtedly worked long, lonely hours, crossing long distances and embedding herself in the Ander's Mission community.

Hospitals in the Ciskei increased their training and employment of African nurses during this time to meet the growing demand for African nurses. Grey Hospital was the geographic center of the King William's Town Hospital District, situated in the same town as district and regional government offices; but by the mid-twentieth century, the growth and changes in the needs of the white population of the town meant that the hospital became primarily a white or "European" hospital. There were some segregated provisions for Africans, but the mission hospitals had grown to cater to the Xhosa population and led in training African nurses, still predominantly women.[115] The number of trainees at the Victoria Hospital increased from four in 1908, to ten in 1921, and fifty-eight in 1938.[116] In 1930 the hospital was declared a Class 1 training

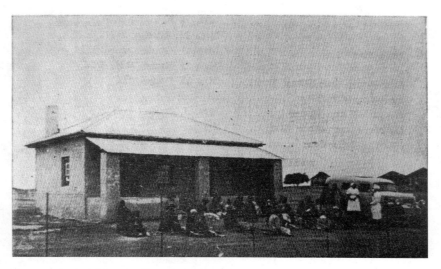

Figure 1. Ander's Mission. "Mount Coke Hospital, The Methodist Church of South Africa, Reports and Statements for the Year 1947," Mount Coke Hospital Reports, Newsletters Quarterly Reports, Methodist Papers, Folder 1, Cory Library (courtesy of Rhodes University, Cory Library).

facility, and one of its trainees, P. Xala, won third place in the national final examinations. By 1931 it had trained forty-nine nurses from around the country and expanded its training to include midwifery.[117] Mount Coke Hospital was recognized as a training hospital in 1937. Within the next two decades, it grew to have forty nurses training in the hospital at a time, with eleven staff nurses of African descent employed permanently. It had also expanded from twenty to ninety-three beds, established five district clinics, and conducted thousands of home visits.[118] St. Matthew's was recognized as a Class 2 training facility in 1938 (meaning it could train nurses for the national qualifying exams). In that year, it had eight nurses in training. It hired its first African nursing sister in 1946, when it already had two African staff nurses (an older term used for enrolled nurses versus registered nurses or nursing sisters).[119] In 1948 it had nineteen trainees, and by the late 1950s it had almost thirty. To this, the state added training of African nurses at Frere Hospital in East London and Frontier Hospital in Queenstown.[120] As the mission hospitals trained their student nurses to take the national council exams, training became more uniform and linked to developments in the profession on a broader scale. The hospitals adopted the three-and-a-half-year training course, with trainees working full-time in the hospitals as well as attending lectures given

Medical Systems and the Rise of African Nursing

by doctors, matrons, and other training nurses. This provided cheap labor for the hospitals and prepared the student nurses to take the South African Medical Council examinations (or qualified them for hospital certificates if they did not pass the national exams). Further significant changes to training for Black nurses came in the 1940s to help support the growing demand for Black nurses.[121] Training hospitals implemented a preliminary course for trainees to allow nurses to try out nursing before further training. The block system gave student nurses alternate periods of practical work and in-class instruction.

As scholars have described elsewhere, student nurses were subjected to a strict moral as well as technical training that resembled military service. Except for four weeks of annual leave, trainees were expected to work in the hospitals full-time, with some compensation that increased each year of their training. They were largely required to live in the nurses' quarters during their training and at times were required to wear their uniforms even outside the hospital, such as at the Victoria Hospital. Nursing students were also expected to maintain "good character" and serve as examples of Christian virtue—with Victoria Hospital requiring references from two "responsible Europeans" as part of the initial application.[122] The religious aspect of the mission hospitals significantly shaped the experience nurses had in their training and work. The major mission hospitals in the Ciskei at the time viewed the spiritual work they believed they were accomplishing as vital to their overall mission. Victoria Hospital's report of 1937 expressed the hope that as more and more people attended the hospital, its spiritual influence was spreading.[123] The Mount Coke Hospital owed its existence to efforts to revitalize the mission through medical care. Its longtime medical superintendent, Herbert Bennett, also served as a chaplain for some time.[124] Like other mission hospitals, Victoria, Mount Coke, and St. Matthew's conducted daily prayers with the patients, held Sunday services (especially for the children), conducted devotionals, and distributed religious tracts. Although hospital reports gave little evidence of the conversion of their patients to Christianity, the hospital staff counted their efforts successful if they merely influenced their patients. This Christian-infused civilizing ideology accompanied the medical training nurses received. Mission hospitals indeed hoped to deepen the conversion of their African nurses as well as their patients. A 1932 Victoria Hospital report noted the hospital's hopes for the religious training of the student nurses: "One of the best services a mission can render is to add to the impulse for good, the conversion, of each young soul such disciplinary training as will make that impulse effective and strengthen character."[125] A 1955 Mount Coke report stated, "The badge for Nurses who qualify at the Mount Coke Hospital, stresses the fact that the Hospital has a two-fold task, namely, not only to heal the sick, but also to preach the Gospel."[126] Hospitals enlisted nurses in their spiritual work with patients, asking them to lead hospital ward prayers and conduct morning devotionals at clinics. Some hospitals required nurses to attend Sunday services if they were on duty, regardless of their personal denominational affiliation. Thus for many African nurses training in the Ciskei, biomedicine was also closely linked to Christianity.

This certainly had implications for the way that biomedical staff and African nurses interacted with Xhosa healers, beliefs, and practices in this era of greater tensions between the two systems. A few European doctors catered to certain Xhosa beliefs about the healing process to appeal to Xhosa patients in the early twentieth century. For example, even as Digby argued that Western and indigenous medicine hardly intersected, she gave the example of a Dr. Murray stationed at St. Matthew's Hospital in the 1920s whom the surrounding community believed to have stronger medicine than a Dr. Hill. Murray succeeded in part because he adapted more to local beliefs by *telling* patients what was wrong first (like Xhosa *amagqirha*) then giving them medicine, whereas Hill *asked* the patients what was wrong first.[127] Xhosa nurses may have taken a similar, more open approach, especially if they worked closely with doctors like Murray. Yet even if the doctors made some adjustments, their ultimate goal in this time period was to convert patients and African trainees to biomedicine and Christianity, from Macvicar's scientific evangelism to religious preaching.[128] Mount Coke reported greater tension with Xhosa health practitioners than other hospitals. In its earlier years, it included sections in annual reports titled "Opposition," where it reported on encounters with *amagqirha*. In 1940 the hospital wrote that it understood that the "witchdoctors" were actively campaigning against the hospital, "sowing distrust" by telling patients that they would not come out of the hospital alive. This led the report to conclude, "We fight not against disease alone, but 'against the rulers of the darkness of this world.'" The 1944 annual report claimed that "witchdoctors and superstition" still held "great sway," and some patients were even taken out of the hospital to be treated by *amagqirha*.[129]

Martin Lunde insightfully points out that mission hospital publications hoping to generate donations may have focused on only part of the story.[130] In fact, some records indicate more acceptance and exchange was perhaps going on among African practitioners from both systems. Hospital records and efforts by African practitioners demonstrated a characteristic willingness to use effective techniques from other systems or practitioners in a way that did not displace their central beliefs and practices. For example, Mount Coke hospital also reported that "witch-doctors" would send their children to the hospital, come themselves for treatment, or even bring patients for diagnosis at the hospital before taking them home to treat them.[131] African herbalists, especially in urban

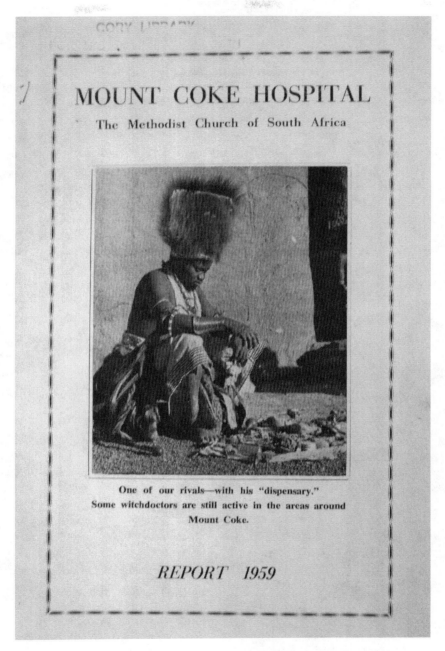

Figure 2. "One of our rivals—with his 'dispensary.'" Mount Coke Hospital Report 1959. Mount Coke Hospital Reports, Newsletters Quarterly Reports, Methodist Papers, Folder 1, Cory Library (courtesy of Rhodes University, Cory Library).

areas in the 1930s through the 1950s, sought to gain professional respect by forming regulatory organizations and seeking legal recognition. Their requests for official government recognition went ignored during this time, but their efforts demonstrate the growing commercialization of African medicine and how some African practitioners used the professional ethos of the time to combat marginalization.[132] Papers given by African health practitioners at a 1954 conference or study course in "African Culture and Its Relation to the Training of African Nurses" also reflect a more open-minded response by African doctors and nurses to African practices and beliefs. For example, while E. C. Jali, a medical aide at the Institute for Family and Community Health in Durban, called African diagnoses simplistic and African treatments "worthless," he stressed the importance of being sympathetic to the beliefs of the patients and nursing trainees to encourage them to discuss them freely in the hospital. Jali also acknowledged the good that *amagqirha* could do for people. Similarly, Xuma gave a paper at the conference pointing out the internal logic of Xhosa beliefs, even giving some examples of successful treatments. In the same talk, Xuma emphasized that biomedicine had changed over time and that Europeans had also believed in witches and good luck charms at one point in an apparent attempt to de-exoticize African beliefs.[133] The interaction between biomedicine and Xhosa medicine would have been more immediate for nurses in rural clinics. Some already may have been ideologically facing the direction of the missions as they would have been educated there. Some interviews and writings by nurses show tensions were there, but they perhaps felt closer affinity with the missionaries than the Xhosa practitioners who were more eclectic.

Conflict within the hospitals and professional organizations reflected tensions of the era. The rise in African nursing came at a time when the profession itself was gaining more autonomy and yet bringing in more racial discrimination. Nurses had formed associations in previous decades but still operated under the South African Medical and Dental Council for the regulation and registration of their profession. The growth and strains in the nursing sector during World War II and the push for a nurses' union by junior and student nurses suffering under the "tyranny of matrons" led to the formation of the South African Nursing Council (SANC) and South African Nursing Association (SANA) in 1944. This set the stage for the future, as unions were rejected as a part of the nursing profession and the profession gained more sovereignty. However, it also left room for racial discrimination to be brought in with the rise of apartheid. The SANC included all races, but its color-blind policies did not recognize or resolve discrimination against Black nurses who, for example, did not have as many leadership roles, received far lower salaries, and had inferior training facilities.[134]

Medical Systems and the Rise of African Nursing 47

Racial tensions in the country and the struggles in nursing training programs manifested themselves in a number of strikes in hospitals in the 1940s. For example, Anne Mager explored the religious, racial, and gendered hierarchical tensions underlying the strike at Lovedale Hospital that occurred in 1949, one year after the Nationalist Party victory that ushered in apartheid. Throughout their earlier years, mission hospitals employed white matrons often from England with only a small number of African nurses serving as heads of wards in hospitals. The Victoria Hospital requirement that potential trainees provide references from two "responsible Europeans" also reflected the racial hierarchy in the hospitals. Similar to other authors, Mager described mission hospitals as "bent on eliminating 'all traces of heathenism . . . in the Black man's concept of disease'" and thus favoring students with particular religious experiences. Tensions also rose between the ideological and practical demands on nurses in the hospital. While the hospital reinforced gendered notions of nurses as subordinate to doctors, Mager wrote that district nurses and midwives working in much more independent roles "desperately needed to develop the qualities of initiative and resourcefulness" that led to "outbursts" of "insubordination."[135] Furthermore, as Afrikaner nationalism rose in the 1940s, so did Black militancy. This spread to the Lovedale hospitals, located in the same town as the University of Fort Hare, a hotbed for Black political activism. Nursing students associated with Fort Hare students, especially connecting around issues of oppression by superiors. In 1949 a probationary nurse was expelled for challenging her superior. In the words of the Native Affairs Department, "a regrettable spirit of indiscipline" gripped her fellow trainees.[136] Feeling the injustice of the overly harsh reprisal, many nurses walked out in solidarity to demand the nurse's reinstatement. They abandoned the hostels along with their duties and camped on the grounds (with support from the Fort Hare African National Congress Youth League branch). The hospital brought in parents and granted the dismissed student the right to appeal in order to gain control, but this only temporarily appeased the trainees. The hospital eventually closed its training sections for the year and blacklisted striking nurses from training at other mission hospitals. It apparently took the Macvicar Hospital a few years to recover from the great loss of trainees who had staffed the hospital.[137]

Tensions persisted as apartheid ironically both limited and gave rise to opportunities for African nurses. Leadership positions opened up for Black women in racially segregated wards in hospitals. For example, by 1950, in the new Baragwanath Hospital, each ward operated under the supervision of a Black nurse, signaling the increasing importance of Black nurses in racially segregated health institutions.[138] At the same time, greater racial separation also developed within the professional organizations. As Marks described in

48   Medical Systems and the Rise of African Nursing

Divided Sisterhood, the Nursing Amendment Act of 1957 brought apartheid into the profession's governance by only allowing white members to vote for an all-white board and creating separate subcouncils for other races. Even after years of training of Black nurses, many white nurses and medical professionals continued to question the abilities and cultural adaptability of African nurses in discussions of the likelihood of their success.[139] Some Black nurses pushed back against these trends. In response to an invitation to participate in the 1954 conference on African culture and the training of African nurses, a number of nurses refused, replying, "We are tired of these people always digging into our primitive background as if we were the only race which had primitive ancestors."[140] In 1958 nurses held another strike at Victoria Hospital that opposed strict hierarchical regimes and severe punishments. After a staff nurse was expelled, 100 out of 140 nurses held a sit-down strike. Political activists at Fort Hare once again supported their sisters' struggle. Similar to a decade earlier, the hospital responded by expelling the rebellious nurses, suspending training, and demanding strict discipline, insomuch that nurses who trained there subsequently remembered feeling like they were in the military during their time at Victoria.[141] Despite the pushback from some, however, the racial and professional hierarchies would continue in South Africa for the foreseeable future.

Conclusion

From the first four female Xhosa nursing aides trained at Grey Hospital as colonial medicine encroached on Xhosa medicine to Makiwane's landmark achievement at the Lovedale mission hospital in 1908, African nurses rose as an integral part of both the Ciskei's and South Africa's health care system. By the 1950s they had gained a well-respected, elevated status in their own communities, and many young African women aspired to become nurses.[142] By this time, working with Xhosa beliefs and practices was more fraught with tension than the mid-nineteenth century, although Xhosa practitioners were likely less combative than European biomedical practitioners. Racial and professional tensions also manifested themselves as the number of African nurses grew and apartheid was imposed. As the apartheid state implemented new initiatives and gained more control in the Ciskei, the health care system shifted to a new era of state control and nurses' work. The system increasingly relied on African nurses to work in their communities, but their racial position in the broader system changed.

CHAPTER TWO

The Politics of Ciskei Homeland
Health Care

THE GROWTH IN THE NUMBER of trained Black nurses working in South Africa in the 1960s through the 1980s was remarkable. By the late 1970s, Black nurses constituted the majority of registered and enrolled nurses. Fully qualified African nurses grew from over 5,000 in 1960 to about 20,000 in 1978 (with an additional 32,000 enrolled nurses and nursing assistants), and to 24,142 by the end of 1983, for an increase of almost 400 percent in just over two decades.[1] An economic boom in the 1960s, greater African use of hospitals, and increased urbanization and educational opportunities led to a bigger Black middle class and more women interested in becoming nurses. One of the great demands for African nurses came from the formation of apartheid homelands. Statistics indicate that at times, over half of African nurses enumerated above worked in the homelands through the 1970s. For example, African nurses working in all the homelands combined numbered 10,725 in 1973.[2] In the Ciskei, numbers available after the establishment of the Ciskeian Nursing Council in 1984 show a growth in all levels of registered nurses of about 52 percent within a seven-year period, numbering 2,420 in 1984, nearly 3,547 in 1987, and 3,668 in 1991.[3]

The morphing political terrain of the 1960s through Ciskeian independence in the 1980s caused a number of shifts in the Ciskei health system. This affected the work of the growing number of African nurses. The 1960s brought a new state commitment to extending district services through rural clinics. During the 1970s, as the Ciskei government gained more self-governing powers, it took over mission hospitals and consolidated the health care system under a government-run, comprehensive approach that emphasized prevention and community health education. South African health department officials implemented comprehensive health care for mainly practical reasons, backed by ideologies of the time. The Ciskei carried this through into the 1980s.

Yet top-down directives did not entirely shape the system. Not all Ciskeian officials and health care practitioners on the ground were implicated in homeland corruption or took political directives. Many nurses, for instance, made the system their own, advancing services with their own commitments, visions, and degrees of autonomy. The paradoxical outcome was that although they acted within the broader problematic apartheid context, they made some improvements to health care services and the health of their people. The Ciskei increased the number of facilities, improved community health services, and curbed some diseases with immunization and feeding schemes. Improvements did not mean the Ciskei system and the health of the people became ideal. The impact was uneven, and some of the programs only treated the symptoms of South Africa's deeply rooted structures of inequality and exploitation. Furthermore, the untenable financial basis of the Ciskei as well as homeland corruption eventually crippled the system. Still, health officials and practitioners such as nurses forged ahead in their small sphere, despite the growing constraints and shortfalls, until the Ciskei fell apart in the early 1990s.

District Clinics into Comprehensive Health Care

Health care in the Ciskei started out in the 1960s with a cumbersome system of four separate but overlapping lines of authority—the tribal and regional authorities under Bantu Affairs, the South African Department of Health, the Cape Provincial Administration, and the mission hospitals. The tribal and regional authorities system replaced the preceding Native Affairs council system that had divided or reconfigured Xhosa chiefdoms under British colonial rule and left headmen to deal with local matters of public works, education, and relief of the sick.[4] Under apartheid, the government instituted "tribal" and "regional" authorities designed to more closely match so-called traditional authority in the homelands. The state split Xhosa territories into the Transkei Territorial Authority (1959) and the Ciskei Territorial Authority (1961), with councils of chiefs, headmen, or chairmen from each tribal authority. These territorial authorities could not change South African law but were given some self-governing powers.[5] Like the previous councils, the local tribal authorities (thirty-eight under nine regional authorities in the Ciskei) had decision-making power about local welfare and community development, including the authority to build clinics and give feedback on hospital and clinic services.

Under the new system in the 1960s, tribal authorities in the Ciskei used their power to increase the number of clinics in the region. White Bantu Affairs commissioners and Ciskei authorities recognized the importance of extending health care to the people through district clinic services, whether for political,

The Politics of Ciskei Homeland Health Care 51

practical, or more benevolent reasons. Out-station clinics certainly served a very important role in delivering care to a large number of people. In 1963, for example, Mount Coke reported that the hospital had attended to 16,694 people, while its five district clinics had attended to 10,000 more, for a total of 26,720.[6] Beginning in 1965, the regional authorities constructed a number of clinics and upgraded existing ones, taking over some clinics from hospitals. In 1965 and 1966, more than a dozen clinics were newly established or upgraded. In 1967 the Ciskei Territorial Authority made R 40,000 available for the erection of twenty more clinics in seven of the regional authorities.[7]

Opportunities and confusion came with the various entities involved, especially as approaches and funding changed. To establish a clinic, a regional authority would submit an application to the South African Department of Health, which would then send someone to inspect the chosen site. Sites were approved according to the number of people they would serve, proximity to the nearest clinic or hospital, potential coverage by a district surgeon, quality of the water supply and roads, and proximity to telephone service (perhaps in a trading post, but preferably in a school or police station). It was also best if the site had space for a demonstration garden and could be fenced.[8] For example, in the Keiskammahoek Regional authority, a clinic was reestablished in 1967 at Gxulu, ten miles away from St. Matthew's, and an entirely new clinic was built a year later in Rabula, serving more mountainous areas nine miles from other clinics and fourteen miles from the hospital. Whereas Rabula required more infrastructure, both had the right geographic position, population density, infrastructure, and coverage by St. Matthew's doctors.[9] Once the clinic was up and running, the local authorities were responsible for the upkeep and supervision of the clinic. However, if they wanted a part refund on the nurse's salary from the South African Department of Health (seven-eighths during this time), the nurse and the clinic had to pass periodic inspections by the department. The result was that nurses had to answer to multiple authorities, and facilities passed between different units. For example, in the Hewu district in the late 1960s, the regional government took over the Shiloh and Hackney clinics from the provincial administration and discussed building three more clinics.[10] Whereas Mount Coke's clinic system had been highlighted as exemplary in the 1950s, in the late 1960s, hospital records indicate that the hospital shut down or turned over all its clinics but Twecu to regional authorities to focus on growing its orthopedic and other surgical services.[11]

The 1970s brought a merging of these multiple systems that mirrored the consolidation of Ciskei territory and homeland political power. The process of restructuring the Ciskei was a contested and complex one that picked up the pace despite the resistance and mistrust the process engendered.[12] The reconfiguration of local authority opened opportunities for new political forces vying for power. The South African government installed A. Velile Sandile as the paramount chief of the amaXhosa of the Ciskei, and the Ciskei Territorial Assembly subsequently became a place for those claiming chiefly authority to gain influence.[13] Lennox Sebe, an educator with a degree in agriculture, claimed a Rharhabe chieftainship through his Tshawe lineage. He was first elected to the Assembly, where he held ministerial positions under Sandile's successor, Chief Justice Mabandla (who became chief executive in 1968). Sebe and Mabandla became rivals, establishing competing parties after the Ciskei gained self-governing status and held elections for a new Legislative Assembly in 1973. Within a few short years, Sebe and his Ciskei National Independence Party (CNIP) made the Ciskei a one-party state as the Legislative Assembly established new government councils, set up departments and ministries, and took over the administration of services.[14] Creating a geographically unified nation became a priority. Land consolidation included boundary negotiations and mass relocation. Unlike the Transkei, which was one territorial unit, the Ciskei was made up of nineteen scattered territories, separated by white-owned agricultural land and towns. As the South African government pushed for homeland independence in the mid-1970s, Ciskei leaders negotiated with the Transkei and the South African Republic to create a single Ciskei territory. When the Transkei was granted independence in 1976, it gained two contiguous districts from the Ciskei, Herschel and Glen Grey. Those who did not want to live in the Transkei fled to Ciskei areas such as Thornhill and Sada in the north.[15] The Ciskei eventually obtained land between its disparate territories, redrawn into eight political districts: Hewu, Seymour, Victoria East, Keiskammahoek, Middledrift, Peddie, Zwelitsha, Mdantsane. The Border region between the Transkei and Ciskei remained white-owned land of the South African Republic and retained towns like King William's Town. Settlements of Xhosa living outside the homelands were deemed "black spots" and targeted for removal (although many residents successfully resisted this). Thousands of people either self-relocated or were resettled in the Ciskei as a result, increasing the population by an estimated 76 percent in the 1970s.[16] Some removed from the Republic's land in the Cape Province also landed in Sada, while others were dumped in Dimbaza, a destination for those forcibly relocated beginning in 1967. Established in the early 1960s, the township of Mdantsane quickly grew as the site for people removed from East London areas or those seeking economic opportunities near East London but restricted to residing in the Ciskei. In 1970 the South African government passed the Bantu Homelands Citizenship Act requiring all Africans to be citizens of a self-governing "Bantu" territory.

The Politics of Ciskei Homeland Health Care   53

As the Ciskei moved toward so-called independence, the South African Department of Health imposed a new comprehensive health care scheme. In 1970 the Department of Bantu Affairs accepted financial responsibility for "Bantu" hospital services. Bantu Affairs then worked more closely with the South African Department of Health to start implementing the new approach in homeland regions. This approach prioritized social medicine, integrated services, primary health care, and preventive and promotive medicine—in other words, comprehensive integrated health care that gave "new life" to the 1944 Gluckman Report on national health services.[17] The Gluckman Report had come from a social medicine and community health movement in the 1940s, exemplified by Drs. Sydney and Emily Kark, who built the Pholela Health Center in southwestern Natal. For a moment, the excitement over community-centered health care caught on, and a number of centers were established. Within the national government, concerns about the declining health of Black populations and the fear of epidemics led to the National Health Services Commission (or Gluckman Commission), 1942–44, a government inquiry into the state of health services in the country. The report proposed a national plan focused on prevention, outreach, and the social determinants of health. While politics within and without the medical profession and the advent of apartheid had stopped the Gluckman Report recommendations from being adopted in South Africa, the apartheid government later implemented a similar approach in the homelands to ensure a healthy Black workforce in a less expensive way.[18] People in rural homelands suffered from malnutrition, TB, and other communicable diseases, but the areas faced a severe shortage of doctors and overloaded hospitals. Department of Health officials hoped shoring up the clinics would relieve some of the pressure on the hospitals.[19] It was partly this necessity that led hospital and health officials to acknowledge on the record that their fully qualified nurses performed outstanding work in the clinics above and beyond their normal expectations.[20] Officials could also look to the World Health Organization (WHO) for ideological backing. Drawing on WHO definitions, they would describe comprehensive health as encompassing the physical, mental, and social well-being of an individual. By extension, at the community level this meant "the prolongation of life; the improvement and enhancement of the environment; the control of infectious and contagious diseases; the improvement of personal hygiene; and the early diagnosis and detection of illness."[21]

Ciskeian politicians and officials readily adopted the new approach for similar reasons, but for their own as well. They focused on clinics, in part to deal with financial and personnel restraints, in part so that politicians could appeal to their constituents, and in part to reach remote people in dire need of care.

Ciskei hospitals did not have the staff to send doctors to each clinic even weekly or biweekly. In fact, they did not even have enough doctors to handle the number of patients coming to the hospitals. St. Matthew's Hospital, for example, had a particularly difficult time retaining doctors for more than one or two years in the 1970s. Ciskei Territory legislative records from the 1970s include numerous statements by chiefs and councilors that the health of the people was of upmost importance. Members of the legislature from rural areas repeatedly asked for services to be improved and extended to those in remote places to answer the needs of their people. These demands evidence the political importance of health care and give the impression that politicians with influence favored urban townships such as Mdantsane and the areas near the political center of Ciskei—Zwelitsha, then Bhisho. They also suggest that some assembly members genuinely cared about the state of health of their people. Ciskei health officials also repeated the more ideological importance of providing "total" care "for the individual, the family, the community and the nation of the Ciskei." This required preventive services as well as curative and environmental services. Subsequent annual reports continued to emphasize this three-pronged approach and the vital role of clinics, social workers, and environmental inspectors in delivering comprehensive care.

Not so different from earlier systems, a major aspect of the new comprehensive system was extending the clinic system with more nurses. Ciskei authorities enthusiastically declared that they would have two nurses at each clinic, on duty twenty-four hours, and that the Ciskei would one day have a clinic in every location.[22] The hospitals were tasked with overseeing a network of three types of clinics: permanent clinics, subclinics, and mobile clinics. The long-term plan also included health centers and various health teams. Nurses working in the clinics and health centers provided primary health care, treating common colds, minor ailments, and cases such as gastroenteritis, hypertension, diabetes, or sexually transmitted infections. Most also dealt with maternity cases, delivering babies and running antenatal and well-baby clinics. Preventive measures included distributing immunizations and vaccinations and addressing malnutrition. Nurses stationed at clinics and subclinics continued the long-standing program of distributing milk powder to malnourished or impoverished children. Weekly subclinics offered basic or elementary services where permanent clinics were not available. Mobile clinics and health teams also took health care directly to people. Plans for school health services started with the appointment of a senior nurse in each district to give health education, detect preventable conditions, and monitor and administer immunizations in schools.[23] The Ciskei also began to involve environmental inspectors as well as social workers to aid in addressing all aspects of the people's

The Politics of Ciskei Homeland Health Care

health. Working closely with mission hospitals, implementation in the homelands began in 1970, backed by financing from Pretoria. In 1971 the Ciskei asked Mount Coke Hospital to act as the controlling body and supervise rural clinics and mobile team assistants. The hospital took over the administration of nine clinics and subclinics built by "tribal" authorities. The hospital superintendent, J. J. Adendorff, set to work organizing and analyzing the system, mapping out where clinics were needed and planning for the future.[24] This change affected two other mission hospitals in the area as well, St. Matthew's and the relatively new Dutch Reformed Church mission hospital in Peddie, Nompumelelo (which admitted its first patient in 1964).[25]

On the other hand, the government built the Cecilia Makiwane Hospital during this time. The state started planning for a hospital in Mdantsane in the late 1960s when the township was growing and the public hospital in East London, Frere Hospital, was overcrowded.[26] The government had big plans for this hospital. Unlike the four former mission hospitals that serviced rural populations, this hospital became a specialty referral and teaching hospital in an urban area. It opened partially in 1975, named after Fikile Siyo (the Ciskei minister of interior and then minister of health until he was driven out by Sebe in 1977). It offered general medicine, surgery, orthopedics, urology, and ophthalmology. It also had radiology and other laboratories. It employed 18 consultants, 37 general duties medical officers, and 553 nurses. The end goal was to house 1,450 beds.[27] It attended to thousands. In 1978 the hospital reported that it treated more than 100,000 people per year since its opening, averaging 8,700 per month.[28] As it expanded, it established a school of nursing that trained registered nurses and midwives and offered further diplomas and in-service training. Ciskei politicians could point to the hospital as a modern facility, housing high-technology medicine and more specialization, just like the kind of medicine developing in South Africa and the rest of the world in the 1960s and 1970s. Yet apartheid politics determined its location in an urban area difficult for many rural people across the Ciskei to access.[29]

As the Ciskei gained more self-governing power, the newly established (1972) Ciskeian Legislative Assembly formed its own Department of Health and Welfare in November 1975. With new authority, Ciskeian officials set out to streamline health care services under African leadership and take over mission hospitals. Mission hospitals had anticipated this move (it had started in the Transkei in 1972). Some, like St. Matthew's, accepted it as inevitable and appropriate that the government take responsibility over health care.[30] Others hoped they could remain church governed, especially Methodist mission hospitals.[31] The Lovedale hospitals had retained church influence after they had become Cape Provincial hospitals in 1950, with the Federal Theological Seminary in

Alice sending staff to conduct services at the hospital as late as 1971.[32] With administrative changes and continued growth in the 1960s, the Mount Coke Hospital administration had reaffirmed its commitment to its spiritual mission. As it expanded its buildings and services, it also hired full-time evangelists.[33] Superintendent Adendorff took the lead in advocating for mission hospitals and resisted government control as long as possible, arguing that the Christian ethos helped mission hospitals run more economically and attracted doctors to rural areas.[34] Some hospitals and doctors joined the Transkei and Ciskei Association of Mission Hospitals in hopes of presenting a united front to the government.[35] Yet the South African state had the financial upper hand when negotiating mission hospital takeovers.[36] The few authors who have written about the mission hospital takeover have lamented the loss of the hospitals' Christian character, argued that the missions gave in to apartheid, or high-lighted how nurses maintained religious practices in the hospitals.[37] Consider-ing the difficulties the hospital had in securing funding and full-time doctors as well as dealing with overcrowding, St. Matthew's Hospital's more practical response made sense. The takeover was completed at Mount Coke in August 1976, at Nompumelelo in February 1977, and at St. Matthew's in April 1977.

Although many hospital staff committed to keeping a Christian witness, "Africanization of staff" prevented maintaining control of that as well. Remov-ing white leadership was a political priority for those promoting the benefits of homelands but a threat to the control and power of the white staff of mis-sion hospitals.[38] In the process of the government takeover, Mount Coke had to submit a list of Black staff and white staff and wait for word from the Ciskei Department of Health and Pretoria on their fate.[39] A number of matrons and doctors left the Ciskei at this time, and the Ciskei indeed continued to find it difficult to recruit more doctors. Later, Mount Coke's superintendent, Dr. Rod Mcdade, was fired without notice and replaced by Dr. Leslie Mzimba. Ironically, a white Ciskei minister of health, Jack Klopper, delivered the termi-nation letter, evidence of the hand of Pretoria in these changes and the politi-cal motivations behind Africanization.[40] It was likely Adendorff who lamented in a Mount Coke newsletter, "There has been a marked decline in interest in the Spiritual work, particularly amongst the nurses, since take-over."[41] At the same time, little in my interviews indicated that hospitals experienced major changes in their operations as they transitioned to the new management. Hull similarly found that nurses continued to carry on Christian practices in Bethesda Hospital in Natal.[42] Overall, the end result was a more unified health care sys-tem that led to more efficiency and opened up the possibility of African con-trol. By the end of the 1970s, the Ciskei included five hospitals, sixty-eight rural health centers or clinics, and forty-one subclinics. The Ciskei oversaw

The Politics of Ciskei Homeland Health Care

this system with 75 professional and administrative officers, 2,803 other employees, and a R16 million budget.[43] Yet these changes also put the hospitals more firmly under apartheid governments, with their accompanying financial and staffing problems.

Challenges and Achievements of Ciskei Health Care

In 1978 Sebe and his CNIP claimed electoral victory in the Ciskei. Soon after, his rival's party dissolved into the CNIP and Sebe declared himself president for life. This essentially secured Ciskei's path to independence. Even though an independent commission of inquiry, the Quail Commission, concluded that the Ciskei did not have an adequate economy or popular support for independence, Sebe and the South African government went ahead with the process anyway. With great fanfare celebrating a manufactured Ciskei national identity, the two governments proclaimed the Ciskei independent on December 4, 1981. Subsequent years were tumultuous ones for the Ciskei and South Africa. The global economic downturn in the 1970s and increased sanctions against apartheid in South Africa led to economic strains. Mass resistance increased throughout South Africa, and Sebe continued to face political challenges, despite his victory at establishing a one-party state and his attempts at agricultural and industrial development. Ciskei ministers and internal enemies changed frequently. Mdantsane residents orchestrated a major boycott of Ciskei busses in 1983 that turned violent at times; Sebe suspected his own brother, head of Ciskei security forces Charles Sebe, of plotting a coup and jailed him in 1984; the Transkei attacked Sebe's palace in 1987; and multiple community movements at times clashed violently with Ciskei forces. Sebe continued to impose CNIP dominance and ruthlessly quash opposition with his security forces but would not last long after Nelson Mandela's release from prison in early 1990.[44]

The yearly reports of the Ciskei Department of Health during this time, however, give little indication that it existed in this politically turbulent time or that there were corruption charges and eight ministers of health in thirteen years (that is, until the written record disappears in 1989, when Jan Pieterse resigned as minister and the Ciskei was in a political state of emergency). Even as opposition to apartheid mounted in the mid-1970s and the economic situation and health of people in the homelands in general declined, the Ciskei Department of Health and Welfare continued to implement initiatives already underway with strong government support. Although it did not reach levels near that of the Republic of South Africa, the Ciskei ended up spending the most per capita on health care among the homelands.[45] The silence regarding politics in health records could be reflective of the commitment officials had to the Ciskei project or indicative of biomedical professionals trained to divorce their work from politics or view health in isolation from social and political forces. These silences and biases in the government records make assessing health care in the period of Ciskei independence challenging. Official government publications from the early years of Ciskei independence celebrate the achievements of the new nation, overstating improvements and taking credit for developments begun before Ciskeian independence. Similarly, speeches and forewords to written reports by ministers overseeing health care often provide glowing praise of the system. Yet considering the more complex perspective of the detailed yearly reports, as well as taking into account legislative debates, independent reports, newspaper articles, and oral history sources, it is possible to get a sense of the overall challenges and achievements of the Ciskei health care system. These records also indicate that lower level officials were less concerned about politics and more concerned about how to improve the conditions on the ground. Many nurses and employees also enjoyed greater autonomy within homeland systems, even though they worked in a limited sphere.[46]

It was no small undertaking to administer the health care system under a new government administration that faced a number of difficult health challenges. Tuberculosis continued to be a major problem, along with malnutrition, resulting in incidents of kwashiorkor, marasmus, and pellagra. People in the region also battled respiratory diseases, gastroenteritis, and other communicable diseases such as measles and typhoid fever (with HIV/AIDS coming after 1988).[47] In 1972 the World Health Organization estimated that 58 percent of rural Black deaths in South Africa were caused by malnutrition and gastroenteritis.[48] Environmental and economic conditions exacerbated these problems. Scholars pointed to a decline in agricultural productivity and overcrowding in the Ciskei in part because of government betterment and relocation and in part because of periodic droughts.[49] Migrant labor and massive relocation also played a role. Dr. Trudi Thomas's study on the correlation between absent fathers and the rates of diseases of malnutrition among children in the area served by the St. Matthew's Hospital poignantly demonstrated the negative effects of migrant labor on health.[50] People suffering poor conditions in relocation areas generally suffered more ill-health than other places and created a need for new health care services. Infant mortality rates for Black South Africans during these times are not entirely reliable, as record keeping was not complete; yet the information available reveals the state of Ciskeian health in comparative perspective. There is evidence that from 1960 through the 1980s, the infant mortality rate for white South Africans decreased from 30 per 1,000 births to around 9 or 13. In contrast, those classified as Africans suffered a rate of up to six times higher.[51] Estimates for Africans in the 1960s and 1970s ranged

The Politics of Ciskei Homeland Health Care 59

from 140 to 180, while other numbers showed the rate remaining steady at 80 through the early 1980s and dropping to around 63 at the end of the decade. Switzer estimated a rate of 250 in the rural Ciskei in the early 1980s, and Digby wrote that the Ciskei had an infant mortality rate similar to most other homelands of around 50 in 1989 (excluding Transkei).[52] Despite the range of numbers, it is clear that the health of Ciskeians was suffering in a number of places.

Comparing reports that bookend the last decade of the government written record, the Department of Health and Welfare report of 1978 and the Department of Health report of 1988, it is clear that the Ciskei did increase health care available to people with the establishment of more clinics as well as with improved hospitals. The increase in clinics was not as dramatic as in the 1960s and 1970s (Digby shows a bigger total increase in Ciskeian clinics from fifty-three in 1976 to eighty-nine in 1985). Yet the number of clinics grew by three or four under most hospitals from 1978 to 1988, and the number of mobile clinics also extended the reach of health services. In some cases, this was a significant improvement in the services available.[53]

In 1988 the Ciskei had the lowest population to clinic ratio among the homelands and South African provinces, with one clinic for every eight thousand people (Venda and the Cape Province had the next closest ratio of nearly ten thousand).[54] Retired nurses who worked in the Ciskei remembered the increase in the number of clinics in rural villages as positive improvements. Their memories likely conflated the time before and after Ciskei independence, but the way they remembered the increase shows that they felt the impact was great. For example, Lulu Zuma, speaking of both the Ciskei and Transkei, said that "clinics started springing up, . . . springing up in all the rural areas."[55] Former clinic nurse and clinic supervisor Victoria Mjikeliso remembered the increase in clinics making it easier for people to access health care: "In the Ciskei, a lot of clinics were built and they were nearer each other. They were at the proximity for people to be able to attend—walking distances."[56] Some

Table 2.1. Ciskei increase in clinics

Hospital	1978 clinics	1988 clinics
Cecilia Makiwane	14	18 (7 rural, 1 mobile)
Mount Coke	18 static, 14 subclinics	28
St. Matthew's/S. S. Gida	13 (static clinics only)	16 (static clinics only)
Nompumelelo	7	13
Victoria	6 (static clinics only, 1983)	7 (rural only)
Hewu District	12 static, 9 subclinics	20 (total, 1986)

nurses also talked of the improved infrastructure of existing facilities. Nobantu Baleni, another former supervisor, claimed, "We had first-class clinics with the Ciskei government. All the clinics were [renovated]. All the clinics had nurse's homes, for the nurses to sleep."[57] Their positions as supervisors may have influenced Baleni and Mjikeliso to take a more positive perspective of the past. Yet even if the clinics were unevenly placed or did not make it to every village as promised, the numbers do show an increase in facilities.

The Ciskei also endeavored to improve hospital facilities. The government inherited mission hospitals badly in need of infrastructure improvements, and some areas were in desperate need of any health care services at all. Three new hospitals were eventually built to address these problems. St. Matthew's Hospital finally made way for a new hospital in the town of Keiskammahoek, named S. S. Gida, completed in 1985. The Hewu Hospital officially opened in 1987 with 250 beds and was linked to the Thornhill Mini Hospital with 25 beds, making the biggest impact for those who had relocated from other territories to the northern Ciskei. The government began talking about upgrading the Mount Coke Hospital in the mid-1980s. Politicians wanted services in Bhisho, the new Ciskei capital, so the Bhisho Hospital was built as a replacement for Mount Coke. It opened in 1991 as apartheid was unraveling.[58] The number of beds offered at the major hospitals increased with this new construction, most dramatically with the Hewu Hospital, and Cecilia Makiwane and Nompumelelo both expanded greatly under the Ciskei.[59] The bed to population ratio tells a slightly different story. This number did not increase significantly in the 1960s and 1970s because of apartheid relocations. The population of the Ciskei almost doubled between 1973 and 1983, from about 350,000 to 630,000.[60] As a result, Switzer pointed out, the proportion of beds to population stayed virtually the same as in the first half of the twentieth century, with 2.1 per 1,000 in 1946 and 2.3 in 1980.[61] With more hospital beds in Mdantsane, Peddie, and Hewu in the 1980s, however, the Ciskei made more gains in more densely populated areas, reporting a ratio of just over 4 in 1988.[62]

The Ciskei expanded its comprehensive health services with more mobile teams. At the end of 1982, the Ciskei announced a change in the type of clinics it would offer. In place of subclinics, the government would provide either mobile clinics or community health centers. The minister of health, then C. H. J. Van Aswegen, also announced that it would work with the Departments of Agriculture, Education, and Rural Development to create a five-year plan for improving comprehensive health care.[63] Despite major challenges in obtaining and maintaining adequate transportation resources, these teams addressed immunizations, or vaccinations, school health issues, TB, and environmental issues. Mjikeliso described the more comprehensive approach to

The Politics of Ciskei Homeland Health Care   61

community health care that sent teams of practitioners traveling around from village to village throughout the 1980s and early 1990s:

> And these outreach services were practiced a lot there because what they wanted, the people mustn't go to the clinic, they must know about the health issues. So they were in place, those outreach teams, in all the areas of the Ciskei. You have a school nurse, a nurse who was dealing with family planning, a nurse who was dealing with TB, the educators, . . . the environmental health officers. We had them at that time. We had the dentist, we had the doctors—doctors were going around the clinics, reaching people. And we also had the mobile services, where people were being seen in those far areas by the nurses. And they were working as a team, doing this comprehensive approach.[64]

Nonzwakazi Gqomfa, who had a career in both mobile and static clinics in the Victoria East areas, similarly praised the comprehensive approach of the Ciskei health services. She remembered the breadth of issues she helped address in the mobile clinic that stopped at the end of long dusty roads or in villages tucked away in hills with low-growing vegetation: "But we used to go out every day and with the primary health care services, we used to render the well-baby clinics, . . . do immunizations, weighing of babies, . . . give them milk supply to help the mothers with the feeding of the babies, . . . the handouts for the elderly, . . . the soups, pro-nutro, milk, to give to the old people and the malnourished." She then talked about the role of the village health workers (VHWs) in reaching the community, saying, "They used to go door to door and come and report to you anything they see so that you go and visit. . . . Those that are not able to come to the clinic, we used to go out to them."[65]

Other retired nurses talked proudly of the multifaceted approach the Ciskei health services adopted. Alecia Phiwo Dubula enjoyed working in the St. Matthew's and S. S. Gida regions with representatives from the Departments of Works and Agriculture to address health issues in communities beyond simple curative medicine.[66] Dentists and agricultural inspectors would descend out of vans with the nurses. Social workers, whether stationed at schools, in hospitals, or with clinics, dealt with cases wherein an individual or family's health was affected by a breakdown in economic or social relations. This made the approach truly comprehensive in the eyes of the nurses who worked in the Ciskei. Again, there could have been an element of self-promotion in the testimonies of these nurses. Yet independent research showed that for some places, the comprehensive health care system worked well. Julia Segar's study published at Rhodes University in 1991 highlighted the coverage the Rabula villages had with mobile clinics, school programs, and TB and psychiatric teams. A fully staffed Rabula clinic served the area along with eleven VHWs who referred patients to the S. S. Gida Hospital for specialized services. The study reported a 94 percent usage of the public health facilities and almost full immunization coverage.[67]

In addition to the Rhodes study, statistics reported by the Ciskei in 1988 regarding immunization showed marked progress with this aspect of preventive care. A major development was the institution of compulsory immunization for school enrollment in 1984. Measles outbreaks in 1983 and 1986 made immunization more urgent.[68] In 1987 the Department of Health further attempted to immunize every child and adopted the WHO goal of immunizing all children by 1990. It reported that by the end of 1988, five districts had finished the first stage, with 99–100 percent of children immunized in Keiskammahoek, Middledrift, and Victoria districts. Thirty-five villages in the Zwelitsha district received the first shots for measles, polio, diphtheria, whooping cough, and tetanus. The Peddie, Mdantsane, and Hewu districts reached over 90 percent coverage. Despite funding cuts, hopes were high that with a little bit of expansion of the program they could eradicate measles, polio, diphtheria, and whooping cough by 1991.[69]

The challenges implementing comprehensive health care in the Ciskei demanded more senior nurses and tutors and more integrated training for nurses. Digby described how apartheid homeland governments and the South African government created various programs and linked with universities to provide the training that was "so desperately needed."[70] The Ciskei increased nursing training through in-service training programs, study leaves, and integrated training linked to the University of Fort Hare. Many nurses I interviewed appreciated that the Ciskei offered nurses in-service training and short courses on a variety of topics to add to their general nursing and midwifery courses. A number of nurses who worked in rural clinics, for example, completed a degree in community health nursing and health administration, either through the new program provided at the Cecilia Makiwane Hospital or through the University of South Africa. Many also completed certificates in psychiatric nursing and obtained training in family planning, two other areas where the Ciskei sought to improve health care coverage.[71] Continuously adding to their skill set with experience and training improved the nurses' abilities to deliver health care. Cecilia Makiwane and the University of Fort Hare both entered into nursing training in the 1980s, with Fort Hare establishing a nursing school in partnership with the hospital in 1984. More nursing programs became linked to universities during this time as they changed the curriculum. This increased opportunities for Black nurses to gain MA and PhD degrees and become heads of academic departments. General registered nurse training grew from three to four years and included psychiatric, community health, and midwifery courses that had been offered as post-basic courses before.[72] As dealt with more in the conclusion, retired nurses criticized the integrated university courses as less practical, but they serve as another example of how the Ciskei expanded personnel training.

The Ciskei also experimented with training VHWs. To answer a huge shortage of doctors and other specialists in the 1980s, the Ciskei relied on foreign doctors and seconded South African doctors.[73] At times the South African Defense Force supplied military doctors to Ciskei hospitals.[74] Moreover, the Ciskei began to lose more and more nurses to the private sector in the late 1980s as the Ciskei could not pay them better wages. VHWs supplemented nurses' work as low-level professionals who monitored patients, kept track of home environment conditions, focused on preventive health care, and provided basic first aid. They had minimal training and little medical authority, but nurses who worked with them praised them for acting as the eyes and ears of nurses in remote villages. They could follow up with patients on a strict treatment regimen, report sanitation problems, register births, and perform follow-up home visits. The Ciskei used VHWs to great effect in some areas. From 1983 the Hewu district, for instance, employed forty VHWs, and VHWs monitored the reach of immunizations for the Nompumelelo Hospital. The following year, they apparently helped clinics and hospitals spread the word about the effectiveness of using salt and sugar as a home remedy to treat diarrhea.[75] Although the impact of the VHWs is not entirely clear, the number of workers in action in the Ciskei and the number of people they reached suggest that they did contribute to the increase in the reach of health care services to remote Ciskeians. VHWs visited at least 23,393 homes in 1988 and made a reported 58,699 health education visits. The Ciskei Department of Health Report concluded that VHWs were "indispensable" in reducing malnutrition, gastroenteritis, and measles.[76]

Like other aspects of Ciskeian health care, however, the impact of VHWs was uneven.[77] A number of elements factored into the uneven reach of Ciskeian health care, but political decisions often led to discrepancies. The inescapable underlying fact was that it was part of a broader apartheid system that resulted in great health challenges and systemic limitations. Politicians knew the power of providing health care in winning over loyalties and favored certain areas where they hoped to have a political influence. The case of two clinics built in the village of Zinyoka (six miles [nine kilometers] outside of King William's Town), provides a striking example. Whereas other more remote locations struggled to have their repeated requests for clinics answered, Zinyoka got two because the government wanted to counter the influence of Black Consciousness activists in the village. Steve Biko and his colleagues threatened the Ciskei government with their political presence in and around King William's Town in the mid-1970s. In 1975 they opened the Zanempilo Community Health Center in Zinyoka, a well-resourced center run by Black doctors and nurses who did not support separate development and yet proved committed to uplifting Black communities. The fact that the Ciskei government attempted to thwart the work of Zanempilo by building a rival clinic in the same village revealed that the government used health care provision as a political tool at times.[78] As another example, one interviewee, Lumka Someketha, spoke very highly of the Mthombe village in the Mount Coke district, where she worked for six months while another nurse was on maternity leave. Even though the village was small and the clinic had few patients ("you couldn't see ten people a day"), the clinic nurses and social worker each had their own accommodation and the hospital kept the clinic well stocked because a Ciskei minister lived there.[79]

The Ciskei also made some progress in fending off diseases of malnutrition; but as Packard pointed out in regard to government efforts to curb TB, this included "little or no amelioration of the underlying causes."[80] Three of the most common cases nurses dealt with in children in rural clinics and hospitals were gastroenteritis, kwashiorkor, and marasmus. In an effort to immediately address malnutrition, the clinics, hospitals, various government agencies, and welfare organizations had long been providing food supplements to those in need, particularly by delivering powdered milk from clinics. In 1978 the Ciskei government stated that it sought to ensure that all preschool children obtained five hundred grams of milk powder per week.[81] A study conducted by the National Research Institute for Nutritional Diseases in 1979 concluded that the weight and height of Ciskei children aged six months to two years was comparable to international standards, but that there was a general lack of protein in people's diets, leading to cases of kwashiorkor and pellagra.[82] This led the government to introduce protein-enriched coarsely ground maize or mealie meal into the region. The Ciskei Republic continued food supplement programs into the 1980s, showing that earlier efforts had not solved the larger problem, even though government reports claimed that the feeding schemes had a positive impact.[83] Certainly, the food supplements helped to sustain a number of people, and nutritional education at clinics did positively change some feeding practices. Yet malnutrition also clearly continued to be a problem. News articles and research reports highlighted the fact that government feeding schemes only scratched the surface and pointed to an underlying crisis.[84] Some practitioners and officials, such as St. Matthew's Dr. Trudi Thomas, recognized the economic struggles of the people as the root cause of malnutrition.[85]

The Politics of Ciskei Homeland Health Care 65

Black doctors spoke out even more forcefully. Dr. Mamphela Ramphele, based at the Zanempilo Community Health Center, argued that the root causes were not just migrant labor but also job reservation, unemployment, low wages, and a lack of educational facilities (not just illiteracy, as other doctors claimed). Unlike other doctors, she disagreed that family planning was a solution. If there was no income, she argued, there would be no food no matter how small the family.[86] Dr. Charles Bikitsha, medical doctor, Transkei minister of health, and advisor to the Ciskei, also was not afraid to credit underdevelopment, exploitation, and neglect with causing these problems in the homelands.[87] A survey done by the Quaker Peace Work Committee and Border Council of Churches for a Carnegie conference on poverty "revealed a grim picture of 'grinding poverty, broken families and general destitution'" in Ciskei resettlement communities in 1984.[88]

The shaky foundation of the broader system is particularly revealed by the frustrations, discontent, and unsustainability of the financial relationship between the Ciskei and the Republic of South Africa. Although it wanted to operate as an independent government, the Ciskei depended on the Republic of South Africa to fulfill its promises of providing funding. Resources given to the Ciskei from Pretoria included direct financial assistance such as annual grants, relief aid, and development loans.[89] It also included aid more difficult to quantify, such as seconded ministers and director generals or hospital superintendents. With increasing self-governance and the granting of political independence to the Ciskei, the financial needs of the Ciskei rapidly increased. In the 1970s, as the Ciskei set up more and more government structures for independence, the budget swelled from R9.9 million in 1970/71 to R118 million in 1980/81.[90] The Ciskei continued to overrely on aid from the Republic,

Table 2.2. Republic of South Africa (RSA) payments to Ciskei

Year	Estimated direct payments from RSA	Estimated from Ciskei internal revenue	Ciskei total budget
1981/82	R121,492,700	R21,095	R146,489,000
1982/83	—	—	R269,735,000
1983/84	—	R59,959,000	R358,443,452
1984/85	R314,789,900	R59,959,000	R509,591,314
1985/86	R325,129,000	R98,375,000	R591,799,000
1987/88	R628,200,000	R136,800,000	R859,000,000
1988/89	R663,107,000	—	R1,068,506,000
1989/90	R748,314,977	—	R1,312,231,000

sparking controversy in South African political debates. After its official independence, total South African direct payments to the Ciskei constituted anywhere from 55 percent to more than 70 percent of the Ciskei's total budget (excluding other forms of aid).[91]

On the South African side, debates grew in parliament about the amount of money the government was putting toward the upkeep of the homelands. Some members of parliament felt that giving almost 9 percent of the 1984/85 state budget to the homelands was too much. Frederik van Zyl Slabbert, the head of the Progressive Federal Party pointed out that the South African economy could not sustain the government's apartheid policies. "Over 30 years . . . we have developed a system of bureaucratic patronage and privilege which is costing us a fortune," he declared. Furthermore, he argued, South African funding comprised 77 percent of the income of the homeland governments, and this benefited the employees of those governments more than the regular citizens. His speech was rightly taken as an attack on apartheid policy, one that bluntly exposed problems with the homeland system. On the other hand, Sheena Duncan, the head of the women's political group the Black Sash, felt that 8.8 percent of the Republic of South Africa budget was much too little, representing "a totally distorted and inadequate distribution of the financial wealth of this country."[92] Debates about the future of homeland funding persisted into 1989 and 1990, when some in the financial media decried the assistance for "self determination" as "wasteful nonsense," while others continued to argue that homeland residents were rightful recipients of South African resources and in fact ought to receive more funding—not as a transfer of funds but as a refund.[93]

Despite the pressure put on South Africa by Ciskeian officials and politicians to pay up, the Ciskei's Department of Health's yearly budget consistently reported deficits. Budget reports in 1986–88 pointed to the allocation shortfall as a problem, with the budget not taking into account inflation. With a large number of nurses and other medical staff at the various expanding facilities, salaries and wages constituted a majority of each year's budget and needed to increase with yearly increments as well. Moreover, taxes and tariffs also increased costs in the late 1980s. With competing demands on limited resources, the legislature voted in some years to maintain the budget of the previous year, or even allocate less money than the year before (see table 2.3).[94]

In some years, the Department of Health asked for more money from the treasury or other government funds to make up for the expected deficit. As in 1984 the department also appealed to the South African government to boost its contributions, either through statutory payments or payments through other government programs such as the Committee for Economic and Development

Table 2.3. Ciskei Department of Health budget

Year	Budget/Actual expenditure	Deficit
1978	R16 million/—	—
1982/83	—/R71,845,000	—
1983/84*	R56 million/R62,882,000	R6,900,000
1984/85	R41,267,000/R55,226,762	R13,959,762
1985/86	R56,620,000/R66,334,946	R9,714,946
1986/87	R63,250,000/R80,680531	R17,430,531
1987/88	R89,300,000/R97,446,300	R8,146,300
1988/89	R105,798,000/R116,987,560	R11,189,560

*Year the Department of Health split from the Department of Social Welfare and Pensions

Co-operation in Southern Africa (or KEOSSA, the Afrikaans acronym).[95] In other years, the department relied on resources and investments from outside the Ciskei and South Africa. Digby argued that the Ciskei and Bophuthatswana were the best financially endowed homelands, with two or three times the per capita expenditures of KwaNdebele and Lebowa. In her assessment, the Ciskei succeeded in this in part by securing private funding or investments to pay workers' salaries and to combat malnutrition.[96] Indeed, like the mission hospitals that struggled financially before, the Ciskei brought in a number of outside resources. In 1982 more than thirty organizations reportedly supplemented Ciskei medical services. Grants and aid continued to pay for VHWs, feeding schemes, and supplies.[97]

The deficit in funding caused staffing and resource problems that hindered the Ciskei's delivery of health care. The problem persisted as doctors and nurses increasingly chose to work in the private sector.[98] The 1983 annual report stated that the department could not fill vacant posts because of financial constraints and instituted a hiring freeze.[99] A tense interaction in 1984 between the Ciskei minister of health, Hennie C. Beukes, and a KEOSSA official led Beukes to complain to the Ciskei National Assembly: "I would like to challenge Mr. Botha to build two 250-bed hospitals with nurses' accommodation and with accommodation for doctors, equipped with the best German equipment . . . for 35 million rand. . . . Maybe he will help us seeing that he says we do not need the Israeli doctors; maybe he will help us to get the 57 doctors that we are still short of."[100] One of the most glaring strains on services caused by financial deficits related to the transport necessary to reach remote rural populations. The environmental services division, immunization teams, mobile clinics, and other medical officers required to travel all highlighted the lack of transport as a major challenge. At the end of 1984, for instance, the St. Matthew's Hospital reported: "1984 was another disastrous year for our transport department; generally poor and undisciplined drivers, inadequate maintenance and repair facilities and terrible roads all contributed to the breakdown of all the transport dependent services—mobile teams, clinic supervisory services, stores and supplies, health education and TB follow up."[101] In 1985 the Department of Health lamented, "Our Community Health Services . . . have practically come to a stand still [sic] due to the lack of suitable transport." It went on to give an astonishing number: 45 of 186 vehicles were in good condition. The rest spent 80 percent of the time in the workshop.[102] Road conditions and "undisciplined" drivers factored into transportation problems.[103] Yet reports and newspaper articles indicate a lack of financial resources and corruption caused many of the problems.[104]

Staff and transportation shortages were made worse by corruption, including a scandal involving Beukes, two other white Ciskeian officials, and an Israeli construction company. The Ciskei's links to Israel proved important in obtaining extra funding—for both the health care system and corrupt officials. With room for officials and politicians to skim off the top, this relationship both benefited and hurt Ciskei health care. Sebe established close relations with Israeli investors in Tel Aviv, where he obtained a Ciskei trade office, and the West Bank city of Ariel was declared a sister city to Bhisho. Israeli doctors went to work in the Ciskei, and in 1985 the Israeli project Degem trained VHWs.[105] An Israeli company, the Gur Corporation, built the S. S. Gida Hospital in Keiskammahoek, modeled after Israeli hospitals. The hospital later received consultations from Israeli health professionals.[106] Upon further inspection, the hospital was discovered to have structural flaws, and news broke that Minister of Health Beukes and the Director General H. M. Mdleleni had accepted money and materials from the Gur Corporation in exchange for building contracts. Two white South African representatives for the Ciskei to Israel had already been fired for demanding 10 percent of the projects of those seeking to invest in the Ciskei. The Hewu Hospital's opening was delayed because it was also being built by the Gur Corporation.[107] Beukes, who claimed he only acted under instruction, resigned and was later convicted by a one-man commission. Considering the corruption taking place in other parts of the Ciskeian government, it is likely that Beukes and Mdleleni were guilty but also scapegoats.[108] In the end, South African aid and other statutory payments remained at inadequate levels that were unsustainable, undermining the Ciskei's comprehensive health care achievements and opening the door for further corruption problems.

The Politics of Ciskei Homeland Health Care

Ciskei Nurses—Independent and Progressive?

Nurses worked in this problematic system. Yet although money and the comprehensive approach were tied to South Africa, Ciskei health care was not just a product of Pretoria with a Xhosa face. Certainly, some top officials were fully invested in the Ciskei project. Politicians looked for everything they could praise to garner support. For example, in the 1988 annual report, the Department of Health enthusiastically welcomed Dr. H. Zokufa back from the United States, where he had completed a PhD in pharmacology. Zokufa was distinguished by the fact that he was a Ciskeian and would be taking over the pharmacology department at Cecilia Makiwane Hospital—all of this made possible by the Ciskei system itself, the report was careful to point out. The report proceeded by naming various other Ciskeians at work in positions of leadership, from directors of health programs to lead carpenters.[109] And yet the minister of health was usually a white person, often tied to Pretoria, which posed a problem for making the case for Ciskei independence. On the other hand, health officials and practitioners at different levels took the health care system as their own and used their own skills and ideas to shape it. Changes in the South African nursing profession more broadly throughout this time reflected growing autonomy of the nursing associations and a greater recognition of Black nursing achievements.[110] By the late 1970s, Black nurses were widely employed in private hospitals as well, and more officials and managerial staff became open to equalizing pay across races.[111] Still, homelands offered nurses an environment less immediately dominated by racial hierarchies. In mission hospitals in the past and in the South African Republic, racial barriers had blocked Black nurses from promotions. In contrast, nurses felt they could fulfill their potential in the homelands.[112] For example, Lulu Msutu Zuma counted her time as a matron at the hospital in Mthatha as the highlight of her career. One of her major successes was the disaster management plan she devised for the entire Transkei. "I was at the top there and I liked it. I so liked it!" she exclaimed. This was not just about reveling in having power over others. In the Transkei, she could carry out her ideas with support and resources. Although she gained most of her management experience in the Transkei, her comments can be applied to the Ciskei. She further explained:

> For the first time we were free to do as you thought was necessary. So if I, if, for instance I got to a hospital and I was employed there and the matron is Black and the superintendent is Black—or even if she's not Black she's in this thing of Black people and so forth—I could just come to a hospital and say, "People, why is it that this hospital hasn't got number one, number two, number three, number

four, because I feel like this would be better off if we had this and that and that." And if they said, "Can you do it?" I would say, "Yes." And they would say, "Do it!" And I could do it, and I could do it without being pointed at as that Black nurse.[113]

Gamase Mtyeku expressed a similar sentiment. After training Black nurses at Frere Hospital for over ten years before she was promoted to be a senior nurse, she left to work at Cecilia Makiwane Hospital. She took in the first midwifery students as the senior tutor. "It felt good," she said of working in a Black-managed hospital. "I was good once upon a time," she continued, "but now it felt you were doing some contribution."[114]

An important outlet for nursing leadership in the Ciskei came through the establishment of the Ciskeian Nursing Council and Ciskeian Medical Council in 1984. Although separate nursing councils for the homelands segregated the broader profession, nurses enjoyed working outside of the racism of the South African Nursing Council.[115] A newspaper article announcing the opening of Ciskeian Nursing Association offices celebrated this change with the title "Goodbye to baasskap [boss-ship]."[116] The Ciskeian councils gave them full control over their nursing and other medical fields. They took over the administration of training, examinations, registration, and regulation of the medical and nursing professions. Constance Nosina Mesatywa, a highly educated and well-traveled nurse born in Alice, was brought into the Ciskei as its chief nursing officer in 1976. She played a significant role in implementing the Ciskei's comprehensive health care, overseeing the introduction of new clinics and hospital services and nursing training. She served on the South African Nursing Council in 1979 and was instrumental in setting up the Ciskeian Nursing Council, where she served as its first president. She also later served as director general of the Ciskei Department of Health. Mesatywa was later praised as the founder of the Ciskeian Nursing Council, where she gained influence she could not have elsewhere.[117] Virginia N. Mkosana became the deputy registrar of the Ciskeian Nursing Council in the mid-1980s and spoke with pride about the work she did to start the council from scratch and raise it to a high standard (claiming it was the best among the homeland councils).[118] Because of the long hours she dedicated to compiling the council's reports, she kept the reports when the Ciskei was disbanded and people were discarding old Ciskei records. She carefully gave them to me to deposit into an archive, along with a booklet celebrating the history of the nursing council, evidence of the fact that many officials involved in the Ciskeian Nursing Council viewed the organization as a great achievement.

In contrast to those who touted the achievements of the Ciskeian system, statements by nurses who did not like the political influence of the Ciskeian

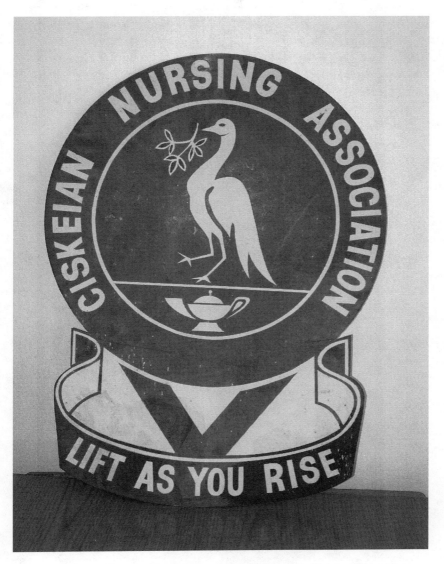

Figure 3. Ciskeian Nursing Association emblem. Democratic Nursing Organization of South Africa (DENOSA), Bhisho office. Photo by author, 2015.

government in health care provide evidence that not all the nurses I interviewed believed in Ciskei propaganda. Rather, their critiques reflect the admonitions of their training that they remain apolitical and that they genuinely wanted to focus on providing health care despite the larger apartheid context. Nine nurses I interviewed talked about the restriction that South African and Ciskeian health care facilities could only serve citizens of their respective nations, believing it to be detrimental. At the discussion I had with nurses about this book, one nurse made the point that they were trained as nurses to be advocates for their patients and yet apartheid blocked them from doing so.[119] Another ten talked about the influence of Ciskeian politics in their work in a way that showed they did not approve of Ciskeian political tactics. Thyra Nomkitha Mavuso, for example, had a problem with the political directives they were given at times when she worked in the Victoria Hospital and its clinics. "And, the government would say, 'On such-and-such a day, we want everybody to go to such-and-such a place for a rally,'" she said. "So that thing now affected the nurses" as they had to leave the hospital. She felt they could not question these orders without repercussion and this frustrated her.[120] Mavis Makubalo also complained of a time when the Ciskei government wanted a choir of nurses she supervised at the S. S. Gida Hospital to sing at a festival, and yet she needed to be sure the hospital was fully staffed. Makubalo's husband worked as a translator and clerk for top Ciskeian politicians. They may have expected her to support any Ciskeian celebration. However, Makubalo showed that her patients and her hospital work were more important than Ciskei political nation building when she refused to let all her staff go to sing.[121] When she was in charge at the Zwelitsha clinic, Beauty Nongauza would argue with the nurses there about leaving the patients to go to the Ciskeian national celebrations held at the Ntaba ka Ndoda manufactured national shrine. As a result, she believed, she was transferred back to the hospital so that she would not interfere with these Ciskeian rituals.[122] Some nurses expressed disdain at the way the government might punish someone by transferring them. Makubalo complained of the favoritism of the Ciskei system that left her and others often wondering when they might be suddenly transferred: "There's a time when if by the twentieth you haven't received a letter which says Mrs. Makubalo, on the first of November you are starting at Whittlesea, you would say, 'Whew!'"[123] Similarly, Cecilia Makiwane Hospital tutor Mtyeku remarked: "Now all of a sudden it was voting day. You had to queue up and you weren't sure how much [impact] this 'X' of yours you've just made is going to make in your life, in your *profession* . . . in your children getting the benefits that were due to them."[124] Joan Mavuso was working in a clinic in 1982 when she was abruptly told to go work in Cecilia Makiwane Hospital, "with immediate effect." She described the reappointment letter as quite harsh, offering no explanation. She assumed it had to do with politics but did not know what it was she had done.[125] A few felt someone could have been sent to a rural clinic as punishment. The suspicion and disapproval expressed by these nurses showed that not all nurses bought into the homeland system, but they worked to deliver health care to the best of their ability in their own limited sphere.

Conclusion

The historical record paints a complex picture of both productive and problematic developments in the Ciskeian health care system, driven by apartheid officials and politicians on one level and committed health care practitioners on another. The Ciskei homeland was an apartheid institution with major problems. Many places marred by relocation and structural inequality continued to suffer, and the Ciskei's flawed politics and finances exacerbated challenges such as staffing, transportation, and budget shortages. Yet from the increase in clinics under the territorial authorities, to the introduction of comprehensive health care and the streamlining of the health care system under the Ciskei Legislative Assembly, various government entities increased the number of services and medical care providers available to their population. A range of teams and practitioners committed to the comprehensive approach helped improve community health in many places, notably curbing some diseases. The Ciskei also offered African nurses opportunities to excel in a system led by Africans on many levels. Nurses stationed in rural clinics in particular continued to work on the ground with their own commitments and goals, delivering care in remote villages in the thick of a myriad of challenges. It is to the details of how these crucial actors did so that the chapters now turn.

CHAPTER THREE

Remembering Clinic Work

I CONDUCTED ONE OF MY FIRST INTERVIEWS with Thembisa E. Nkonki and Zotshi Mcako. Mcako had worked most of her career in the Ginsberg township clinic, near King William's Town. She took me north of the town to Tyutyu Village to meet her friend, Nkonki, who had been stationed in rural Ciskei clinics and worked as a district clinic supervisor during her career. Nkonki and Mcako told me of the weighty responsibilities nurses carried in rural clinics. Nurses in charge of these clinics could never be young nurses, fresh from training, they argued. Major urban hospitals may have had nurses working nonstop in overcrowded wards, but it was comparatively easier in hospitals where doctors were available. Nkonki remarked, "If you find out this is a breech [birth] then you call for a doctor and within minutes he's there." In rural villages, on the other hand, nurses had to get used to the conditions and "the work that is there, . . . because you stand for yourself, there is no doctor."[1] Other nurses who spent their careers in rural clinics similarly compared working in a hospital to working in the rural clinics. Nombeko Cecilia Tunyiswa explained that in the hospital "you treat the patient according to doctor's instructions and the patient gets well." When talking about being placed alone at the Ann Shaw clinic, she said that in the community, "the patient comes to *you*. . . . You are a general nurse, you are a midwife, you are a doctor!"[2] As one who relieved nurses on leave in various clinics and worked in newly established Victoria East clinics, Penelope Ntshona stated that rural clinic nurses had to deal with everything "immediately and effectively [because] you are independent."[3] Thus, Alecia Phiwo Dubula said about working in a number of St. Matthew's and S. S. Gida clinics, "You must have a big breakfast so you can stand up for the day."[4]

The retired nurses I interviewed shared stories and descriptions of their work that were seared into their memories because of their intensity or regularity.

Remembering Clinic Work

These memories of both the daily grind and dramatic incidents indicate what was significant to these nurses. They reveal what it took to deliver health care in the rural Ciskei in the 1960s through the 1980s. Although working in rural mission hospitals involved similar cases and patient dynamics (especially if nurses assisted with home deliveries), working in clinics in the villages presented unique circumstances. Like those quoted here, many nurses emphasized the heavy responsibilities they carried as the sole biomedical care providers in remote villages. With a lack of equipment and transportation challenges, this required technical skill, stamina, and sharp thinking. Working in rural clinics also involved the less frenzied labor of cultivating relationships with rural communities as nurses became intimately involved in their patients' lives. Not only did they visit patients in their homes, but they also sought to address TB, gastroenteritis, malnutrition, family planning, and psychiatric health through community health education. Working in areas where many able-bodied men had migrated elsewhere for work, they delivered babies at the beginning of life and treated those with diabetes and hypertension at the end of their lives. The vivid stories nurses told of handling maternity cases in particular encapsulate many of the challenges of rural nursing as well as the nurses' training and commitment. This training and commitment contributed significantly to their success, along with their endurance and a sense of personal fulfillment. Their collective memories paint a picture of the vital work these nurses performed to implement comprehensive health care on the ground.

Conditions of Service

Nurses who worked in rural clinics throughout the 1960s, 1970s, and 1980s were expected to dedicate most of their time and energy to their patients and the surrounding communities. Their work hours and residency requirements were demanding. They were expected to present spotlessly clean clinics and happy faces despite long hours of work. Although the independent Ciskei kept their medical supplies well stocked and improved the clinic infrastructure, nurses worked without certain supplies and equipment and at times struggled to obtain emergency transport. They tended to have good relationships with their colleagues while working in these conditions, although few elaborated on these relationships or their pay.

At times nurses applied directly for clinic positions. At other times, when hospitals had more control over clinic staffing, they might be allocated to a clinic in the monthly change list that announced nurses' assignments within the hospital. In any case, employment contracts drawn up in the 1960s set the standards for clinic work into the 1980s. Nurses were typically contracted to open the clinic Monday through Friday, from eight o'clock in the morning until half past four or five o'clock in the afternoon. This amounted to an eight-hour day with a lunch break. On Saturdays, they were to open from eight o'clock in the morning until one o'clock in the afternoon. However, one nurse was expected to always be on call and live within half a mile of the clinic if she did not stay in the nurses' quarters attached to the clinic itself. Contract guidelines drawn up by the South African Department of Health provided for different types of leave. Clinic nurses were to have one to two weekends off per month (beginning at five o'clock on Friday evening and ending at eight o'clock on Monday morning) and could acquire annual leave of up to thirty days (which was to be taken at once and not by "piecemeal"). Special circumstances allowed for other types of leave. For example, a nurse would have time to attend refresher courses after five years of service, could have up to four months of maternity leave, and could receive disability leave. Otherwise, the nurses were expected to be readily available for the community at any time of day or night. Any absence of more than forty-eight hours was considered a leave requiring prior approval. Nurses were paid for this work by salary at the end of each month, with annual raises possible depending on their performance.[5]

The nurses were expected to adhere to a high standard of conduct while living within the community and were scrutinized while on duty. As the guide to contracts read, "The nurse must at all times be an example to the people to whom she ministers. This must be reflected in her personal neatness and appearance, her attitude to her work, the handling of her patients and in her moral standard and general living habits." This applied to their housing down to the details of their uniforms. Indeed, a nurse's appearance was dictated by strict protocol in the nursing profession—with student nurses sometimes required to wear their uniforms when off duty. In the clinic contract guidelines, nurses were given a uniform allowance of forty South African rands per annum and given specific instructions to wear their appropriate epaulettes marking their rank "*at all times*" or face a fine. The contracts included the color of the uniforms the nurses could wear along with the accessories. The gray or blue uniforms were the most practical for district work, although nurses could wear their white uniforms. They were not allowed to wear jerseys or sweaters over their uniforms, only a simple coat or cape, and they had to wear "proper duty shoes (black or brown lace type)" along with their starched white hat.[6] One can imagine that clinic nurses felt independent and free until the supervisor came around. Under the Tribal Authorities, when the South African Department of Health was paying seven-eighths of the nurses' salaries, the department would send a supervisor to check conditions of the clinic and the nurse's work. When a Sister J. Korsch conducted inspections in the mid-1960s, she almost always started her reports by commenting on the appearance of the nurse: "She was

Remembering Clinic Work

in clean uniform and the clinic reasonably tidy," "[She] was out visiting and later returned to the clinic. She was in clean uniform, looking neat and professional." She might write something more detailed if the nurse's appearance was amiss: "On 3.10. I found nurse in a black skirt fastened with safety pins and a greenish ¾ length overall edged with frills on which she wore very tattered epaulettes. This was covered by a dirty embroidered apron for protection."[7] Supervisors also checked the cleanliness of the clinic and the state of the nurses' accommodation, inspected the equipment and records the nurses kept, and reported on the number of different cases the nurses saw and how much time they spent out visiting the community and running educational initiatives.

These conditions of service felt more difficult to some nurses than others, depending on the workload, family situation, and interests of the nurses. None of the nurses I interviewed complained about the inspections or strict standards of conduct. Rather, they lamented recent changes in uniform requirements, indicating that they believed that wearing a clean and official uniform signified the dignity and high standards of nursing. While a few nurses felt working in the rural areas was less demanding, with no required night duty and fewer complicated patients, most talked of the demanding hours as one of the major challenges facing nurses who worked in rural clinics. If a clinic serviced a large area and had one or two fully qualified nurses, a nurse could be on her feet the entire day and after hours—the reason Dubula said a clinic nurse would need a big breakfast. Linda E. Ngoro remembered that when she worked at the Perksdale and Qibirha clinics, she would not have time to take a tea break if she had patients lined up outside. "You cannot go to tea. They shout there, 'It's a long time we are here! We are very sick.'" Some patients may have come from far. The Perksdale and Qibirha clinics were located in the often dry and flat terrain about twenty-two and twenty-eight miles (thirty-five and forty-five kilometers), respectively, from their referral hospital, S. S. Gida. At times she would be working alone after having a sleepless night attending to patients. Yet she had to work until the clinic closed. The patients did not understand: "Now those people there outside . . . do not expect you to go to lunch." If there was another nurse on duty, the nurses could take turns having a lunch break, but otherwise, Ngoro said they could "never, never, never close the clinic. Our clinics were *never* closed."[8]

Mobile clinics in rural areas could also present a heavy workload. Constance N. Thoto described how long her days could be running mobile clinics for the Victoria Hospital catchment area, where they ran weekly programs and treated general cases. Her descriptions give the impression that she faced a long line of all sorts of patients waiting at the vehicle. "You saw about seventy, eighty [patients per day]," she remembered, "because now you were taking

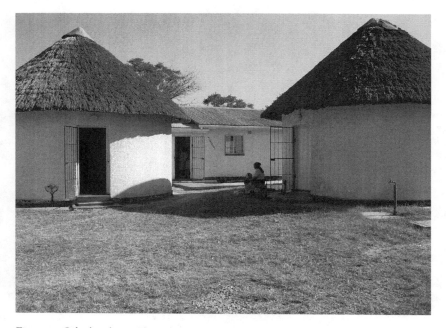

Figure 4. Qibirha clinic. Photo by author, 2016.

them the well-baby clinic where you immunize. You had to palpate antenatal patients. You had to see minor ailments and all that." This work could extend into the evening: "And you would not leave the area until you have attended to everybody. . . . At times used to come home about six o'clock or seven o'clock in the evening." She could not leave patients for the next day "because some of them have walked to [the] site" and she did not want to leave them stranded.[9]

The on-call system was taxing for many nurses who were stationed in the villages. Unlike working in hospitals, the nurses did not differentiate between day duty or night duty; they were always on duty.[10] Although she worked at St. Matthew's Hospital in the 1970s, Nontsikelelo Biko remarked, "I mean, those days a nurse was just a nurse twenty-four hours around the clock. There was no time you would say, 'I'm off.'"[11] Those who worked in the clinics in the various districts shared similar sentiments. Some nurses commented that communities did not recognize or respect the operating hours of the clinic, especially when a nurse lived on the clinic premises or in a house nearby. Evelyn Magodla said, "They would never keep time, . . . and the people are demanding."[12] Yet some cases just sprung up after hours. Nomali Bangani related, "There was that thing called the 'on call.' You work during the day. You work

Remembering Clinic Work

during the night. You are on call when somebody comes to deliver a baby, when somebody had an accident, you wake [to knocking on the door]. *Nkqo nkqo nkqo.* 'Nurse. Nurse!'"[13] Nomabali Mbombo expressed strong feelings about the stress of being on call: "We used to do a lot of terrible, terrible, terrible, terrible time at the clinics where you used to go to do what was called a call system. . . . You have to wake up from the nurse's home and attend to those people. It was horrible."[14] And Weziwe Tsotsobe emphasized that they had no overtime pay for this work, saying, "We were just given hours to [take off] as day offs."[15] Understandably, as Nomathemba Ncukana remembered, the on-call system would drive some nurses to request to be moved from the clinics to the hospitals.[16]

Being on call was made worse when a nurse had to deal with cases all by herself. Vuyiswa Sodlulashe worked in the Ann Shaw clinic and other clinics in the Middledrift district before working as a supervisor of family planning. "Whatever comes in the after-hours, it's yours . . . and you'd be all alone," she explained.[17] At the standard smaller clinics, the ideal was to have three fully qualified nurses. This would allow one nurse to rest or take leave when needed. However, many nurses found themselves to be one of two or the only fully qualified nurse at clinics, with an auxiliary or assistant nurse to assist them at times.[18] In clinics that did not have hired cleaners or gardeners, nurses would also have to perform janitorial tasks and work in the garden. It could be physically exhausting and nerve-wracking to deal with cases as the sole nurse in charge. Those who staffed a clinic as the only fully qualified nurse had very little time off. Longtime clinic nurse and clinic supervisor Nobantu Baleni explained that when she was the only one stationed at rural clinics, she usually had only one weekend off per month. "Even then," she continued, "it was only Saturday, you come here [Zwelitsha] Saturday. Sunday you go back, evening. Saturday, Sunday. The whole month you are there. Because you don't have somebody to take your place."[19] At the Lenye clinic in the Keiskammahoek district, Thembeka Gantsho remembered two fully qualified nurses who took turns taking the weekend off. This meant that one would always be left alone on the weekends.[20] Celiwe Mbie struggled in a similar situation at the Gxulu clinic. She worked with only one other nursing sister: "No assistant nurse, no nobody else. Two sisters. The other member of staff was a cleaner, and a gardener. Only. So now if the other sister . . . is on leave, most of the time you are left by yourself. So there's no second opinion on whatever. You are all by yourself. You either send the patient to hospital or you take that risk."[21] At bigger clinics, there were at times three or four nurses, with some focusing on special services such as family planning or psychiatric services. With a bigger number of staff, one nurse could even be allocated to run the clinic at night, easing the

Remembering Clinic Work

burden of the on-call system. Yet even clinics with four nurses could end up with only one available. Makubalo talked about working at clinics like Masicedane under St. Matthew's or S. S. Gida, where the staff could seemingly dissipate: "We were only four registered nurses. She's on leave, you are three. She's sick, you are two. She's off duty, you are one."[22]

Two nurses told of specific times when they broke under this pressure. One lashed back at a local authority and the other boycotted. Bangani remembered one day when she was working at the Ann Shaw clinic and an impatient Middledrift magistrate showed up in the morning after she had spent the night helping deliver a baby. "Man!" she exclaimed, "the clinic was two rooms because the other two rooms was my residence. . . . I was still washing because it was just after seven. I was just finished delivering a patient." The magistrate stood at the clinic entrance just on the other side of the house: "He stood there and got impatient. And he said, 'Where is this nurse?' And then, hey! I was so furious." In response, she took her time getting ready. "And then at long last I came out and I said, 'Mr. Xhamela, . . . unless you as the magistrate in this area—and you are responsible too to have a word—you send a second or a third nurse here. Otherwise I'm not going to divide myself into two.'" Bangani admitted she was wrong to react in an angry way. But she just could not maintain her composure, because "there's only one nurse. And I've never been late. It's only this day."[23]

Lungelwa F. Mhlambiso worked as a nurse for years at the Amathole Basin clinic. Nestled in the Amathole Mountains, the clinic was situated about fifteen to twenty miles (twenty-five to thirty kilometers) of gravel roads from Alice and the Lovedale Hospital. She managed to secure this post to be stationed in her husband's family village. This meant she was always around. For years she worked all by herself in the clinic. She vividly described her exhaustion, which led her to decide to "boycott."

> You will be called during the night. You went off maybe at six o'clock and yet you are supposed to be off at four. You went off at six o'clock. At eight o'clock, when you are starting to sleep [*knocks on the table*]. You are needed. There's a midwifery [or] maternity patient outside. You have to wake up and come and attend to this maternity patient. Maybe you'll deliver two a.m. in the morning. You are there but eight o'clock, the people are outside, waiting for you to attend. You were not asleep throughout the night. I say that person maybe delivered at two a.m., so you made that delivery at least by four a.m. and it won't go during the night. It's you who'll wait until tomorrow, still under your care. Eight o'clock it's full up. Maybe child health—child welfare day. [*clapping*] It's full up with mothers with children. They are needing your help. And once you are feeling—

Remembering Clinic Work

at times you feel very tired. You are sulky. "Heyi. *Hayi mntakabawo*, nurse is very sulky today." They don't know that no, it's not that you are sulky. You are tired.

Mhlambiso became so exhausted that she told her supervisor that she needed to go attend to a family member who was sick at home but instead locked herself inside her house. Her supervisor called a replacement, Buyiswa Vakalisa, who came with the supervisor to check on her. Mhlambiso's husband had not approved of her deception so let out her secret. "So, [*laughs*] so it was bad," she continued. "I told them, no I was tired. I cannot concentrate to the people anymore. I'm full up." They decided to have Vakalisa work at the clinic for at least two months to relieve Mhlambiso. Even though Vakalisa eventually had to leave, "they saw the need that really there must be somebody to help. Otherwise you are working under very, very strenuous conditions with no money."[24]

As time went on, the personal safety of nurses stationed at clinics during the night became a concern for some. A few nurses expressed that they felt vulnerable when they stayed at the clinics at night without any security guard. Evelyn Magodla, who worked in St. Matthew's and S. S. Gida clinics during her career, remarked, "And worst part about all in the clinics—there was no security. You were left there, nurse, alone with no security."[25] Nurses kept money from fees people paid during the day and would transfer the money periodically depending on the system they had set up with their referral hospital. Small as the monies were, nurses feared that *tsotsis* (thieves or criminals) would attempt to steal the money or attack the nurse. Mbie remembered hearing of a break-in at a clinic near Gxulu where she worked. This incident heightened her fear of nurses being victims of ill-intentioned characters. "And then we became afraid now," she said. "That if there is a knock there during the night you would wonder, 'Oh God, I wonder if it's really a patient or if it's just somebody.'"[26] Bangani expressed a similar fear of responding to a knock during the night: "You open the door and there's no caretaker. There's no security. You are all by yourself and your children."[27] Nkonki told of a nurse who was hospitalized after being physically attacked at the Dimbaza clinic. Her face was so swollen from being hit with an iron rod that she could not open her eyes. Attacks appear to have been rare; still, the threat of dealing with *tsotsis* alone at night instilled fear in some nurses.[28] Eunice Lulama Mkosana even claimed that nurses chose not to stay in her village clinic, the Mgwalana clinic, because of it.[29]

Accommodation and transportation to remote villages posed challenges for clinic nurses. In the 1960s, on average, the clinics consisted of four-roomed houses. Just like Bangani's description of the Ann Shaw clinic, these small clinics had two front rooms that served as waiting and consulting rooms, while the back two rooms housed the nurses stationed there—one as the sleeping quarters and the other as a kitchen. Many clinics also had a small yard outside the clinic, which ideally would be fenced to keep roaming cattle or thieves out. Others may have had up to three rondavels. Bigger clinics built in later years may have had up to six consulting rooms and an official pharmacy room. The clinic employing body—at times a tribal authority, at other times a hospital or the Ciskeian government—was expected to construct the buildings and provide equipment and accommodation for the nurses as well as set the terms of her salary. Once built, the employing body had to equip and maintain the clinics (although according to 1960s South African Department of Health reports, that did not always happen). Nurses could expect the mission hospital

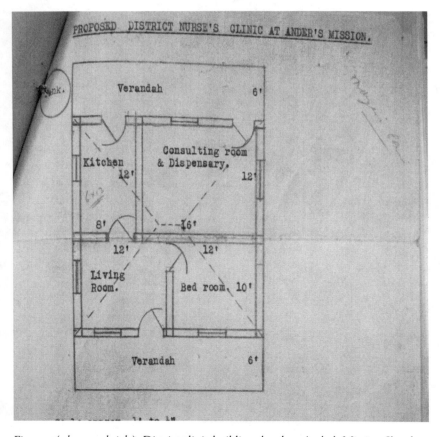

Figure 5 (*above and right*). District clinic building sketches. Ander's Mission Sketch, Box 509, Ander's Mission Location Clinic Folder, Eastern Cape Archives and Records. District clinic blueprint, Box 539, June 1965–December 1966 Folder, Eastern Cape Archives and Records.

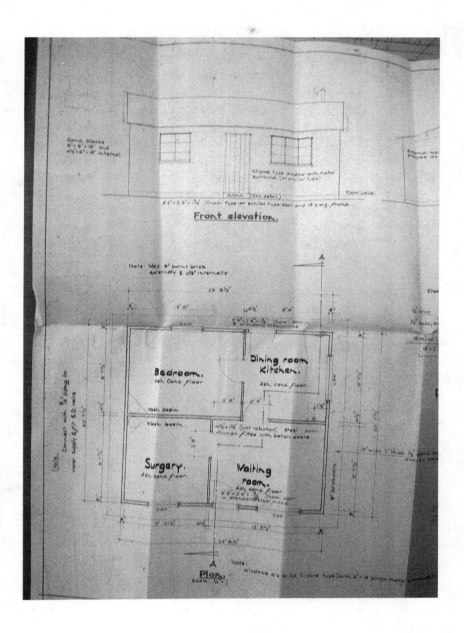

or state to provide the medical equipment, including medicines, a maternity bag, cleaning materials, record-keeping books, and a safe for collected fees. The employing body was even mandated to furnish the nurses' living quarters or help the nurse find other accommodation. If other accommodation was provided for the nurse, she would be required to pay rent and, "considering that the nurse must always set a good example to her people," contract guidelines stipulated that "she cannot be allowed to live in over-crowded quarters herself."[30] Some clinics offered nurses very little space for patients or accommodation. "The space was too small," Pholisa Nombulelo Majiza pointed out. "There were no waiting rooms because when it's raining, the people are staying outside."[31] Majiza managed to secure the post in her husband's village of Burns Hill, where she worked for ten years out of a building that followed the standardized model. Mjikeliso, former Ciskei clinic supervisor who worked at clinics in the Middledrift and Keiskammahoek districts, remembered, "It was so bad," with the two rooms in front serving as the clinic and only two rooms for the nurses at the back.[32]

If nurses had multiple children whom they wanted to stay with, arranging for accommodation could become particularly difficult, although conditions improved over time. As discussed more in chapter 5, health care officials worried more about overcrowded quarters becoming a bad example than ensuring nurses had adequate housing for their families.[33] If a clinic had two full-time nurses, the women would have to squeeze into the accommodation or secure a bigger place to stay. Women who worked in clinics where their families were already based stayed at home but would sleep in the nurses' quarters when they were on call.[34] While some nurses (eight) found that living in the village allowed them to stay with their children or newborn babies, others housed their children with family members who lived elsewhere. If this was the case, obtaining adequate transportation to travel to and from the clinic caused stress for nurses who would end up staying away from their families most of the month. Nine nurses commented on the lack of public transport that could take them to the clinic, making transportation a major challenge for them. Two remarked that this deterred women from remaining in jobs at the clinics.

At the same time, when asked to comment on the Ciskei health care system in general, many talked about the improvements made to clinic buildings and nurses' homes during Ciskeian independence. Baleni called Ciskei clinics "first class" and remembered that under the Ciskei, many of these clinics were renovated and upgraded: "All the [Ciskei] clinics had nurses' homes, for the nurses to sleep. We had a really beautiful nurses' home with lounge furnished, with beds, you know, wardrobes, and everything. You felt being at home, you felt being at home."[35] Baleni spoke as a former clinic supervisor, proud of the

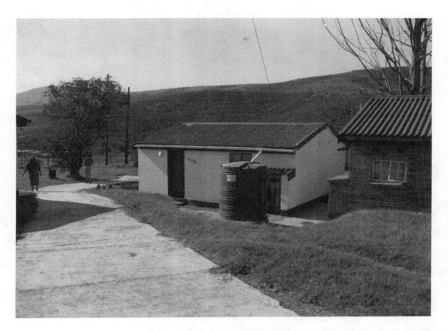

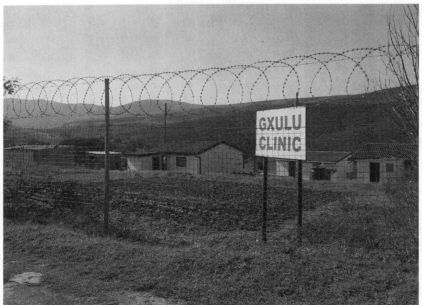

Figure 6. Original Gxulu clinic (*top*) and expanded clinic complex (*bottom*). Photos by author, 2016.

Ciskei system for which she worked. Yet she was not alone in speaking positively of the nurses' living conditions in rural areas. Others gave supporting evidence. For example, the Gxulu clinic, built in the late 1960s, eventually had a four-roomed nurses' home that Mbie remembered having two bedrooms, a lounge, and a kitchen.[36] Tunyiswa, who had worked in Ann Shaw and other clinics in the area, also talked about the convenience of nurses' homes being where nurses could house their children so that they could stay with their children full time.[37]

Memories of the conditions the nurses worked under were thus not all negative. Someketha, who spent much of her career at Mount Coke and Bhisho Hospitals, spoke very highly of the Mthombe village, where each clinic employee had their own fully furnished accommodation and the clinic was well supplied with a good connection to the hospital.[38] Some assured me that, unlike present-day clinics, their clinics had a well-stocked supply of medicines and sterilized equipment, the Ciskei services were well organized, and health care reached many Ciskeians. Nonzwakazi Gqomfa, who had a career in both mobile and static clinics in the Victoria East areas, said, "I should think the Ciskei government had the best health care system. It was well organized, well, well organized." For her, this was evidenced by the fact that nurses rotated out to clinics, which helped them get to know the people. Practitioners held health education days, clinics had well-stocked medicines, and the system offered in-service training. Others, like Mjikeliso, talked of the increase in clinics: "In the Ciskei, a lot of clinics were built and they were nearer each other. They were at the proximity for people to be able to attend—walking distances."[39] As noted in previous chapters, not all villages or regions enjoyed equal resources. Still, a number of nurses praised the government for the support it gave them. Bangani felt that "the Ciskei government really boosted the [community] nurses" by giving them the backing they needed in the communities. Local headmen would introduce them to their communities and ask their people to listen to them. Different government departments worked with them in planning meetings.[40] When asked about how things changed with the dissolution of the Ciskei, Baleni stated that they were better off under the Ciskei because "the Ciskei paid attention to the villages."[41] As a former clinic supervisor, Baleni may have been speaking more out of pride in the work that she had accomplished in the Ciskei period, yet these comments do correspond with archival evidence of real improvements to clinics in a number of areas, if not to an ideal level.

Of course, the clinics did not have the same infrastructure and equipment as the hospitals—some nurses wished they could have had oxygen tanks or sterilizing tools at the clinics. Nurses also remembered their everyday work being challenged by a lack of resources such as linens, electricity, and phone lines. To compensate for the lack of linens, Nkonki and Thoto said they instructed pregnant women who attended the antenatal clinics to start collecting newspapers to serve as a protective draw sheet for the day they gave birth.[42] Most clinics in the Ciskei in the 1960s through the 1980s had no electricity, similar to the villages where they were stationed. This caused difficulties when nurses had to attend to patients after sundown or if they needed to keep certain supplies refrigerated. A few nurses mentioned that they had gas refrigerators wherein to keep immunizations, while Mbie talked of taking immunizations around with coolers packed with ice and the hope that the temperature would remain adequate.[43] Others talked of the difficulty of using paraffin lamps or candles at night. "And you used to struggle during the night with a patient," Majiza remembered. It was difficult to do detailed work in the dim light with shadows bouncing around her Burns Hill clinic: "Sometimes you have an assaulted patient where you have to stitch the patient before taking the patient to the hospital. Or you have a delivery where you are going to deliver with candles. [*laughs*] With candlelight! *Yho!*"[44] Mbie said things got better when they had gas lamps in the St. Matthew's and Nompumelelo clinics where she worked. Still, the nurse would have to ask whoever accompanied the patient to hold the lamp while she delivered the baby.[45] This arrangement caused problems when a rainstorm had flooded the bridge from the Ginsberg township to Grey Hospital in King William's Town and Mcaku had to deliver a breech baby at a home. As soon as the first leg came out, the woman holding the lamp was startled and ran away![46] Thoto commented that some of the lamps were so small "one could cough or sneeze and blow it out."[47] Understandably, Mhlambiso described delivering patients with candles as "primitive." "No, no, no, no. We never had electricity. No, we never had electricity at all," she said. "Mind you, you are delivering [a baby]. If your gas has stopped, you'll have to light very many candles."[48] At least they were "still young with good eyesight," Mbie remarked.[49]

Communicating with and traveling to the referral hospitals could also pose a major challenge for those stationed at rural clinics. Few clinics had direct telephone lines to the hospitals. When clinics were built in the 1960s, one of the considerations for choosing the location was its proximity to a phone line already established at a trading station, post office, or a local authority's office. Before the clinics had phones, Hilary Mnyanda, who worked in a variety of clinics and later in an HIV/AIDS provincial office, said they would send a relative to call the hospital from one of the phones in the village.[50] Eventually, the clinics received hand radios. Most of the nurses who talked about these radios affectionately called them the "over." Having worked for a number of years in the Tshatshu clinic near King William's Town, Thandiwe Mkwelo remembered, "There was a radio but you'd call—you would press and then call. And you say, 'Come in, come in.' . . . 'Over. Come in. I've got a patient here to be fetched.'"[51] Sodlulashe remembered the radio being much faster than the telecom phones that some clinics in the Middledrift district subsequently had because they could call an ambulance directly. She also highlighted the usefulness of the radios for nurses calling for help from other clinics.[52]

In communicating with the hospitals, some nurses found their referral hospitals responsive and attentive while others reported major struggles. Baleni fondly remembered her supervisor in Mount Coke clinics, J. N. Sishuba, coming around to spend some time with the nurses and understand how they were faring so she could help improve conditions.[53] Some commented on how the hospital or medicine depots kept their clinics well supplied as they submitted orders. Some remembered ambulances arriving quickly—or within the expected thirty to forty-five minutes it would take to drive from the hospital. A few said that things improved under the independent Ciskei when there were more vehicles. Yet other nurses struggled with transportation to the hospitals, especially in emergencies. As discussed previously, the Ciskeian Department of Health reported recurring problems with transportation, which certainly affected the availability of ambulances. Waiting on the ambulance was worse when a village was an hour's drive from the hospital or when the nurse had a difficult pregnancy case. "Oh, the problems!" Nkonki exclaimed, "No transport to take [sterilized packs at the hospital] straight to you, you have no medicines, there is no transport to take the medicines to you. You phone and phone and phone until sometimes you send a junior nurse or junior somebody to go to the hospital and collect."[54] The distance from the hospital and the terrain the ambulance had to negotiate factored in to how much nurses at certain clinics could rely on the ambulance. For example, nurses who worked at Rabula and Gxulu clinics talked about the difficulties the ambulances had reaching these remote clinics in the hills near Keiskammahoek. In the Rabula village, about seven to eight miles (twelve kilometers) from Keiskammahoek, nurses sometimes sent people to the hospital on horseback.[55] Bad roads, rains, and a high demand on the ambulance made matters worse. The ambulance from St. Matthew's reportedly was "so unreliable" in the early 1980s "that it is not unusual to wait nine hours for it to arrive, and in bad weather it does not attempt the journey."[56] Mkwelo said that with the shortage of vehicles, they may have had to wait for an ambulance to finish fetching someone in Dimbaza before coming to the Tshatshu clinic, today likely a thirty-minute drive. In some urgent cases, nurses had to carry their black bags and walk to deliver care or use privately owned vehicles to transport patients. More than ten nurses reported

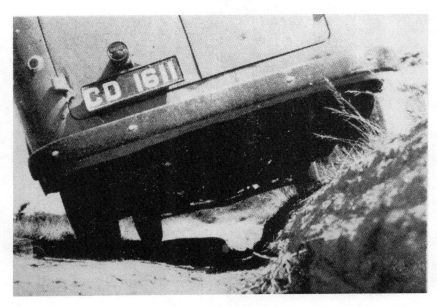

Figure 7. "No tarred roads here!" Mount Coke Hospital Report 1954, Mount Coke Hospital Reports, Newsletters Quarterly Reports, Methodist Papers, Folder 1, Cory Library (courtesy of Rhodes University, Cory Library).

that they would advise patients to use their own transportation or that they would "grab any" transportation that was available.[57]

Among all these conditions of clinic work, nurses did not address two particular topics as much as might be expected: relations with their nursing colleagues and their pay. Nurses did not volunteer much information about their relationships with the nurses they worked with in rural clinics. A number of the nurses worked alone, thus did not have as many experiences with colleagues to share. Sodlulashe also said that in some places nurses were changed often, with people going on leave or being allocated back to the hospitals, giving them less time to build relationships.[58] Yet some had to live and work closely with one or two other nurses stationed in the clinics. Apparently, these relationships generally did not cause many problems that stood out in their minds years later or nurses worked as a team out of necessity. When another nurse joined those who had been working alone, the nurse could have appreciated the company and second opinion rather than focus on interpersonal conflict.[59] At least ten nurses said that they had experienced good or very good relationships with their fellow nurses or expressed gratitude for training given by senior clinic nurses. Eight commented on how important it was to work as a team for the good of the patient. As Dubula explained, "When you are two, you don't have problems because you must love each other for the progress. If you want work to happen, . . . you don't keep on fighting, don't waste your time by fighting." Weekly evaluations of the work and their relationship helped her check to see if there was a problem: "Because all of us, the goal is the patient care."[60] Mkosana, who worked for years in the Mgwalana clinic, acknowledged that it could be difficult to work with people: "Working with people is not easy. Because each person has his own character. But," she noted, "we have to work together."[61]

Sodlulashe was the only one who told a story about working with her colleagues. Her memory of how well she worked with nurses at the Ann Shaw clinic illustrates how they all worked together for one goal. One day, a man from Radio Ciskei came to visit the clinic, by then a slightly larger building with a short hallway and multiple rooms. Just as he arrived, one of the nurses yelled for help with a patient who was reacting badly to some treatment. Sodlulashe excitedly described the way they all sprang into action: "Everybody ran [*claps*]," she narrated. "One passed here into the treat—the office. Some in the office, some in the treatment. The one who's got the key for the drug cupboard went for the drugs, and then took out the drug, was closing, was giving to somebody straight to the patient and the patient was alright." They did not notice the tall man who had come in until things had calmed down. It was then that he said he was from the radio and was impressed with the way they interacted.[62] With similar fond memories, Pumla Kwatsha said it was the "best thing working hand in hand" with her fellow nurses in places like the Twecu clinic. She followed that comment with "I loved nursing," indicating that her relationships with her colleagues were one of the things that made her enjoy her career.[63] When I saw many of these nurses interact years later, they demonstrated the same fondness for each other.

On the other hand, a few comments indicate that giving correction was not always easy or that nurses of different ranks felt differently about their interactions. Nonfundo Rulashe felt her perfectionist character, which led her to strictly follow protocol, meant that some nurses who worked under her in Nompumlelo and Keiskammahoek clinics did not like her.[64] Sheila Sonjica, who worked as a clinic inspector and family planning supervisor, said it was "nasty" to be reprimanded at times, and Tsotstobe emphasized the importance of learning to accept and respect others, even across the different levels of nursing.[65] Tsotsobe's comments about the different ways senior nurses could treat more junior nurses indicate that she witnessed or experienced some friction herself in Mount Coke and other clinics: "And then if you respect a lower categories [*sic*] he or she will in turn respect you. And he or she will listen to you better than the one who despised them. . . . Don't underestimate whether she's of a lower category than yourself because you are a team. You are working as a team." Tsotobe's observations also reflect what others said about feeling that nursing taught them interpersonal skills. As a nurse in charge, Dubula learned to pay attention to people's behavior and tried to understand them to make sure they could focus on the patients.[66] Vakalisa, the nurse who worked in the clinics around Middledrift and relieved Mhlambiso after her boycott, said that nursing helped her learn how to study and understand people so that she could work well with them. "So," she said, "working with people, *ikwenza uba ufunde*, you know what to say, you know their moods, you know their exposure to—this one you delay, this one—because each one is unique."[67] Overall then, while relations with fellow nurses were not something nurses talked much about, for the majority, those relationships were an enjoyable part of their careers, even if they took some work at times.

Some nurses made comments about their salary and pensions, but otherwise the pay they received for their work did not receive as much attention in the interviews as would be expected for this significant part of employment. It was difficult for some nurses to remember exact pay across the years with inflation, raises, and different grades changing the amount over time. Some nurses remembered the exact numbers of their pay because of how little it was—some were paid six or seven pounds per month during their first year of training in the 1940s through the 1950s. Nurses were paid as soon as they started their training, and the pay increased every year. For employed, qualified nurses, the salary went up to more than R100 or R200 in the 1950s. In the late 1960s, a district nurse could enter into a contract for R660 a month and could increase her pay with increments up to between R800 and R1,000.[68] This increased over the 1970s and 1980s, with some nurses remembering that they retired in the 1990s with between R2,000 and R4,000 take-home pay per month. For a point of comparison, the estimated average income for African men in South Africa in 1973 was between R13 and R32 per week (that is, R52 to R128 per month), and 61 percent of African female workers earned less than R10 per week (less than R40 per month).[69] These estimated incomes would have barely provided for basic needs. The *Daily Dispatch* reported in 1974 that the fixed monthly expenses of a nurse living in Mdantsane with her husband and two children totaled R90. She and her family budgeted R65 for food, R12 for rent and electricity, R3 transportation, and R10 to pay a domestic servant.[70] Any other expenses for education, travel, or entertainment would have easily pushed them beyond R100. A decade later, in 1984, Market Research Africa estimated the average monthly household income for Africans at R273.[71]

Although nurses' pay alone did not make them feel entirely secure or rich, they were earning a sizeable salary compared with the majority of average Africans. The comments nurses made about what they could do with that money is perhaps more telling than the exact amount of their checks. Of those who worked in rural clinics, twenty-two commented or answered questions about their pay. Ten characterized it as low. Three said it was enough to allow them to buy household goods, help other family members, and help pay for their children's education, among other things. Indeed, nurses were considered part of the Black middle class because of their salary, professional status, and the education they could provide for their children. They joined salaried traders, entrepreneurs, teachers, social workers, and professional politicians who held the hope of new social mobility, especially in apartheid homelands where they were promised new and exciting opportunities.[72] Single, divorced, and widowed nurses supported themselves, their children, parents, or other extended family members with their earnings. For husbands and wives running an independent household during this time period, that extra income could make the difference in the kind of education their children received. Tsotsobe's comments capture the overall impression of nurses' pay when she said the pay was worse in the homelands than in other places in South Africa at the time, but it was "enough."[73]

At the same time, there were aspects about a public nurse's pay that caused some consternation. A few talked about nurses seeking jobs overseas because of the promise of a bigger salary, and the most-cited reason for others wanting to quit the profession was the pay.[74] One nurse said the pay in the Ciskei "wasn't wonderful," and securing a good education for her children required extra effort.[75] It is possible that some nurses did not focus on their salaries because they were taught to view nursing as a calling that required some sacrifice or because they were socialized into the profession when striking for better pay was considered inappropriate. Five nurses who worked in rural clinics felt that current nurses had the right to earn more money than in the past; yet some also chided present-day nurses for entering the profession for money and not for other altruistic reasons. The few more forceful comments about a nurse's salary related to the racial discrimination in nursing pay in South Africa and the loss of pensions for nurses who worked for multiple governments. Racial discrimination in pay began in training and continued if nurses worked in South Africa. Marks wrote that in 1979 the starting salary for African nurses was two-thirds that of white nurses with the same qualifications.[76] Some nurses still felt the sting of this injustice years later. One nurse who worked at Frere Hospital her whole career was so bitter about the racial discrimination in her pay that she declined my interview request because it was too painful to

Remembering Clinic Work 93

remember. Other nurses highlighted the injustice of the fact that they lost their pensions because they switched from the Transkei government to the Ciskei government or to the South African government. This left many retired nurses in the lurch.[77] The conditions of service the nurses worked under were in part shaped by the Ciskeian government and apartheid politics; but nurses "were always told that you must be apolitical."[78] This caused resentment among some. A woman who attended my dialogue with retired nurses in November 2018 remarked that they were told they should not be political, but that this frustrated her because the whole profession was shaped by politics in the racial segregation that plagued the broader system. While very few talked about Ciskei or apartheid politics in detail, some did lament the interference of politics in nursing in general. Nine nurses I interviewed mentioned the deplorable segregation of patients between South Africa and Ciskei, and another ten made comments about the interference of the Ciskei government in nursing staff activities and appointments as discussed in the previous chapter. Three talked about certain clinics being built for political reasons. The fact that the nurses interpreted these things as politically related shows that at least these nurses recognized that the broader political context affected their work and their salaries. Still, as the profession dictated at the time, most nurses did not talk about politics and there were few very strong trends in the way the nurses talked about their pay. Instead, the nurses spoke more readily about issues such as their work hours, accommodation, equipment, transportation, and the common cases they dealt with, leaving the impression that the broader context and their salaries were not fully satisfactory but that other issues made for more prominent memories.

The Daily Grind

In the interviews I conducted, I sought to understand what occupied the nurses' time and attention while on duty. At times I asked about everyday aspects of the nurses' work—their routines, the common cases they saw each day, how the work compared with hospital work. While stationed in the villages, nurses were expected to perform all necessary tasks for running a clinic, ranging from baby clinics and immunizations to distributing milk powder and sterilizing equipment. They provided primary health care, treating common colds, minor ailments, and cases such as TB, gastroenteritis, hypertension, diabetes, or sexually transmitted infections. They addressed some cases on certain days of the week—the antenatal clinic on Tuesday, a well-baby clinic on Thursday, and chronic patients on Wednesday, for example. In clinics that did not have hired cleaners or gardeners, nurses would also have to perform janitorial tasks after their work was done for the day. They may even have looked after the clinic garden. Nurses listed the cases they dealt with and talked about their daily or weekly routines, especially when I asked; but they narrated more stories about the types of cases that took more of their time, energy, and thoughts. These included prevalent diseases and health challenges or aspects that a nurse specialized in treating as well as the work of understanding and educating communities. They also tended to talk more about cases that were intertwined with other issues I asked them about, such as engaging with Xhosa medicine.

In addition to treating general minor ailments such as fever, flu, and injuries, the most prevalent cases that nurses mentioned as common at rural clinics included TB, diarrhea or gastroenteritis among children, chronic cases such as hypertension and diabetes, and malnutrition. Some said that diarrhea was a seasonal problem, along with pneumonia and bronchitis. This corresponds with hospital and Ciskei government records from the time. Few mentioned typhoid or the measles, even though these two diseases were of concern to the Department of Health at times and the Ciskei pushed to immunize against measles in the 1980s. This could indicate real success on the part of the health care system in curbing these diseases in rural areas or prevalence in some areas over others. Yet the common cases listed by the retired nurses also were those that occupied much of their time and energy, especially in their health education efforts. For example, not only was TB one of the most common diseases, but treating it also required much attention on the medical practitioner's part—a nurse or a VHW was expected to trace the TB patients to their home and through their travels to make sure that they traced affected people and that patients continued taking their medication. As discussed further in the next chapter, they also worked to change prevailing beliefs about the origins of the disease in home visits and health education talks. It is no wonder then that many nurses readily talked about TB as a main issue they dealt with in their work. Nurses similarly dealt with conflicting beliefs about diarrhea and gastroenteritis in children. Many people indeed suffered from those ailments, but the attention nurses paid to those cases in not only curative but preventive efforts made these cases more prominent in the nurses' memories.

The cases the nurses remember as the most common reflect the social determinants of health in the area at the time. With many able-bodied men seeking work in urban areas or mines, the population of rural villages often consisted of the elderly, women, and the very young. Poor economic and agricultural conditions in many of these areas led to a mixture of diseases related to poverty and aging. Thus nurses readily remembered childhood ailments as well as cases of hypertension and diabetes among older populations as most common. Diseases of malnutrition among children also stood out in nurses' minds along with diarrhea and gastroenteritis. The most common disease of malnutrition mentioned by the nurses was kwashiorkor, followed by marasmus and pellagra. Kwashiorkor is caused by a lack of protein in a person's diet, even though the person may have a reasonable caloric intake. The most visible symptom of kwashiorkor is swelling of the stomach as the lower parts of the body retain fluids. Marasmus is a more severe form of malnutrition caused by a general lack of calories that results in a rapid wasting away of muscle and fat. Pellagra, caused by a deficiency in niacin, is associated with an overreliance on maize and results in dermatitis, gastrointestinal ailments, and mental disturbances. Diseases of malnutrition were linked to the way women fed their children as well as the state of local food sources. One of the most moving accounts of the high rate of malnutrition came from Nontobeko Moletsane, a nurse who had worked in the village of Zinyoka near Bhisho, at the Black Consciousness Zanempilo Community Health Center in the mid-1970s. So many children suffered from malnutrition in the village that she claimed the people had funerals on the weekends and in the middle of the week. In her investigations of the root of the problem, she discovered that many women who relied on their husbands to send money from urban areas or mines had resigned themselves to poverty. One woman she visited boiled water in big pots so that her children would be calm as they anticipated a meal until they fell asleep. The mother broke down and cried to Moletsane about her predicament. Similar to St. Matthew's Dr. Thomas, who started a cottage industry program for women in the hospital's catchment area, Zanempilo addressed malnutrition by creating a women's craft group but also provided budgeting and gardening classes to address the problems.[79] Nurses in other areas used baby clinics and health education days to teach nutrition principles to villagers. In addition to the fact that impoverished families lacked protein and relied on mealie meal, a number of nurses talked about how they also urged mothers or grandmothers feeding babies formula to not skimp on formula because it chronically deprived their babies of nutrition. Some used the clinic gardens as a way to engage women in producing their own vegetables. They also acted as the agents of the milk-powder scheme that ran for years in the region. Yet since their work only treated symptoms of an underlying inequitable economic system, they continued to deal with malnutrition.

Nurses stationed in the clinics were expected to spend a significant amount of their time engaging in community outreach and home visits to address topics such as nutrition and disease recognition. Some nurses indeed viewed this as an important part of their work, emphasizing its significance, detailing the praxis, and commenting on how they enjoyed the comprehensive nature of this kind of health care. For example, Gqomfa told how she would investigate households in Victoria East communities. After she saw a patient at the clinic, she would go to the house to assess the situation, checking on all those who lived there and their general conditions.

> And then when you go to the household, maybe you are going to see an old lady, but it's not the old lady that you are going to see. You see everything when you go there. If there is a child, you must [check] the card, the well-baby clinic card, if the baby has had all the immunizations. If there is an old lady, you check if they are not taking any chronic medication, if the chronic medication is taken properly. If there is a TB patient (because they will come and report to you that there is a TB patient discharged maybe from the hospital), you go and check if the follow-up is being done—if there are no other people that are contacts [of the infected person], that the [one who is a] contact should be treated, and the [other] contacts should be told. You trace everything.[80]

This practice led them to gain intimate knowledge of the lifestyles and living conditions of the people in their communities. Nozokolo Hono, who worked in clinics in the Middledrift and Peddie districts, described the same process of inspecting a patient's living conditions after the patient came to the clinic. "Say, for instance, a mother brings her child to the clinic for one complaint," she began, "like for instance, diarrhea. You begin to wonder, 'Why is this child having diarrhea now and again?' You go there because you want to see how they prepare feeds. How are the utensils they are using? And then you correct."[81] Nurses would correct by teaching mothers individually, demonstrating cleanliness and hygienic practices. Sodlulashe talked about how home visits helped her learn more about the impact of a person's environment on her health so that she would know to advise women on spending the money their husbands sent from the mines or urban areas on children's food instead of making beer for his return.[82]

A number of nurses liked this type of involvement in the community because it allowed them to understand the patient as a whole person and to offer more effective health care. Dubula commented, "And those home visits, that you go to their homes so that you can see somebody in totality. So you don't just take what she's saying to you. . . . So I used to pick up such things [social problems at home]. So I enjoy the clinic more than anything."[83] Bangani remembered the considerations that went in to following up on a patient after she or he had been referred to a doctor and discharged: "But when the patient is discharged, you've got to visit that patient, see how she lives. You see? You study, *ukuthi*, how does she live. *Ithini imeko yakhe? Isupportwe njani la* patient? *Iphila kanjani?* [What are her circumstances? How is the patient supported? How does she live?]" Bangani explained that it was not enough to deal with the physical symptoms the patient presented because sometimes "there's an underlying cause." Maybe the patient was lonely, worried about something, or unable to afford to do things for herself and thus not eating well. "So as a community nurse," Bangani said, "you check all those things. See that somebody needs a support." Once she understood issues shared among the community, she could gather the community together and address the issues on a broader scale or teach people to garden. "So it was nice like that," she concluded, expressing the satisfaction she felt in understanding and then effectively addressing a patient's whole situation.[84] Some of these nurses took such an interest in community health that they decided to complete a diploma or certificate in community nursing even though they had worked in rural clinics for some time.

Nurses remembered other ailments or community health issues because the Ciskei Department of Health emphasized them or because the nurses had specialized in addressing those cases. For example, Lulama Nkani went through the ten steps a hospital should follow to promote breastfeeding with me because that became her specialty at the Bhisho Hospital.[85] Whereas most did not have much to say about HIV/AIDS because it surfaced in the region at the end of their careers, eight nurses talked about it because they worked directly with HIV/AIDS programs in the 1990s. Among the other health issues mentioned by the nurses I interviewed, psychiatric cases and family planning were the most prominently discussed. Beginning in the mid-1970s, the Ciskei Department of Health focused on improving and expanding services in these two areas, requiring nurses to pay more attention to these cases and obtain further training. The region already had some mental health resources. There were two psychiatric hospitals—the Tower Hospital in Fort Beaufort and the Komani Hospital in Queenstown. As the world paid more attention to mental health, the Ciskei itself also promoted psychiatric health care more. Other hospitals added psychiatric nursing managers, and psychiatric nursing became part of the new four-year general nursing training course introduced in the 1980s. Psychiatric nurses also began to become integral parts of mobile health teams and health centers and clinics. In 1984 the department created a new position in the Ciskei head office and proposed a new Mental Health Act, adopted in 1986, that outlined procedures and policies for the care of mentally ill patients.[86] Sixteen of the nurses I interviewed received training of some length or another in psychiatric nursing, and a dozen mentioned that psychiatric cases became a regular concern in rural clinic work. Most of these nurses talked about psychiatric cases as common—with Baleni, who completed an advanced degree in psychiatric nursing, saying the most common cases were TB and psychiatric cases. Yet Vakalisa, who worked in clinics around Middledrift, admitted they were not so common where she worked.[87] Those who talked about specific mental ailments mentioned schizophrenia and drug abuse of dagga (or marijuana) as the main problems, while others talked of the importance of educating the community and making sure patients did not default on their medication. Other substantial discussions about psychiatric cases came when nurses talked about differences between Xhosa medicine and clinic medicine, as analyzed in the next chapter. Thus, the combination of a greater emphasis by the state, specialization by nurses, and conflicting approaches to psychiatric cases in the community made those cases relatively prominent in the memories of a number of interviewees.

The Ciskei Department of Health also promoted family planning in the mid to late 1970s. The introduction of birth control pills sparked debate about their ethical use in the *Daily Dispatch* newspaper in the 1960s through the 1970s. During this time, government and medical professional proponents in South Africa and international advocates increasingly argued that family planning was an answer to addressing poverty and malnutrition in places like rural South Africa.[88] The South African government adopted a program in 1974 to provide free birth control to Black women. Pills, injections (Depo-Provera), and other contraceptives became available at rural clinics.[89] The Ciskeian Department of Health promoted family planning as a way to encourage the spacing of children as well as provide education about sex and sexually transmitted infections. Nurses could earn certificates and diplomas in family planning. Cecilia Makiwane Hospital offered short courses in these subjects. Some Ciskei politicians and community members were skeptical about this in the 1970s, questioning the cultural propriety of family planning and the motives of those promoting it among Black Africans. Evelyn Magodla said they suffered when they implemented family planning at St. Matthew's Hospital in the latter half of the 1970s because people "knew nothing about family planning, *ne*, and they were against it."[90] Department of Health officials had to justify the adoption of family planning to Ciskei legislators in 1975, arguing that it would not stop the population growth of their emerging nation or break down families and support selfish behavior. They argued that people actually wanted it, and the "poor" and "ill-educated" would like to know about it to help them deal with their problems and make rational choices.[91] Subsequent legislative debates included suspicions that the promotion of family planning was supported by white people because they wanted to decrease the Black population.[92] There was a basis for these fears as it was later revealed that some South African government officials promoted birth control as a way to curb Black population growth.[93] Dr. Mamphela Ramphele's critique that family planning was not a solution when the majority of the population could not feed their family no matter how small took into account the larger apartheid context in a different way.[94] Health officials in the Ciskei worked through the skepticism, however, and by the late 1970s family planning in the Ciskei was "taken as a service itself," as Hono put it.[95]

The nurses who promoted family planning adopted the medical profession's stance on the merits of family planning for helping women take care of their children and their own health. Sonjica became supervisor of Family Planning Services for the Ciskei in 1979, where she was expected to work closely with clinics in promoting family planning. In a newspaper article she wrote to address "confusion" about family planning, she stated, "The right interpretation of family planning or its intentions are that individuals or couples adopt a life style to have the number of children they can afford to bring up, love, clothe, and educate." Sonjica went on to argue that Xhosa people had always engaged in contraception, so people should not be afraid of new methods that could help prevent illegitimate births, abandoned babies, and malnutrition.[96] Other nurses who held similar views occupied special posts such as hospital matrons in charge of family planning or family planning nurses in community health centers. Interviewees who dealt with these programs talked about counseling women about spacing their children and using birth control. Some even conducted gynecological exams and performed contraceptive procedures. Others very much enjoyed advising adolescents about their bodies, sexual activity, and pregnancy. Many gave talks at community health education meetings and in schools. According to a Ciskeian government report, people in the communities began to accept family planning as promoted by nurses.[97] A 1985 Rhodes University study similarly concluded that the work of nurses in rural clinics did increase family planning among the people in the Amathole Basin; however, the study argued that the impact was not dramatic and did not reach outlying communities as much as the village where the clinic was based.[98] Just as family planning had an uneven impact, fewer nurses (about sixteen) talked of family planning more than other health issues. The nurses who did were mostly those who specialized in it or felt it was extremely important to promote. Thus, while it may have been the focus of some nurses' work, others may have seen it as part of their usual procedures or a less significant aspect of clinic work.

Maternity Cases

Although the different aspects of childbirth were part of the regular work of clinics, maternity cases often featured in the interviews as emergencies. More than thirty-five talked about maternity cases. Many told detailed and dramatic stories with emotion and animation because of the intensity of the situations. These were high-stakes cases with two lives at risk that demanded a nurse's full attention and precision, especially when complications occurred. Working in the clinics or assisting with home deliveries, nurses largely had to deal with complications alone, making them even more stressful. Difficulties in childbirth were compounded by other challenges already outlined of working in the clinics. Yet the rewards were great. Bringing life into the world and using their skills and instinct to save a mother and her child brought nurses joy and fulfilment. Six women even proudly reported that they never had a death in childbirth. Statistics indicate that if asked, more women interviewed would have reported the same. These kinds of successes occupied a prominent place in many memories.

Although giving birth could seem like a routine procedure, many things could go wrong in the process, and the nurses did not want to lose any patients or cause any problems themselves. Making a mistake could mean the loss of a completely healthy person. As Nkonki remarked: "*Yho*, you must be very much alert. Otherwise you will have either dead mothers or dead babies at the clinic. . . . Remember, the mother is not ill, she is hundred percent right. The baby is also first class when they come in, and you tell somebody that somebody's dead now, one of the two. *Hayi, ah-ah. Yho, hayi.* [No, ah-ah. Yho, no.]"[99] Similarly, Ann Shaw nurse Tunyiswa commented, "You feel this child must come to the world being all right with no injuries. It's your responsibility."[100] Former clinic supervisor and Middledrift region nurse Bangani said maternity cases brought her closer to God because when she was alone and responsible for two lives, she had to ask God for help: "But when you are dispersed to the clinic or [ward] . . . and you are responsible for that patient, you always said, 'Oh God help me because I'm looking after two souls— the mother and the child.'"[101] Heated exchanges and sharp words were more likely to come when nurses were anxious about the lives of their patients in these stressful cases. Although Feziwe Badi worked most of her career in Grey Hospital, she offered insights into the intensity nurses felt when dealing with maternity cases. She explained that nurses may have come across as harsh in dealing with childbirth not because they were unkind but because they were anxious about the "two lives there that you need to save."[102] Nombeko Hewana worked at Mount Coke Hospital, the Debe Nek clinic, and in family planning throughout her career. She told four stories of times when she had disagreements with people involved in complicated maternity cases—one with a white nurse who ill-treated a patient about to give birth, one with a doctor who did not come to help with a first-time delivery, one with a patient who believed young female nurses did not have the experience to deliver her, and one with a woman giving birth who did not want to push (wherein Hewana finally resorted to slapping her to motivate her).[103]

Remembering Clinic Work

Having "two patients in one" posed many complications that required nurses to think quickly and employ all their training and stamina. They could not just focus on what one patient needed but had to deal with the other simultaneously, as well as the effects the two patients had on each other.[104] Each moment counted.[105] Nkonki described the concentration and analytical skills required to evaluate a mother about to give birth: "So if you are there, you don't know exactly what are you feeling? You look that way, you are using your brains now and your fingers, what is this? What is this? Sometimes you have to use this . . . fetal scope to locate the [fetal heart] so that if you, in most cases, if you feel it below the umbilicus somebody must be on labor, if not on labor there is something wrong with there."[106] In performing their evaluations, nurses had to be precise and vigilant so that they could successfully deliver a patient or transfer a patient to the hospital in time if necessary. Tshatshu nurse Mkwelo talked about how crucial it was for nurses to correctly monitor patients and make the right decision to deliver the patients themselves or transfer them to the hospital: "You observe the patient immediately. When she lies there on the table, you observe the patient. Everything. Everything! You are near the patient, *near* the patient all the time so that you don't get complications— so that she doesn't get complicated." Mkwelo described some of the signs and symptoms that she looked for in more detail in her years at Tshatshu clinic and elsewhere, while hovering over maternity patients.

> You must make a decision because you must have those signs and symptoms. The pulse is like this. The fetal heart, you don't hear the fetal heart. Maybe the patient is draining lycra, the green stuff. Then you see that this child needs an operation, this one. [She's] got a fetal distress once he has *le nto*, greenish discharge to say, no, it's fetal distress. Then he must go to hospital so that he can go for operation. So you must make an assessment that this one can go home, this one can remain, this one I can supervise. I can sit. I can manage for her to give birth here in the clinic. But if we have no facilities in the clinic, you transfer the patient immediately to Mount Coke because you'll be in for it.[107]

Similarly, Nkonki stated, "You must detect these things early when there is still time for the patient . . . to be saved by being taken to hospital." Mcako added, "You must be very alert, you must be very alert." This went all the way down to nurses taking care to give a newborn baby the correct medicine when they had to read drug labels by lamp or candlelight during the night.[108]

Much of this work was all the more difficult because a nurse more often than not worked all alone delivering a baby—either at a clinic or in a home. Nurses stationed in hospitals who assisted in home deliveries had similar experiences, even having to walk long distances to reach patients.[109] Evelyn Magodla's memory of her first maternity case at Rabula clinic exemplifies the pressure these nurses felt as sole biomedical practitioners attending to maternity cases. It was her first case out in a rural area, and she had to go up a mountain to help a woman in labor.

> There came some of the people, . . . that somebody is going to get a baby. "So nurse, take your suitcase, there's the horse, go to the mountain." So I took my suitcase, I climbed the horse, go to the mountain. And I was panicking like mad. . . . I phoned St. Matthew's. . . . You know, I was so scared . . . because it was going to be my first experience. But you know—no ambulance came. I have to deliver that woman there, at her house, *ne*? Then when I've already delivered her, only then the ambulance came. . . . I was so scared. When I got [to the hospital], those nurses—those old nurses—they were laughing at me, "Wooh, you're so panicking!" *Ha ra ra*, I was just nice and fed up. Because—I'm panicking. . . . If that person died, who's going to be at fault? It's going to be me![110]

Whereas the nurses at the hospital who laughed at Magodla's panic had other nurses, doctors, and equipment to rely on, Magodla had gone alone to deliver someone at home, far from the clinic in a place difficult to reach. As she rode the horse to the remote home, she felt the great weight of that responsibility. Even though she called for an ambulance, she was completely responsible for any mistake that might be made or for dealing with serious complications until she had other support.

Other nurses told stories of specific difficult cases that stood out in their memories because of the intense stress and emotion involved or the extraordinary circumstances. These stories included births that occurred in unusual places, breech births and retained placentas, or complications made more dangerous by transportation challenges. The timing of maternity cases posed many challenges. Women could rarely control or predict the exact time of a birth those days. A pregnant woman would "just [turn] up when she's in labor."[111] Tunyiswa and Sodlulashe both talked about having to deliver a baby on Christmas day.[112] Mkwelo told of a woman who came at the last minute and delivered in the waiting room.[113] Sodlulashe also remembered delivering twins at the stream below the Ann Shaw clinic because the woman could not make it to the clinic. Another time, she delivered a premature baby at the public transportation stop on the way out of her home village of Madubela.[114] Nurses attempted to meet with patients to provide antenatal care and watch for cases that may need a doctor's referral, such as first pregnancies or women who had many pregnancies. Antenatal clinics made up a major part of a rural or district nurse's work in large part for that very reason. Nurses also stressed to their antenatal patients that they must come as soon as they felt labor pains. They should not wait until they are about to deliver. As Theresa Nonceba Ntonga put it, "When they are in labor, they will wait until they are really in labor late. And then you must go outside in that car and deliver in the car." Indeed, Ntonga had to rush to deliver a baby in the small space of a car outside the Amabele clinic, one of the many clinics where she worked.[115] Still, many mothers might not come for antenatal care or would not make it to the clinic or hospital in time.

Those who attempted to deliver at home until circumstances forced them to call a nurse presented greater difficulties. Nkonki explained that some would rely on the help of traditional birth attendants or older women experienced in assisting in childbirth; yet when these women could not deal with complications, they would call the nurse, when the mother was well into the labor.[116] For example, Hono, who spent a lot of her time in Middledrift and Peddie clinics, told of a time when an advanced breech case showed up at the clinic one morning: "And the leg was already out. . . . And you know it was navy,

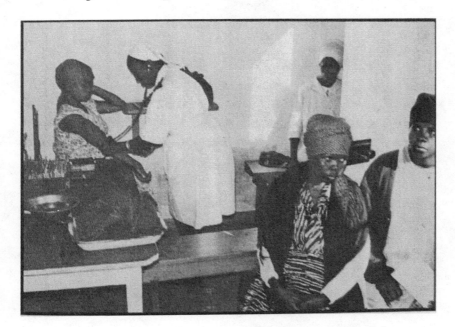

Figure 8. Sister V. V. Matthews attending to antenatal patients. Mount Coke Hospital Report 1969, Mount Coke Hospital Reports, Newsletters Quarterly Reports, Methodist Papers, Folder 2, Cory Library (courtesy of Rhodes University, Cory Library).

proving that it has long been out. So, you said no, immediately proceed to hospital."[117] Mbie talked about the complications she encountered in the areas around Nompumelelo where people preferred to deliver at home. The 1985 Ciskei Department of Health report estimated that only 10 percent of child-bearing-aged women attended antenatal clinics and family planning clinics in the Nompumelelo district.[118] According to Mbie, some well-known *amagqirha* lived in the villages around Nompumelelo and would give women in labor a type of Xhosa medicine designed to ease birth. Yet this medicine could not address all issues, and some would end up having long, complicated labors. Women with breech births or retained placentas often did not notify a nurse until it was too late. It was under these circumstances that Mbie "once encountered" a stillborn with a woman who came "very late with fetal distress and she was so swollen and down below because she was made to push before time." The ambulance did not make it to her in time to save the baby. In another incident, Mbie went to a woman who had long been pushing a breech baby, "but God helped me to maneuver and deliver a live baby." Another time, she helped a woman deliver premature twins at home. Unfortunately, both babies died because, according to Mbie, the mother had not been attending the clinic and thus had not received adequate monitoring.[119]

Other complicated cases may have started with the help of a nurse but had grown more distressing with transportation challenges or when multiple cases presented themselves at once. Rulashe, who worked in clinics around Nompumelelo and Keiskammahoek, related a very stressful delivery of a mother who had not booked in at her clinic. "She delivered and then when I examined, she didn't stop bleeding. It was a twin pregnancy," she narrated. She called for an ambulance and waited and waited. The delay heightened the danger of the case.

> Eventually when the ambulance came, just when she was about to [be carried out] . . . at the door, when the ambulance man was there with the stretcher, she bled heavily. I was mad. I was mad. Ooh but God's mercy, God's mercy. I was praying all the way to hospital. I accompanied the patient to the hospital, all the way to hospital. Ooh man! That one. But she made it, together with the twins.[120]

Majiza remembered just one particularly difficult case she dealt with at Burns Hill—a woman with high blood pressure who came in during the late afternoon. "I had to do my best," she related. She phoned the hospital and then raced the patient to the hospital in her husband's car. Waiting for an ambulance was too risky. "So I had to drive like mad to the hospital. And she had eclampsia, and she was fitting on the way to the hospital. But fortunately for me she survived and the baby too," she concluded.[121] Baleni remembered times she dealt with a retained placenta in the Bhisho area. One incident occurred when she was working at the Tilden clinic. Her patient would not stop bleeding after the baby was born, so she sent two men to find the community van to take the woman to Grey Hospital. Unfortunately, the two men came back saying they saw the van near the school where a function was going to be held, but no one could find the driver. Baleni had to leave the woman with her relatives and walk more than six kilometers to find the driver. In another incident, Baleni was working all alone, relieving a nurse at the Peelton clinic. While she was with a woman about to deliver, a boy of around ten or eleven years old came to the clinic with a cut that needed suturing at the hospital. "Now what do I do?" Baleni recounted, "I've got a delivery this side, . . . I've got this boy this side, . . . I don't have a phone in the clinic." Luckily the nurse she was relieving, a Mrs. Vena, had not left the village yet, so Baleni sent a note to Vena, who came running to help. Vena allowed Baleni to walk to the railway station to phone for the ambulance.[122] Otherwise, calling for the ambulance could have resulted in much more complicated results.

A number of nurses commented on the difficulty of spending time with a birth and then having to immediately attend to other patients, especially after a nighttime delivery. Mgwalana village nurse Mkosana described the time it took to help with a home delivery: "Sometimes you stayed at that home for a couple of hours not delivering. Oh! Hey. But we have to be . . . patient. Don't leave that patient until she delivers." After the delivery, the nurse would then need to monitor the mother and the baby to make sure they were both well before she left. "Now when you come back, you find the clinic is full of other people," she continued. Similar to nurses already quoted in this chapter, she said, "You have got to attend [to] those people again; but you must [be] nice, don't be funny. And finish them because others who are here, they are going far back at home. So [you] got to attend those people. You don't say . . . 'I'm tired now. I didn't sleep. I was busy delivering that patient.'"[123] Even if a clinic had two or three fully qualified nurses, when it was one nurse's turn to be on call, it often happened that she would spend the entire night with a patient, then be expected to open the clinic at eight o'clock the next morning. Mjikeliso talked of sleepless nights when she worked at clinics in the Middledrift and Keiskammahoek districts, when she had to deal with multiple patients: "Maybe you will see three maternity patients delivering at the same day. If you have finished with this one, then there will come another one then after that, that means you will not sleep."[124] Not all nighttime cases related to childbirth, but maternity cases were particularly strenuous because of the time and attention they required throughout the night, into the early hours of the morning.

One of the more dramatic maternity cases was shared by Nkonki, who told of a time when she was working at the Tyutyu-Bhisho clinic when a young woman went into labor prematurely. Nkonki had been called to the home by the family, who thought the daughter had a bad case of diarrhea. It did not take Nkonki long to discover the daughter was pregnant. When Nkonki realized the baby was about to come out, and "I am not even in the clinic," she placed two of her fingers on the baby's head to prevent its birth: "Because if this baby could be delivered here, no incubators! So she would get cold, shiver, and die because it is long before time." She sent someone to call an ambulance and kept her two fingers on the baby's head all the way from the home, on the stretcher, into the ambulance, and into the labor ward. She only moved her fingers when the nurses at the hospital told her they were ready to take over. Nkonki concluded the story: "So that child was saved and was given my name."

Despite the high stress of maternity cases, Nkonki talked about her satisfaction in taking them on. "Hey, though it would put one in jail, . . . it's so nice," she remarked. When I pressed her more about why it was "so nice," she talked about how her skills were sharpened and her confidence boosted when working with these cases. Nurses were completely responsible for things that could go wrong but also completely responsible when they did things right. "Nobody is going to help you, that's the thing. Unlike in the hospital, . . . you are using your brains now." Nkonki explained, "You don't depend on anyone there." She continued, "You know you must do things the right way and do proper findings."[125] It was a time to use their good technical and quick problem-solving skills. When speaking about her experiences in the Lenye clinic and others around Keiskammahoek, Gantsho stated similarly, "The clinic is far from the hospital. So you are alone, you don't have an advisor now to do this, to give advice that the patient should be transferred to the hospital."[126] Nurses thus learned to rely on their own judgment and abilities. The more experience they gained, the more accurate, skillful, and confident they became. Even though there were terrible aspects about working at the clinic, like the on-call system, Mbombo said working in the clinics "was the best thing that happened" to her because of the way she developed her skills as a nurse: "I grew professionally and I was able to work independently in assisting the patients without having to rely on the doctor all the time. You tend to acquire a lot of experience in different conditions of the patients." She learned which patients needed a doctor's referral and to make "a good diagnosis of all your clients and be able to treat them quite effectively."[127] Ncukana, at one time an Ann Shaw nurse who also worked in Victoria and S. S. Gida Hospitals, commented, "Seeing that you have live births and you could be able to detect any complications before a child is born. That was what was very interesting."[128]

Multiple nurses I interviewed expressed the humble delight they felt when they learned that patients named their children after them, the nurses who successfully delivered the children. Ncukana remarked, "You know, helping somebody to deliver a human being on earth was something that was appreciated." Giving the child the nurse's name was a profound expression of that gratitude. Other nurses talked of the pleasure of running into former patients years later and being introduced to the grown child they had delivered. Ncukana related,

> And when you see [them] in years to come, you say, "I delivered you." That was—that is most encouraging. And even some of the community would remember you for that. They would come and say, "You know you delivered my twins. You helped me when I was pregnant. You delivered my babies. You know so-and-so who's now so much old, who's now employed somewhere, is your product?" That was very good.[129]

Speaking of a time she worked as a midwife in Springs in the Gauteng Province, Nosipho Jantjies said, "I would be in town walking, and then you'd see somebody greeting you, a lady greeting you and saying, 'Sister you know your child is doing grade so-and-so now.' Or 'Your child is doing this and that and that,' . . . [or] 'Do you know this young lady? This is your product.' That makes you feel good."[130] Nkonki and Mcako laughed as they reminisced about people bringing maybe a five-year-old child to the clinic and expecting the nurse to recognize that they had delivered the child. "They even tell you, 'It's your baby,'" Mcako added.[131] Many of the nurses loved bringing children into the world or "catching babies" because they loved children. The stress and strain that came from working alone in difficult conditions made the success of a safe delivery sweeter. These feelings of joy made maternity cases that much more memorable and rewarded nurses who worked under strenuous conditions.

Training and Commitment

The very low death rate in childbirth at the hand of these nurses is remarkable considering the conditions they had to work under, with no electricity, ambulances taking time to arrive, or women coming in at the advanced stages of a complicated labor. "We were doing excellent work in spite of all that," Mhlambiso said. "We never had a problem, we never had deaths during child birth."[132] Ngoro also said she never had a death in childbirth, even if it was twins. She worked for many years at the Qibirha clinic. A maternity register dating from 1976 to 1995 recorded only fourteen child deaths out of 756 total births at the clinic during that period.[133] Other available clinic and hospital records indicate a similar success rate. Maternity registers kept between 1983 and 1991 at Peelton clinic registered two hospital transfers and no deaths out of 378 births, and the Tyutyu clinic reported two stillbirths and eighteen referrals out of 544 total cases.[134] The Lovedale hospitals reported only one stillbirth out of 81 births recorded in its district services in 1971.[135] The training nurses received during this time, particularly in midwifery, was a major contributing factor in their success in providing biomedical health care in the rural Ciskei—even if it meant knowing when to transfer a patient to the hospital. Full-time nurses who ran rural clinics were required to have midwifery training. Before changes in training in the 1980s, South African nurses had a minimum of three years of training for general nursing and nine months to a year of midwifery training as a separate program. Many nurses who worked in the Eastern Cape trained at hospitals known for their high standards, such as Livingstone Hospital in Port Elizabeth, King Edward VIII in Durban, McCord's Zulu Hospital, as well as hospitals in the region. With such a high demand for limited training spots in these hospitals, those who were accepted had already shown great potential.[136] Their training honed their sharp intellects and practical skills. Mcako trained in midwifery at St. Monica's in Cape Town, where her instructor spent extra time ensuring she understood procedures. Looking back, Mcako felt "it was wonderful the way they used to care for us."[137] Others who trained at big urban hospitals like Baragwanath Hospital in Soweto, or who trained in rural mission hospitals, remarked that they gained experience in treating a variety of cases or dealing with rural conditions.

Nurses who worked in rural clinics also often added further training to their general nursing and midwifery certificates. Many nurses appreciated that the Ciskei government offered nurses in-service training opportunities on a variety of topics or allowed study leave to gain further qualifications such as psychiatric nursing and family planning. Many also completed a degree in community health nursing and health administration, either through a new program provided at the Cecilia Makiwane Hospital in Mdantsane or through the University of South Africa. Continuously adding to their skill set along with experience and on-the-job training by older nurses improved the nurses' abilities to deliver health care in rural communities.[138]

These nurses' commitment to nursing in rural communities was just as important in helping them persist under strenuous circumstances as their training. Even with their training, the long hours, on-call duty, and lack of resources could have had a crippling effect on the nurses' work—why Mhlambiso went on her boycott. Of the forty-one who commented on why nurses would quit, some indicated that nurses would leave clinics to work in the hospital, while fourteen (speaking about nurses generally) said a nurse would quit because of the difficult working conditions and six said a nurse would quit if she did not have the "calling" to be a nurse. The need for a strong commitment was indeed a theme in the interviews I conducted. When asked to give advice to new nurses, Perksdale clinic nurse Nontsikelelo Mfengqe and Ann Shaw nurse Ncukana both asserted that for a nurse to be successful, she had to be dedicated, patient, and diligent.[139] Mbombo remarked that a nurse had to have experience but also had to care about people enough to motivate her to do further investigations into community health issues.[140] Hono explained that if a nurse liked the community, then she would learn a lot, helping her be a more successful nurse.[141] When asked what kept them going despite the long hours, lack of equipment, and difficult cases, most nurses talked about their love of nursing and their desire to help their people. Gqomfa said, "Because when you work at the clinic as a nurse, what's your desire? You want the people to get healed, to come and say, 'We thank you. You've helped us.'"[142] When asked why she stayed in the rural clinics, Mjikeliso replied, "I decided to help my people because I knew that there was no other alternative because I was trained and I made a pledge that I will work for my community."[143]

Thoto's comment that the community owned their nurse reflected the dedication she had to her work as well as the particular demands of working and living within a community. She described why she liked rural community work: "With the community work, you work in the community. You conduct visits to the homes, you know how they stay at their homes. You happen to know their problems, and so on. . . . In the community, you are involved with them. . . . They own you!" She then went on to describe how a nurse must put her patients first.[144] Some nurses talked about the difficulty of being "owned" by the community or working at a clinic in one's home village. Ncukana said, "Being known by the community, there were too many demands. . . . You would find that at times people couldn't differentiate between emergency and general illness."[145] Yet she focused on her main goal, which helped her deal with such cases: "But what was most important is that you could see the progress of the nursing we were giving to people. You were able to change them from the detrimental practices to good practices." In the first few years of her career, Ntonga worked in strenuous circumstances in three different clinics as she acted as the main provider for her family. In the Mgwali clinic near Port Alfred, she even had to do janitorial work. But she said she was committed to her work and that sustained her.[146] As Victoria East clinic nurse Ntshona said, "When you love a thing, when you are there, you wonder why you were afraid [to do it before]."[147]

Individual personalities, training, and perhaps gendered roles of women as caregivers all may have strengthened the commitment these women had to their work. At least twenty-one of the nurses I interviewed told me that they became nurses because they had always enjoyed helping or nursing people from a young age. Most emphasized that nursing was a "calling," not simply a job or a career. Those trained in mission hospitals would have been taught that the nature of their work was special or sacred, while others who were already religious may have inscribed this onto their demanding yet people-centered careers, looking to Florence Nightingale as their noble forerunner.[148] A few nurses I interviewed even used the term "mothering" to describe their work, indicating that they also saw nursing linked to their natural role as mothers. For example, when explaining why she loved her career, Majiza said when a child came in "helpless, crying in pain and we have to mother that child, . . . you see the fruit when that child gets better."[149]

Expressions of satisfaction in working with communities reflected the commitment these nurses had to their patients, which motivated them to work through difficult circumstances. Even before she trained, Middledrift and Peddie nurse Hono wanted to be a public or community nurse because she wanted to educate the people: "So what I liked was to [enlighten] people, so that they know more, how to care about their own health. And to encourage them to want to be healthy. . . . Because having finished your training, the mission is not complete until you practice that."[150] Majiza told of the joy she felt when she saw her patients improve: "You look after a patient, looking back at the condition they were in when this patient came into my hands— I looked after him or her, I did this for this patient, I did that," and then "you see that patient now becoming a human being again, you do have that feeling inside you that 'I am also a part. I have played a part in this person's health.'"[151] Similarly, Gqomfa said, "If you understand your patients and they understand you, you know their problems, you visit them, they come, they talk, and they are open with you, and the staff is open with you. It's nice working at the clinic. . . . At least you know I've done something for the day, I've solved a problem for somebody."[152]

Still others talked of the joy of working with patients in their own environment. This allowed them to really see the cause of ill-health and address it at its root. Mjikeliso talked about how interesting it was to watch the children grow from the baby clinic, to child immunizations, to family planning sessions as a teenager. "You even go to their houses and visit them at the house and you will see everything there," she explained. She concluded, "It's so interesting to work in the community because they will know everything because you are always there with them and you will see their problems immediately and you will be able to refer."[153] This kind of intimate work with communities led Rulashe to get "attached" to her people: "When you work with the people you relate to them, you get used to them, you get used and attached to each other. So it was nice—it's nice to work with the people in the community."[154] The nurses needed that attachment and desire to "plant what [they] have learned" in the communities, to sustain them in their work, even with their high-quality training.[155]

Conclusion

Nurses' work in rural clinics could be difficult and complex as they carried heavy responsibilities. They dealt with intense emergencies on top of their regular clinic days. They treated common cases such as gastroenteritis, TB, hypertension, and diabetes or diseases of malnutrition and struggled to transport more dire cases to the hospital. After delivering a baby in the middle of the night with no electricity, they still had to wear a smile and a clean uniform in the morning as they attended to clinic patients, made home visits, or spoke at community meetings. The range of work they performed, their demanding contracts, remote locations, and limited resources required great skill and dedication. Those who had the internal drive and commitment survived and found joy in this strenuous work. Interacting well with communities was also a key to successful delivery of biomedical health care in these rural areas. A significant part of that was balancing the promotion of biomedicine with respect for the beliefs and practices of the people.

CHAPTER FOUR

Engaging Xhosa Beliefs and Practices

THE CLINIC WAS JUST ONE OPTION for people seeking medical care in the rural Ciskei in the 1960s through the 1980s. Ciskei residents also had access to home remedies, Xhosa practitioners, and Christian faith healers. Although many people relied on a combination of sources of healing, the two main medical systems they turned to were the Xhosa system and the biomedical system. Nurses were fully aware that people continued to consult *amagqirha*. They recognized the strength of the people's belief in Xhosa practitioners. Mount Coke and Bhisho Hospital nurse Bell Memane declared matter-of-factly, "It's their belief. . . . And we must remember that our health care came all of a sudden." She continued, "In the olden days they've been having these traditional healers, you know? And they were healing them, and they believed in them, mm? So we can't stop them. . . . They must go where they want to be healed."[1] Others similarly acknowledged the autonomy of their patients. Yolisa Ngqokwe worked in a Ciskei clinic and hospitals in neighboring regions. Speaking of patients seeking out *amagqirha*, she remarked, "It's their culture and their right."[2] After a career of working in different clinics in the current Gauteng province and the Ciskei, Jantjies observed, "Otherwise, traditional healing is there to stay. There's nothing that you can do."[3]

Nurses working in the rural regions of the Ciskei contested, shared, and negotiated the beliefs and practices of their patients. Being Xhosa themselves, they had a good understanding of the worldview and values of their Xhosa patients and thus could translate biomedicine linguistically as well as conceptually. Not all the nurses respected the views of their patients. These women also had to deal with notions about gender roles that restricted the influence they had. Yet many nurses I interviewed learned that more success came when they took a cooperative approach. Most importantly, they saw that a sure way to discourage patients from coming to the clinic was to challenge their strongly held beliefs. As former Ciskei clinic nurse and supervisor Baleni explained, if a nurse sat down with a patient who has seen *igqirha*, "you do not contradict her beliefs because you're not going to get anywhere."[4] When addressing divergences in healing practices and beliefs, nurses took two main approaches. First, they concentrated on motivating their patients to take both Xhosa and clinic medicines, without seeking to change or challenge Xhosa beliefs. Second, they attempted to change particular beliefs and practices through various levels of education, including individual informal counseling, community meetings, and cooperation with Xhosa practitioners. In doing so, they worked to have collaborative relationships with local community leaders. When dealing with Xhosa notions of appropriate gender roles, they found ways to reason with patients or reach a patient indirectly. Taking these approaches allowed both healing systems to adapt and persist in the same region. The nurses' work thus resulted in shifts rather than challenges to whole systems, with some changes in the understanding of certain diseases and the types of cases *amagqirha* focused on, plus increased cooperation between nurses and *amagqirha*. Although this history comes primarily from nurses' interviews, careful analysis and evidence from written sources supports these conclusions.

Being Xhosa and a Nurse in the Ciskei Health Care System

Many of the nurses I interviewed straddled two worldviews in their position as Xhosa women and nurses trained in Western biomedicine. The majority understood the Xhosa worldview and would have had a familiarity with Xhosa medical practices and beliefs, even though they had varying types of experiences and beliefs themselves. Some of them had grown up in communities and families that frequently used *amagqirha* and *amaxhwele*; some drew upon both biomedicine and Xhosa medicine themselves; while a few grew up in Christian families that did not use Xhosa medicine at all. On the other hand, the nurses trained and worked in systems opposing or seeking to change Xhosa medicine, even if its stance was turning more cooperative into the 1980s. These experiences influenced the worldviews the nurses adhered to and the approach they would take when working in Xhosa communities.

It is difficult to generalize about how much Xhosa women had their own beliefs challenged during their nursing training because only twenty-seven of the women I interviewed discussed their experiences with health care while growing up. It is safe to say, however, that most of them were at least familiar with the Xhosa worldview regarding health and healing, even if they did not fully adhere to it themselves. Over half of all I interviewed were born and grew up in rural areas where people would have likely had easier access to *amagqirha* than clinics and hospitals. Of the twenty-seven who talked about their childhood experiences with health care, fourteen said they, their families, and their community members attended a clinic or hospital when they needed care, but twelve talked about the difficulties of accessing biomedicine. This, some said, led people to first consult *amagqirha*. Only six or seven discussed using *amagqirha* themselves, and about that same number talked about the herbal remedies that people used, including some who had family members who were *amaxhwele* or were skilled in using herbs to treat ailments. Yet even fewer talked about being unfamiliar with or rejecting *amagqirha*. Four of the twenty-seven said that one or more persons in their family did not like *amagqirha* or did not believe in them—some of them said they were Christian or grew up near a mission station as a way to explain their lack of exposure to *amagqirha*.[5] Even then, as Mount Coke and Bhisho Hospital nurse Someketha explained, nurses encountered medicines in various places in the community, just walking around. "I mean, [you] grew up in the rural area where there are these medicines, and they are being sold even near the shops," she said. "You can see them if you go to the [taxi] rank, and you'll see all different types of medicines put on the floor, written 'this is for *ukuhlamba* [to wash],' . . . [to sleep], . . . to drive away this *impundulu*." As for *amagqirha*, they could be people the nurses grew up with or went to school with. "It's the people around, they are not foreigners," she remarked.[6]

Although the Xhosa believed in natural causes of ill-health similar to that of biomedicine and engaged with biomedicine as demonstrated in earlier chapters, the nurses entered the Ciskei health care system at a time when officials saw the system as antithetical to Xhosa medical systems. At the opening ceremony of the Gxulu clinic in 1967, a Bantu Affairs Commission representative celebrated the event as a mark of progress. With community members and officials gathered around the small, four-roomed building nestled in the hills, he began his speech by stating, "It has been a long struggle against superstition—over a hundred years—to persuade the Bantu people to accept the White man's methods of healing." He then urged the people to not view the nurses with suspicion but as people there to help.[7] Newspaper articles promoting health around the same time spoke of Xhosa practitioners as greedy and exploitative, with one woman writing, "For the love of Michael never [consult] the 'Witch Doctor' or 'Herbalist.'"[8] The Christian civilizing mission of certain hospitals and training programs also persisted through the 1960s and 1970s. At least thirty-six women I interviewed trained in mission hospitals, and at least forty worked in a mission hospital or former mission hospital at one point. The mission and biomedical staff at these institutions often came out in direct opposition to Xhosa practices and beliefs, characterizing Xhosa systems as completely different and backward. Although mission hospital staff believed in a divine

Engaging Xhosa Beliefs and Practices

power beyond science, they did not leave much room for Xhosa beliefs. As discussed in previous chapters, they saw the introduction of biomedicine as a way to convert people away from *amagqirha* and hoped their treatments would prove the power of their religion. In 1966 Mount Coke reported that the "never ending battle against disease, poverty and heathen darkness was carried on during the year," and in 1971, that "with the aid of the Bible, the text-book and a bottle of medicine, that uncultivated African was introduced in the accepted norms of civilization." The hospital saw it as progress when it reported that the patients adhered to the Western biomedical custom of the patient telling the doctor what was wrong instead of expecting the doctor to tell the patient, like the *amagqirha*.[9] Mission hospitals also hoped to make deeper Christian converts out of their student nurses, who could spread the gospel among their people. Even as the Ciskei government took over mission hospitals in the mid-1970s, the hospitals and their staff continued to hold regular prayers for staff and patients. The rhetoric in government and hospital records that placed cleanliness and biomedicine in stark contrast to the superstition or heathenism of the Xhosa also continued.

For some nurses, training in biomedicine and Christian conversion led them to reject Xhosa beliefs and practices all together.[10] For example, when describing the rise of midwifery training among Black nurses, Grace Mashaba took a disparaging tone regarding rural populations, writing: "The Black population was predominantly rural. Ignorance and superstition were still rife."[11] Yet other nurses found ways to reconcile the two systems. They believed in their biomedical training, but several also retained elements of the Xhosa worldview. Furthermore, understanding that the Xhosa believed in natural causes for illhealth and that Xhosa medicine was open to incorporating other effective methods helps us see that the two systems were not always diametrically opposed. Indeed, scholars have shown that patients, and even biomedically trained nurses, could view the two systems as complementary.[12] The limitations of biomedicine also left room for people to accept explanations of ailments and forces that biomedicine could not address.[13]

The way that nurses themselves used or talked about *amagqirha* suggests that training in biomedicine did not necessarily lead them to reject Xhosa medicine altogether. A doctor in the Transkei remembered overhearing nurses talking among themselves about their cousins who were healed by *amagqirha* but noted that they only talked about this while they were off duty. Digby and Sweet call this hidden acceptance of other healing systems "latent pluralism" and suspect that a large majority of nurses also thought this way.[14] A study of nurses' views of African practitioners conducted by Marc Simon Kahn in the mid-1990s adds further evidence of this pluralism. Kahn reported that 80 percent of his respondents believed "traditional healers have been given power to heal by the ancestors," and another large percentage participated in performing "traditional customs."[15] Comments by nurses I interviewed reveal an acceptance of the possibility of the effectiveness of Xhosa therapies, ranging from believing in herbal treatments to seeking help with promotions or protection from ancestors. When speaking of patient choices, Burns Hill nurse Majiza voiced the possibility that Xhosa medicines could heal people. "And sometimes you wonder," she said, "if really it is the mixture of the real medicine or the herbalist. You are not sure. But you always say, 'Thank you. The person is healed.'"[16] Others, like Dubula, who worked in a number of St. Matthew's and S. S. Gida clinics, saw certain remedies as based on herbal knowledge. Dubula reasoned, "You know even tablets originate from the herbs. That's another thing that you must not forget. So it's very difficult to criticize too much." She then shared an example of when she used Xhosa medicine to address a severe stomachache. An older man in her community brought her *umnonono* or leaves from the mountain hard pear (*Olinia emarginata*). "Nurse, chew this," he said, offering it to her. "I did, and I was well," she testified, "so there's nothing bad, there's nothing that is too bad, *uyabona?*"[17] Former clinic supervisor and Middledrift region nurse, Bangani, related a story of a woman who obtained some herbs from an *ixhwele* that helped her recover from a stroke. The woman was relatively young, about fifty years old, and could not walk or speak after her stroke. Somebody known in the community who was good at curing strokes "immediately" showed up and gave her a mixture. "That lady got a bottle there on the third day and she's right now," Bangani related. "She talks, she walks, she's doing everything." Bangani then talked about *sutherlandia*, a mixture advertised to cure many things but that she used to ease her arthritis. She concluded, "We do buy them. Because we believe they might help since they are from under [God's ground]."[18] Similarly, Thyra Nomkhitha Mavuso, a nurse who worked at Victoria Hospital and its clinics, talked about the African wild potato or *hypoxis* plant, believed to heal many different ailments if crushed and poured into a drink. She wanted to plant it in her own garden to help with her arthritis.[19] Although these herbal remedies did not necessarily require a diagnosis by *igqirha*, they were seen as presenting effective alternatives to biomedicine.

As some of my interviews and the work of other scholars have indicated, some nurses went to *amagqirha* for help with issues related to social relationships that biomedicine did not address, such as gaining promotions, having protection when traveling or moving to a new place, or finding something one has lost. St. Matthew's and S. S. Gida clinic nurse Evelyn Magodla said, "Even the nurses, they believed witchcraft. If they are looking for a job they will go

Engaging Xhosa Beliefs and Practices

to a witchdoctor *kuba*, 'Witchdoctor give me medicine because I want to get promotion,' or 'I want a job,' or 'I want to *thakatha* [bewitch] somebody.'"[20] Advertisements from African practitioners in *Imvo Zabantsundu* appealed to those having trouble conceiving children, seeking to increase their fortune in life, seeking protection from witchcraft, or longing for the return of a lover. These advertisements give the impression that the *amagqirha* in the latter part of the twentieth century focused more on individual care, as opposed to their political and community role of the past, and emphasized the more spiritual and social powers they offered that biomedicine could not.[21] For cases that seemingly rested on good fortune or the protection of deceased family members, some nurses, like their patients, might have also petitioned their ancestors for help or sought certain medicines. Elliot Wexu, executive committee member of the South African Herbalists' Association in the late 1960s and 1970s (based in Duncan Village, then Mdantsane), stressed to the *Daily Dispatch* that he and members of his association did not practice witchcraft. They helped people seeking work or having trouble with romantic relationships, including the uneducated as well as "teachers, ministers of religion, nurses, traders and other professional people."[22]

Others more pragmatically resorted to *amagqirha* when biomedicine failed them. Baleni described in detail her experience with such a case. Although she was a proud, committed nurse who believed in biomedicine, she credited her ancestors for solving a health problem that biomedicine did not. She explained to me before our interview began that she had needed to postpone our appointment because she was helping with a family ritual. The same ritual had been performed for her when she was young. She had fallen ill every month when she menstruated. She went around to multiple doctors, searching for a solution— "Every month attending to this doctor, changing this doctor, going to this one." No one found a remedy. Her father resorted to consulting an *igqirha*. "And this tradition healer said," Baleni narrated, "No, your daughter wants this, must do this [ritual]." "No medicine?" her father asked. "No medicine! It's only this. She wants this," *igqirha* replied. Her father hesitated. He told *igqirha* that no one in the family had done such a ritual. *Igqirha* replied, "Yes, I agree, but this one wants it. I hear what you say. You say your sisters and your grandmothers didn't have this and this and this. But this one needs this [ritual], she doesn't need medicine to drink. No." The ritual involved slaughtering a goat and then making a necklace of materials from the goat and oxtails from the family's herd—a type of *intambo*, or necklace with protective powers.[23] Wearing the necklace invited her ancestors to always be with her. Baleni kept the necklace with her throughout her life. When she showed it to me in 2012, she testified that she had never been sick since the ritual had been performed

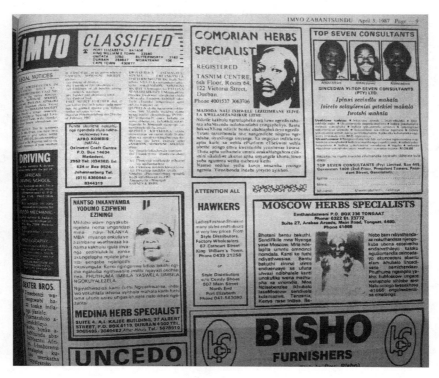

Figure 9. *Imvo Zabantsundu* classifieds, April 3, 1987. Amathole Museum Library. The Comorian Herbs Specialist ad reads "MEN, HERE'S A POWERFUL TRADITIONAL HEALER FROM ZANZIBAR, HE SAYS: I have heard a lot about the hardships of the country, about the diseases of Black people and those that are incurable. People of the Xhosa nation, I'm here for all those who are suffering."

fifty-three years earlier. In this case, her family had called upon the power of the ancestors to address an illness biomedicine could not. However, Baleni's use of the oxtail necklace did not require that Baleni replace belief in one system for another. Although Baleni told me about the effectiveness of the necklace with confidence and pride, when I asked her if there were certain Xhosa medicines that worked well that she might use herself, she replied, "No, . . . no, . . . not that I know of, not that I know of."[24] The plurality of forces influencing one's life that the Xhosa worldview allowed meant that Xhosa nurses could have an eclectic set of beliefs themselves even if their training or the health care system within which they worked took a more absolute one-or-the-other approach.

The rhetoric and stance of the Ciskei government softened in the late 1970s and into the 1980s. When comprehensive health care came in during the 1970s,

THE MOST FAMOUS HERBALIST TAMIL WHO HELPS EVERYONE WHO NEEDS HERBAL MEDICINE

The following are all other herbal medicines that we supply:

1. We have *Mageqa*, which is used when you cannot conceive 7.00
2. True manhood enlargement herbal medicine 5.00
3. We heal seizures completely 5.00
4. We also heal palpitations completely 5.00
5. We also stock *Madudula*, which cleans your body inside and out 6.00
6. Medicine for quitting alcohol and cigarettes 4.00
7. Herbal medicine to chase away evil spirits even if they are hell-bent on making your life unbearable—we chase them away successfully 6.00
8. We have a book that explains every dream and we also have winning numbers for racehorse races 2.00
9. Faa-Fee is also available in all languages 2.00
10. We also remove crab lice and other kinds of lice in the body 3.00
11. Medicine to stop bad dreams and nightmares 3.00

There are lots of other medicines that we have not listed. You can choose the one you want and place an order. You can pay at the post office when you receive the goods via the C.O.D. plan. Another option is to send cash to: TAMIL & COMPANY, P.O. Box 92, MOBENI, NATAL

EZAMAYEZA – HERBAL & TRADITIONAL MEDICINE

When you need traditional and herbal medicine, you can get them from your 100% real traditional healer called Manzolwandle (Seawater) from the area of Soshangane. We can heal every common illness known to man with our medicine. The following are some of the medicines that we supply:

1. We heal and remove crab lice completely R5.00
2. We have medicine that removes white and red parasites from your body R2.00
3. We also have Phindamshaye, which is medicine for someone who is trying to bewitch you so that whatever they are doing returns to them R3.00
4. True manhood enlargement herbal medicine R5.00
5. We remove poison completely from your body R5.00
6. Medicine for chronic backache R2.00
7. We have a book that explains every dream and we also have winning numbers for racehorse races and Faa-Fee R5.00
8. Medicine for removing bad dreams and nightmares R4.00
9. When your urine is bloody and stings, we heal the problem completely R3.00
10. Medicine to strengthen your house from unwanted evil spirits R8.00

There are also lots of other medicines that we have not listed. You can choose the one you want and place an order. You can pay at the post office when you receive the goods via the C.O.D. plan. Another option is to send cash to: MANZOLWANDLE , P.O. BOX 242, MOBENI, NATAL

Figure 10. *Imvo Zabantsundu* advertisement, June 12, 1971. Translation by Hlumela Sondlo.

it did not have a policy about working with African practitioners. In fact, reports and official announcements of the Department of Health and Welfare in the self-governing Ciskei in the mid to late 1970s hardly mention *amagqirha* or *amaxhwele*. The focus was on extending biomedical services, curbing disease, and addressing environmental and sanitation problems—and changing the people's behavior and beliefs in the process. However, some of the historical roots of the comprehensive health care system the homelands adopted had accommodated African medical practitioners. Doctors Sydney and Emily Kark reached out to African medical practitioners at the Pholela Health Center in Natal and made efforts to understand the cultural, social, and psychological aspects of health in the community.[25] This approach gained greater acceptance later, with the international community recognizing the importance of pluralistic medical systems in the late 1970s.[26]

Some Ciskeian politicians raised the possibility of working with Xhosa practitioners in the late 1970s and early 1980s. This reflected the reality of practices and beliefs on the ground but also a growing acceptance of Xhosa medicine in public institutions. Chief Sipho Mangindi Burns-Ncamashe was an educator, Xhosa language and literary leader, and also a Xhosa healer and member of the Ciskei legislature.[27] In May 1976, as legislators discussed the Department of Health and Welfare report, one member praised the department for showing them that TB could be cured and was not caused by *impundulu* or the lightning bird. On the other hand, Burns-Ncamashe raised the question of how patients might feel if certain Xhosa practices were not followed, such as pregnant women being given a protective necklace, or *intambo*. Taking the approach of overlooking Xhosa medicine to focus on biomedicine, the minister of health at the time, Fikile Siyo, replied that "we do not prohibit such African customs" but explained that the hospitals focused on their own treatments.[28] A few years later, in 1980, Burns-Ncamashe called for a dialogue between the government and *amagqirha*. "If [the herbalists of Xhosa Land] are recognized by the Government, why then are there no plans that they be tested and their abilities for curing certain diseases ascertained?" he asked in the legislative debates. At the same time the chief celebrated the training of Ciskei nurses and doctors, he pointed out that the minister had left Xhosa practitioners out of his policy speech. Yet he argued that some of the *amagqirha* could cure cancer. He advocated that they should be taken to universities to analyze their treatments. He said specialists from Cape Town even came to discuss how to deal with psychiatric patients and cure *amafufunyana*, a spirit possession or psychological disorder.[29] In contrast to the condescending attitude expressed by mission hospitals and Ciskeian government officials in prior decades, he couched this in terms of Ciskei national achievements. He said, "The Ciskei nation would be proud if people who had knowledge about medicines and disease came forward so that their knowledge could be harnessed to the benefit of all people." So, he concluded, they should make *amagqirha* feel comfortable going public.[30] A year later, the minister of health, then B. R. Maku, said Ciskei healers were competing with medical practices in the homeland, "and if we can't beat them we must make them join us."[31] Although this did not result in an actual policy, it indicates greater political acceptance of Xhosa practitioners in the Ciskei.

Whereas during this time local newspapers often reported sensational stories of how Xhosa practitioners swindled and stole from people or bewitched or accused people of bewitching others (which at times led to mob violence), less threatening herbalists attempted to forge a more accepted space for themselves within South Africa.[32] As Kirsten Rüther has argued, the popular print media "took a vested interest in stories and news about healers" in the 1970s into the 1990s, which elevated their social standing.[33] This was the case with Wexu's South African Herbalists' Association, which garnered attention in the *Daily Dispatch* and *Imvo Zabantsundu*.[34] It sought to operate as a modern professional organization, imposing regulations, awarding certificates, and ensuring its members obeyed the Witchcraft Suppression Act of 1957 (which consolidated all the laws to apply to the whole country and made accusing others of witchcraft, engaging in witchcraft, or seeking help in sniffing out witches punishable by law). It held annual conferences that included public and celebratory beauty contests, "Miss Herbalist," and dance and best traditionally dressed contests. When troubles within the association arose, its president, Harry Willie, appealed to members of the association to all be truthful and strictly follow the law, for a few dishonest members could bring down the whole association. For good measure, the association periodically donated money toward anticrime efforts.[35] It eventually gained recognition from the Ciskei government and even hoped to establish a college for herbalists in the Ciskei.[36] This college did not materialize, but its proposal is evidence of efforts by African practitioners to professionalize their vocation as a modern one. Similar efforts by various types of practitioners culminated in the founding of the African National Healers Association in 1989.[37]

Training in community health nursing and some efforts by the Department of Health to work with *amagqirha* in the mid-1980s also show a greater willingness to recognize and collaborate with Xhosa practitioners at that time. There were efforts within South Africa by both the biomedical and African medical communities to raise the profile of African practitioners at the time, particularly as it related to psychological health.[38] The Ciskei Department of Health reportedly reached out to *amagqirha* in 1984 to enlist their help in referring

122 Engaging Xhosa Beliefs and Practices

psychiatric patients to hospitals and to encourage those patients to continue to take their medication.[39] However, as in other places in Africa, these efforts were often made to facilitate biomedical initiatives rather than to promote the adoption of Xhosa medicine, and there is no evidence that the Ciskei adopted an official policy regarding *amagqirha*.[40]

Even if training and some department initiatives were more open to Xhosa medical practitioners, without a clearly defined policy, how this was to happen on the ground was largely left to the practitioners who worked in the clinics and hospitals. As one nurse put it, the mere circumstances of working in rural communities forced them to work with *amagqirha*. It became an accepted practice.[41] Whether or not nurses had a background steeped in Xhosa medicine or shaped heavily by Christianity, or whether their training in Western biomedicine had radically changed their worldview, they had a familiarity with and experience in both medical systems that put them in a position to act as intermediaries between the two. This position was amplified when they were engaged in rural community health care.

"You must handle that with forceps"

Some nurses looked down on Xhosa beliefs or the unsanitary practices of *amagqirha*. Others simply viewed the primary problems with *amagqirha* as a lack of medicinal standardization and technical diagnostic tools. Nurses might warn patients, especially mothers, against using Xhosa medicines for children because the *amagqirha* may not measure the dosage correctly.[42] However, the most common theme in the interviews I conducted was the importance of encouraging rather than discouraging patients. In other words, rather than taking a negative approach and dissuading their patients from Xhosa treatments and *amagqirha*, nurses more often openly acknowledged the use of Xhosa therapies and persuaded patients to continue taking both Xhosa and biomedical treatments. This came from a desire to see patients achieve good health but was also a recognition of the power of the beliefs of the patients. In cases where Xhosa therapies or treatments clashed with biomedical teachings—such as with gastroenteritis, TB, and psychiatric cases—nurses then sought to change beliefs or understandings through education and cooperation with both community leaders and *amagqirha*.

Like other places where so-called traditional healers continued to work, the use of *amagqirha* in the Ciskei was tied to people's beliefs as well as practical reasons. In some areas where clinics and hospitals were scarce, people turned to more accessible Xhosa practitioners simply because they were there. Some nurses remembered that when they were growing up, clinics and hospitals were far away and obtaining adequate transportation was difficult, so people

Engaging Xhosa Beliefs and Practices

only attended the hospital when there was an emergency or something that *amagqirha* could not address. This seems to have been the case in the 1960s through the 1980s as well. Even with more clinics built under the Ciskeian government, clinics were generally scattered ten to twenty miles from each other, requiring some patients to travel long distances for clinic care. As was quite common across Africa, many others took a pragmatic approach by trying out different medical systems in their search for solutions. This kind of patient pluralism could mean patients would consult Xhosa medicine before biomedicine, vice versa, or draw on various systems simultaneously. Many times, the clinic and hospital were the last resort for patients who began treatment with Xhosa practitioners. Nursing instructor and head office supervisor Gamase Mtyeku stated, "But those who've come to hospital it means they had already exhausted that tap. That's where they start [with the *amagqirha*]."[43] Eighteen nurses talked about seeing cases of people coming to the hospital dehydrated and weak after unsuccessful Xhosa medical treatment. Some may have come coughing up blood and pieces of their lungs in advanced stages of TB or developed complications from labor allowed to go on too long. Nurses at times rescued patients by delivering the breech birth or coaxing out a retained placenta; however, some cases turned into emergencies that required hospitalization.[44] This made things difficult for the nurses, who at times did not have a good chance of healing the person. Nurses expressed the helplessness they felt as they remembered tragedies they encountered, such as when they could not save a woman who had been in labor too long or a sexually transmitted disease turned to cancer because Xhosa medicine had been ineffective.[45]

Even if biomedicine was readily accessible, patients utilized both Xhosa and biomedicine as they shopped around for the most effective cure. Julia Segar's 1991 Rhodes University study reported that 20 percent of the people surveyed in Rabula said they consulted Xhosa practitioners, 21 percent said they consulted religious healers, and 40 percent said they used some homemade medicines. All bought medicine from local shops, and others said they would use traditional healers when the ailment was perceived as outside of the purview of biomedicine.[46] Some Western pharmaceuticals and vaccinations proved to be powerfully effective, so many Africans relied on Western medicine to treat diseases such as diabetes or influenza. Catherine Burns estimated that 50 percent of patients from all of South Africa had shifted from home-based childbirth to hospitalized childbirth by 1950.[47] By the end of the 1980s, biomedical practitioners had successfully encouraged the majority of women to use biomedical services for the natural process of childbirth. Thus, there was a demand for some types of biomedical health care among the various options for healing therapies. Furthermore, like the nurses discussed above, seeking out biomedicine did not necessarily mean that patients had rejected another belief system entirely. Biomedicine and Xhosa medicine failures left room for people to try other approaches. Some of my interviewees confirmed that patients could see both systems as complementary. For example, Ginsberg clinic nurse Mcako said that some of her patients would go to a Xhosa healer for help in conceiving a child but go to the clinic to deliver.[48] The patients would appeal to spiritual powers to help them with the more mysterious, unpredictable process of conception and draw upon the knowledge and equipment of nurses proven to handle the more apparent and predictable physical process of giving birth.[49]

Nurses were well aware that their patients often consulted both *amagqirha* and biomedically trained nurses and doctors. They noticed cuttings from an *igqirha* on a person's skin or stumbled across powders and aromatic dried leaves in a patient's pockets as they packed clothing in a hospital locker or consulted them in a clinic room. They knew that boiling herbs and washing with them or visiting *igqirha* with a group of family and friends to "clap hands when they sing" and divine the cause of ill-health was common.[50] "It's our culture. We want to know why we are sick," Dubula explained.[51] At times, family members or even *amagqirha* would visit a patient in the hospital, bringing mixtures in bottles. Nurses may have also asked the patient what efforts they had already made to seek healing, or the patient may have come with an advanced problem as discussed above. Thandiwe Mkwelo said she would overhear patients waiting at the Tshatshu clinic, for example, talking to each other about their ailments and visiting the *amagqirha* before coming to the clinic. "What is *umlambo*, Mama?" Mkwelo remembered one patient asking another as she listened in while going about her work. "*Amagqirha*, they say it's *umlambo*."[52] A few nurses I interviewed indicated that they took a hard stance against Xhosa beliefs and practices. This approach turned people away rather than converted them to biomedicine. Eunice Mkosana, a nurse who most prominently worked in her home village at the Mgwalana clinic, told me she would scold her patients for using Xhosa medicines and tell them not to go see *amagqirha*.[53] Ciskei family planning supervisor and clinic inspector Sonjica described how nurses may have rebuked patients: "Initially people used to get fed up and say, 'We are busy treating you and you are busy bringing your own drugs.'"[54] In the various Ciskei hospitals and clinics where she worked to provide for her family, Ntonga noticed that if patients sensed this kind of disdain for Xhosa medicine, they would "hide it." "When they know that this is supposed to be wrong, they don't expose it to you nurses," she explained.[55] When engaging patients and communities who they knew consulted both biomedical and Xhosa practitioners, nurses learned of the need to work *with* rather than *against* Xhosa beliefs.

Dealing with patients who took both Xhosa and biomedical treatments was a delicate matter. Referring to the tools used to carefully pull a baby through the birth canal, Ciskei clinic and S. S. Gida Hospital nurse Makubalo put it, "You must handle that with forceps."[56] Baleni further explained that even though she would visit a patient at home or sit down with a patient and "you teach her, teach, educate, you educate the person," she would still take care to balance that education with respect for the patient's belief: "But, don't say anything adverse to their traditional medicines because she has been taught by that traditional healer as well, you know? Just try and squeeze yours."[57] Similarly, when speaking of working with women in the Middledrift and Peddie districts to change their cooking habits, Hono said she would not tell them to stop cooking maize porridge, but rather tell them to add milk. "So you introduce something from what they know," she concluded. "Because once you start by discouraging their own ways, they won't listen to you. At least you introduce some of the things bit by bit."[58] In other words, nurses would not just "take [the bottles of Xhosa medicine] and throw them away."[59]

One way to work with Xhosa beliefs was to motivate patients to take medicines from both systems. Just over half the nurses who talked about dealing with Xhosa notions of health and healing described how they took this approach. Nurses saw that certain Xhosa therapies were not inherently harmful, especially if they addressed natural causes of ill health. Many talked about the virtues of herbal remedies, highlighting for example, the efficacy of *umhlonyane*, the leaves of which were used to make an herbal tea taken to ease coughs and common colds. Some, like Virginia N. Mkosana, who became the deputy registrar of the Ciskeian Nursing Council, acknowledged that there were many ways to heal minor ailments like a boil.[60] Demonstrating more of an openness to Xhosa healing, Sonjica said, "They were doing it. I mean we are Black and there are drugs that are there that can help."[61] Bangani remembered protective medicines given to children that had no harmful effect, along with the black crushed leaves of *umhlabelo* (likely the *Nidorella* plant) rubbed on the wound to help with a child's broken leg.[62] If they saw no harm, nurses would encourage the patients to take both medicines, saying things such as "go to the traditional healers and take that [drug], that treatment, but don't stop taking our tablets. You can take both together, at the same time, there won't be any harm."[63] Baleni described how she would find out that a TB patient had defaulted on her regimented treatment if the patient was gone visiting *igqirha* when she went for a home visit. In such cases, Baleni would find a way to sit down with the patient and counsel her in a way that welcomed her use of the *igqirha*'s medicine: "Advise her that you know these tablets, they are not going to do any harm even if you take this medicine, traditional medicine." Of course, Baleni believed "TB can only be cured by tablets, and not by traditional [methods]." But she would not say that to the patient. Instead, she would gently say, "You take them both. If you feel that this traditional medicine helps you, it's alright to take it. But don't leave these tablets, also take these tablets. They don't fight."[64] Dubula explained that in encouraging patients to continue with both medicines, the patients might not know which medicine really healed them: "You know when she's healed, she'll say the Xhosa medicine maybe has helped her. . . . Meanwhile it's the tablets." Yet for Dubula, "it doesn't matter as long as they're healthy. That is what is important."[65]

In urging patients to take both medications, the nurses did not challenge Xhosa therapies or beliefs but they did not necessarily promote Xhosa beliefs and practices either. Instead, they were ensuring that their patients took the medication the nurses believed to be most effective—their own biomedical prescriptions. As Baleni said, she believed TB could only be cured by tablets but would still tell her patients to take both to ensure they indeed took the clinic medication. A Nompumelelo nurse who also worked closely with VHWs, Ntombentsha Anjelina Figlan, qualified her encouragement of patients taking Xhosa medicines by saying, "But we discouraged them to leave the tablets and just concentrate on the traditional healers' treatment."[66] Talking about working in communities under the Nompumelelo and St. Matthew's Hospitals, like Gxulu, Mbie similarly remarked, "So at least [encouraging them to take both] would make things better because they would rather stop the tablets and go for the traditional medication."[67] It was particularly important for patients on medication regimes to continue to take their tablets so they did not risk interrupting their TB treatment or allow their blood pressure to fluctuate. Victoria Hospital and mobile clinic nurse Thoto said that at first "Western medicine did not allow them to drink this medicine from the *sangoma*," but then they later realized they should "give them the tablets and ask them also to drink the *sangoma* medicine, knowing that in your mind . . . the tablets are going to help. But because they believed in the *sangoma*, you made it a point that they used both."[68] Thus, the seeming acceptance of Xhosa medicines was not necessarily an endorsement of Xhosa healing but a way to promote biomedicine.

Hono remembered her community health training focusing on understanding the dynamics of the communities. She explained, "Because now when you are trained as a community health nurse, you study the community work in so that you could know which services are best for that community. Is it composed of old people? Is it composed of young people?" Having visited people's homes, talked with individual residents, dealt with ill-health, and generally observed the communities, they could then adapt the services they offered:

"If it's composed of young people, then there are services that you need: family planning, [sexuality] clinics, adolescents' clinic. So you know that you have to prepare yourself if there's child-bearing age, for the midwifery services. Whereas if it's old people, it's different."[69] Throughout the 1970s and 1980s, community health nursing education in-service training and certificate and degree programs promoted respect for patient beliefs, encouraging nurses to orient their services toward the people they served. This included Xhosa beliefs. Like others who worked in community health care, Mount Coke Hospital and outpatients clinic nurse Ivy Hermanus indicated that her training included advice on encouraging patients rather than discouraging them when she remembered, "What we were taught that we must never say to the patient, 'Don't go. Don't do this.' But just mention the advantages and disadvantages and the wrong things that may happen, you know? So that the patient—it's his own decision."[70] Nurses who did not gain this sensitivity through their training may have learned this through experience, coaching by other nurses, or through their own intuition. It is also possible that nurses acknowledged and encouraged Xhosa therapies because they themselves believed in both medical systems.

Hono's and Hermanus's comments correspond with the training manuals developed for district clinic nurses of the All Saints' Mission Hospital in Mthatha in 1971. If these manuals reflect trends in community nursing training, it is evident that it involved training nurses to show the communities that they respected their beliefs and then to use careful education to change some of those beliefs, employing "similarity and association" along with factual information.[71] Indeed, at the same time nurses were careful not to discourage their patients, they also felt it imperative that they change Xhosa remedies they viewed as very problematic. The three main challenges nurses talked about in this regard included the use of enemas to treat gastroenteritis among children, purging TB patients, and the extreme treatment of psychiatric patients. When the underlying beliefs behind the cause of illness led *amagqirha* to use therapies or medicines that caused damage or clashed with biomedical treatments, nurses tried to educate patients individually and through clinic programs, worked with local leaders to educate the broader community, and attempted to cooperate with *amagqirha*. In doing so, they sought to change the understanding of the causes of illnesses and to involve *amagqirha* in referring patients to what they believed was the most effective treatment.

A common clash occurred regarding treating diarrhea in children. Gastroenteritis was an oft-cited health problem for children in the Ciskei. Biomedicine believed the infection of intestines that led to diarrhea, cramping, or vomiting was caused by bacteria, viruses, or parasites. In most cases, gastroenteritis could be allowed to run its course without clinical treatment, as long as the patient

128 Engaging Xhosa Beliefs and Practices

was kept hydrated. While the Xhosa also recognized that diarrhea or vomiting could result from natural contaminants, many Xhosa also believed that certain symptoms signaled the presence of harmful pollutants with more spiritual origins. Infants were more vulnerable to these elements.[72] Gastroenteritis could be caused by the effects of evil winds, *imimoya emdaka*, sent by jealous people, or other harmful substances put in someone's path. Some types of diarrhea were believed to be caused by a snake that had entered into the body, evidenced by relaxed rectal muscles as well as the color of the feces.[73] Many *amagqirha* used enemas in the form of a medicine to drink to stop diarrhea triggered by gastroenteritis if they believed a snake needed to be expunged. Purging the body, however, often ended up leading to severe dehydration, which could even cause death, especially among babies and small children. If a baby with a sunken fontanel and flabby skin was brought to Thoto at Victoria Hospital or one of its mobile clinics, she knew she had to send it to the doctor so the doctor could give intravenous therapy and oral medicine to rehydrate the baby. Otherwise, "That is what was killing most of the children, diarrhea, this herbal enema," Mbie concluded. Some, she said, even developed liver problems.[74]

Enemas given to children with diarrhea caused so many deaths and other problems that nurses worked to explicitly change the beliefs of the people and *amagqirha* about the treatment. Through one-on-one patient consultations and community health meetings, nurses stressed the negative effects of the enemas and encouraged people to come to the clinic for rehydration kits. Some education and persuasion required careful, attentive, individual attention—a "special interview" or home visit. Dubula described how she would explain to people in the St. Matthew's and S. S. Gida clinics where she worked the problem with using an enema to treat diarrhea.

> They like enema, those people, they like enema. So you must give them examples that, if . . . there's a rain that is falling in your garden you don't go and spray your garden with water, because you are wasting. So that child has already had a running stomach, why should you give enema? So they used to understand it, after you have quoted incidents of children who die because they were given enema when they had diarrhea.[75]

Using "similarity and association" as the training materials encouraged, and supporting her arguments with evidence, Dubula explained the negative side effects of using an enema. Nurses might also explain why *amagqirha* treatments could be dangerous in a way that did not undermine the entire system but constituted a warning. For example, Hewana said she used to tell patients who came

Engaging Xhosa Beliefs and Practices

to Mount Coke Hospital or the Debe Nek clinic, "No, never take chances with your baby because traditional healers they are going to give you medicine, the strong medication. And that strong medication can kill your child."[76] As Hewana put it, it was the strength of the medication that was the problem and not that the *amagqirha* were flawed altogether. Nurses also met with *amagqirha* one-on-one to persuade them to cooperate with the nurses on dealing with diarrhea. Hermanus talked of the importance of "educating" the *amagqirha*, but in a positive way: "That we don't say, 'You must not treat people,' but you tell them that you can't give enemas to children that they must induce it, diarrhea. You can't do that." Like others, she remembered explaining the physical process and giving evidence to support her claims: "And because now when you make them vomit they lose more fluid. And sometimes they come with abdomen— their tummies would be distended like this, would be inflated because of that additional medicine that they have given. Sometimes other babies survive or people survive. Others they don't. They die."[77]

Amagqirha used expectorants to treat TB in a way that also clashed with the efforts of nurses. Biomedicine understood the illness to be caused by a bacterial infection, spread by airborne droplets that caused lesions in the lungs (and in some cases spread to the brain and spine). When active, TB in the lungs caused a person to be sick for a number of weeks with a severe cough. If left to grow, the person may even cough up blood, have chest pain, fatigue, fever, night sweats or chills, and unintentional weight loss and loss of appetite. Similar symptoms would often be described by Xhosa people as the effects of being "kicked by the bird," or *impundulu*—wasting away and coughing, even to the point of coughing up blood. Others might explain it as a poison given by evil spirits, blocking their lungs and causing them to cough.[78] Some *amagqirha* treated patients with TB by expunging *impundulu* or its effects from inside a person. For biomedicine, treatment at this time constituted a regimen of up to twelve months of chemotherapy via ingested medicines. In the nurses' view, the Xhosa therapy could counteract the nurses' efforts or cause further damage. It was worse when Xhosa medicine induced vomiting and expelled biomedical pills from the body. Baleni described how she would delicately coach individual patients taking medication from the clinic along with this kind of Xhosa medicine so as to ensure they would get the benefits of the tablet regimen.

> They usually give medicine to swallow and again to vomit, you know such things. So then you just ask, "When do you do this, when do you take this medicine, traditional medicine?" She'll tell you maybe early morning. "Oh you take it early morning. Okay, so please take these tablets in the evening, yeah, take the tablets

Engaging Xhosa Beliefs and Practices

in the evening." If she says she takes the medicine in the evening, you say to her, "Take these tablets in the morning."[79]

Attempting to work with these competing treatments was not something that many nurses wanted to continue, however. If a person was coughing up blood, making them vomit could cause further damage and weaken them. Furthermore, this did not stop TB from spreading through the air to those in close contact with the TB patient, and interrupted treatment could result in untreatable mutations of the bacteria.[80]

Nurses, other biomedical practitioners, and the Ciskei government made a number of different efforts to convince both patients and *amagqirha* that the correct diagnosis and treatment for TB came through biomedicine. Whether during a one-on-one clinic consultation or a home visit, nurses might explain the biomedicine treatment to their individual patients to help them believe in that treatment. Qibirha and Perksdale clinic nurse Ngoro put it simply: "You won't say 'Don't!' to a patient. You must just advise."[81] Baleni described how one might advise: "You teach the person that: why you are coughing blood, you've got cavities in your lungs. That is why you are coughing blood. So these tablets are going to help . . . sealing, closing those holes, cavities."[82] Education about TB detection and treatment featured as part of community health education, and some nurses reached out to *amagqirha* to change the way they understood and treated the disease. Baleni described going to visit healers in their homes, talking with them about TB and its causes and treatments and leaving pamphlets. She recognized that most nurses came and went in the villages as their jobs changed. *Amagqirha*, on the other hand, lived in the community and knew the people well. So she had to "try and be friendly with them." She would show respect for their work by going to visit them in their homes. After explaining how she understood and tested for TB, she would ask for their cooperation. "We educate, give them pamphlets about TB," she said, "and we get cooperation from them, . . . insomuch that they used to send patients to us. You see? To say that, 'This one is coughing blood, is coughing blood. I think she needs some treatment.'"[83] Former clinic supervisor Mjikeliso remarked that they talked to the *amagqirha* about what they could treat and what needed immediate clinic or hospital attention. In doing so, they showed the *amagqirha* they were not discounting them but hoping to work alongside them. "As a result," Mjikeliso said, "they know that if one is coughing for three weeks, they must be taken straight to hospital or to the clinic because there they will get some bottles for coughing, for [testing] sputum."[84] A number of the nurses I interviewed claimed that *amagqirha* and clinics ended up cooperating in diagnosing and treating cases such as TB, and that some *amagqirha* even

Engaging Xhosa Beliefs and Practices

came to the clinic to be treated for certain ailments themselves.[85] Although existing government reports do not document it, some nurses claimed that the Ciskeian government spearheaded a program to cooperate with *amagqirha* on diagnosing TB. Considering the eclectic nature of Xhosa medicine, this certainly could have occurred. Furthermore, it resulted in a change in some *amagqirha* practices and the types of diseases they focused on.

Nurses I interviewed also highlighted psychiatric cases as needing reeducation and the cooperation of *amagqirha*. The Ciskeian government made a concerted effort to address mental health with an increase in psychiatric nursing training into the 1980s. Psychiatric nursing, along with community health nursing and midwifery, were all incorporated into general nursing training in South Africa as it shifted into universities at the time.[86] Many nurses I interviewed had in-service training or took study leave to gain more expertise in the field. The biomedical psychiatric community in South Africa was also increasing its efforts to expand mental health services and research on African understandings of mental illness.[87] Burns-Ncamashe highlighted the specialists from Cape Town who had come to examine *amafufunyana* (spirit possession or a psychological disorder), and psychiatrist M. Vera Bührmann wrote a book, first published in 1984, where she compared analytical psychiatry to the training and treatment of *igqirha* initiates.[88] As nurses engaged more with the communities about psychiatric cases in the late 1970s and into the 1980s, they sought to extend their training and education to the communities.

The difference in the approaches that Xhosa practitioners and the nurses took to treating mental illness reflected what biomedicine saw as a fundamental divergence between the two medical systems. Nurses I interviewed told me that when someone had schizophrenia or epilepsy, Xhosa people often believed it to be the work of a witch or someone seeking to cause them harm. As Nompumelelo nurse and VHW supervisor Figlan said, "Especially with the mental health, they really associated it with something to do with witchcraft and all that, . . . because people will see things that we don't see, will hear voices, will feel that there's something moving in their stomachs and all that. So such things make them—they are quite weird, so they thought they are bewitched."[89] Harriet Ngubane and Julie Parle described *ufufunyana* among the Zulu as a form of malignant spirit possession that was said to have come to South Africa from the north in the early twentieth century (a time of increasing migrant labor and competition as international interest in an industrializing South Africa grew during the Great Depression). Those struck by the worst form of *ufufunyana* would "behave as if mentally deranged," becoming hysterical, throwing themselves on the ground, perhaps attempting to commit suicide, or reacting violently to those who tried to calm them.[90] Others would

132 Engaging Xhosa Beliefs and Practices

hear voices speak in growling tones as if different voices came from inside them, or perform physically incredible acts in a state of frenzy. The Xhosa had similar understandings about what they referred to as *amafufunyana*, a plural term perhaps reflecting the belief that multiple bad spirits could possess a person and speak in different languages. They believed that this was caused by evil or "dirty" medicine or spirits from other lands.[91]

Although the Xhosa did not always diagnose epilepsy and schizophrenia as *amafufunyana*, the nurses I interviewed and other psychiatric biomedical practitioners saw a correlation between the two diagnoses.[92] Biomedicine would consider the symptoms of *amafufunyana* as expressions of something wrong in the workings of the brain or nervous system. For example, epilepsy is described as a central nervous system disorder that causes unpredictable seizures or abnormal behavior. While the exact cause of schizophrenia is still not identified by biomedicine, it is described as a disease of the mind, with symptoms including distorted thoughts, hallucinations, and paranoia. Alternatively, biomedical practitioners may see the symptoms similar to that of *amafufunyana* as something related to extreme mental and emotional stress such as depression or a nervous breakdown, characteristics of what the Xhosa would view as a call to become *igqirha*. While Xhosa practitioners differentiated between the evil causes and a call from the ancestors, all the biomedical explanations were rooted in the belief that there was a natural cause within the body or a person's environment.

The different understandings of the cause of mental ill-health led to very different therapy approaches. If the problem was diagnosed as *amafufunyana*, treatment required driving out the harmful spirits and could include installing benign spirits into the person. It could involve holding someone down while they inhaled therapeutic smoke or drank medicine.[93] Nurses observed that problems arose when patients resisted treatment and people took extreme actions to contain them, especially if they became physically violent.[94] At times, clinic nurses would be called when the patient could not be constrained. Ann Shaw nurse Tunyiswa remembered walking to "those houses" where she would find an agitated person tied down because they had become violent. She would have to give the patients some treatment, most likely an injection, to calm them down. She would then find a way to transfer them to the hospital.[95] Mavuso and Someketha described how they would calm psychiatric patients down by talking with them, complimenting them on clothes they were wearing—"*Yhu*, the way you are so smart. Where did you buy this jacket?"—or making a social connection to their home village or family—"I'm also staying there, where do you stay?"[96] Then they could administer treatment or get them to a hospital. There a biomedical doctor would prescribe tablets, further injections, or possibly electroconvulsive treatment. Most nurses I interviewed who talked about psychiatric cases implied it was better to address the physiological ailment or malfunction in the person's body rather than to try to dissuade people from believing in evil spiritual forces. They focused on changing the way people thought about these issues through community health education as well as consultations with the families of individual patients. They also stressed the good results that came through hospitalization. Longtime South African National Tuberculosis Association (SANTA) TB Hospital nurse Thandiwe Mtanga talked about the importance of reassuring patients and their family members that they would be okay until they could see for themselves how effective biomedical treatment could be. Sufficient proof would come when patients recovered after some time in the hospital or relapsed as they defaulted on their medication.[97] On the other hand, some nurses encouraged people to adhere to Christian beliefs. Mdantsane clinic nurse Bulelwa Ramncwana advised, "You've got to convince her that, 'Take this medicine. Don't think about one is jealous about you. . . . If one is jealous about you,' I used to tell them, 'Pray to your God. God will look after you.'"[98] With a strong Christian influence in the Eastern Cape, this appeal to another spiritual power that could be stronger than witchcraft might possibly have been effective.[99] Just as with other cases, nurses knew that persuading and reasoning with people rather than harshly reprimanding them for their beliefs would allow them to continue to work with people.

As with gastroenteritis and TB, some nurses described talking with Xhosa practitioners in order to change Xhosa practices and work together to help psychiatric patients. For example, if Tunyiswa met *igqirha* in a home or at the clinic with a violent psychiatric patient, she would take the opportunity to talk *igqirha* through her treatment as they calmed the patient and took the patient to the hospital together. "And when he's there with him, . . . you talk to the healer," she explained. As with her patients, to show the *igqirha* she wanted to work with him or her, she encouraged *igqirha* to continue with both medicines. She would tell *igiqrha*, "Let him take the treatment from the clinic. You can give him your treatment but with this one, don't discontinue. Don't discontinue." When they were not dealing with urgent patient matters, they called *amagqirha* to meet with the nurses. "And we used to have group discussions with them," she described. "Come as a group, nurses and them. . . . So there was no problem. They got used to it." And at least from her perspective, "it was harmonious."[100] Mbombo worked at the Mount Coke Hospital and its various clinics as well as on a community health training project run by a doctor out of Cecilia Makiwane Hospital. She particularly worked with *amagqirha* to bring them into community clinic committees. She and the people she worked with to establish these committees also took a positive approach to *amagqirha*. "At first when we tried to work with them, they had

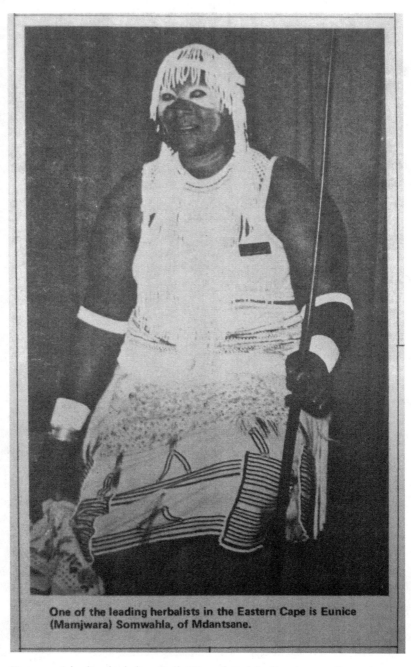

Figure 11. A leading herbalist. *Daily Dispatch*, Indaba Supplement, December 21, 1973. Amathole Museum Library.

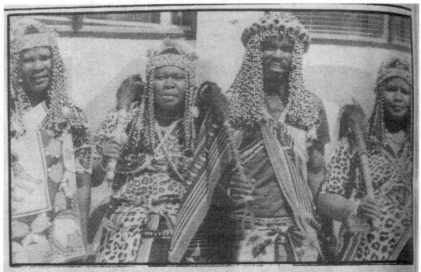

Ukusuka ekhohlo nguNkosk. Marry Njoko, Nkosk. Veronica Hlatshwayo Mnu. Mithwa Thusi noNkosk. Nonasi Tyhilani. Abantwana bokugula babhaqwe zinthatheli bejikeleza bejoja umhlola.

Figure 12. Group of *amagqirha*. *Imvo Zabanstundu*, November 6, 1987. Amathole Museum Library.

that—they felt threatened," she said, "but we reassured them that we're not going to stop their beliefs and their traditional way of treating people, but just to help each other to make it more . . . safer for their patients."[101] Many nurses observed that there has been more cooperation with *amagqirha* in recent or current times than there was before, reflecting an acknowledgment of the continued importance of *amagqirha* in health care delivery in South Africa and greater efforts in the postapartheid period to incorporate indigenous healers. Some also specifically mentioned government efforts to work with *amagqirha* regarding HIV/AIDs.[102] Although this cooperation came mostly after the dissolution of the Ciskei and most of the nurses I interviewed had retired, nurses drew on their experience and training to change beliefs about the cause of this disease and educate communities about prevention and treatment.

Nurses cited community health education as key to changing ideas more broadly about what they viewed as damaging practices. Drawing from her experience working in St. Matthew's and S. S. Gida clinics, Dubula stressed, "If you want your health services to be strong, stick on health education. . . . Health education is *the* thing."[103] In line with the primary and promotive health

136   Engaging Xhosa Beliefs and Practices

care emphasized by the homelands, nurses held health education clinics at the clinic itself and presented information at community meetings sponsored by chiefs and headmen. Working in cooperation with community leaders and VHWs, community health days could be exciting events that even included *amagqirha*. Amathole Basin nurse Mhlambiso described the health education days they held in villages as special occasions where the nurses, VHWs, and other health officials would visit a village. Village leaders called everyone together in an open meeting, then would turn the meeting over to health officials. She remembered: "Then we met together, they give us *ii-reports* from their villages. So somebody must come and give a report. 'Are there toilets in your village? Are there pigs? Are they not roaming around?' And all that." In an effort to use the culture of the people to educate, nurses or VHWs might use songs to send messages. Mhlambiso painted a picture of enthusiastic practitioners singing the songs in hopes that their messages would catch on.

> So they were to come together. And form songs that need you to listen on this health music. So it was a very, very nice thing. It was wonderful . . . with these health songs. . . . [People] must have toilets, must lock up their pigs because pigs can spread dirt, and infect your children in a way—in a nursing way. So, your children will get worms, please, you must keep your pigs away from the area, keep them locked. It was a very—it was, it was a nice time then, then.

Nurses attempted to foster good relationships with Xhosa practitioners by including them in community health meetings. Mhlambiso, for example, enjoyed seeing them attend, wearing their official garb of various skins and white beads: "It was wonderful. . . . In our occasions, they used to dress the Xhosa attire. So the *amagqirhas mos*, liked the attire. It's theirs. So, it used to be nice then."[104] Others took a form more like a lecture. Baleni described health education as speaking at community meetings, "to tell them they must take their treatment as prescribed, you know; and they must not run away from the clinics, they must go, they must immunize children, all those things. That was health education."[105] Mjikeliso described health education as covering "a lot," because their goal was that people would not need the clinic. Thus they touched on "good sanitation, good water supply, . . . good nutrition—you educate them on that, how to behave, not abusing liquor, dagga, drugs, and all those things—you educate them on that."[106]

    The support of local leaders was key in running these events and in giving the nurses some authority. As Dubula remarked, "You must work with the chief, the headman, and other influential people. Make use of them, because they're lead people." With the backing of the local leaders, the people were more likely

Engaging Xhosa Beliefs and Practices

to believe the nurse.[107] Bangani remembered that they "used to conduct meetings with the headmen. And try and sell nursing *yethu i-health* [our nursing and health] to the people." And it worked because, as Bangani said, "We were known. We were recognized, in other words, that nurse so-and-so—nurses would be coming on such-and-such day. *Amanurse athi masithi. Amanurse athi masithi.* [The nurses say this, we must do it. The nurses say that, we must do it.] We were recognized really." This in part led her to claim that the Ciskei government really boosted the nurses.[108] Sodlulashe also talked about how headmen and chiefs serving on community clinic committees could protect nurses if someone in the community were giving them problems or help them with plowing the clinic garden.[109] Working with local political authorities was particularly important for those running mobile teams or conducting outreach to villages within a clinic's catchment area. When Baleni worked as part of a mobile TB team, for example, they went from village to village to dispense medication and immunizations. "That's when you had to approach the headman to have an *imbizo* [meeting] time to educate the people," she explained.[110] Thoto attributed her community nursing training to helping her understand the correct protocol when entering a community. She described her approach when she was assigned to work with a mobile clinic based at Victoria Hospital in 1981: "But before you started it, you had to go to the chief. You had to discuss it with the chiefs first and tell them what you are going to bring and discuss it and see if they approve of it. You wouldn't just walk there and say I'm doing this." Thoto even remembered that when she worked as a community health supervisor, she selected VHWs in conjunction with the chiefs so that they would choose the best people to be trusted in the community.[111] If the nurses did not have the official sanction, they would risk offending the community, such as when Mbie and her colleague on a new HIV/AIDS team heard of a community meeting in a remote village and went to ask for some time and were almost driven away: "The first question was, 'Who told you about our meeting? Who told you? Who phoned you to come and come to our meeting?' For a long time, they were saying we must be driven away." Drawing on previous experience delivering health education, they managed to persist and take their HIV/AIDS talks to these communities.[112]

Finally, interviewees also talked about the importance of a nurse building trust within the community and knowing the home environment of their patients in order to succeed in spreading health education. Some clinics relied on VHWs to perform community outreach in remote villages. Scholars have argued that since most VHWs resided within the communities, they reached people more effectively. Similarly, Digby and Sweet argued that a nurse's success in changing beliefs was linked to whether or not she was "in and of the local community" and had support from local authority rather than her distance from her own cultural beliefs, as mission hospital trainers believed.[113] Indeed, if a nurse socially connected with her patients and understood how they lived, she could more effectively motivate them to receive her care. If the people did not trust her, they would avoid the clinic. Mjikeliso said it was "so interesting to work in the community" because a nurse would always be "there with them" and "see their problems." Dubula remembered how this engendered trust.

> And you do also a home visit, you see what type of background is she from, their beliefs, their . . . all those things. You stay, you become part of the family, you want to observe them. And then you know which are the loopholes here that you're going to cling on, so that they understand. Immediately that they believe in you, they'll take what you're saying. The community must have trust. If they don't trust you they won't tell you anything. You must build that trust. Build a rapport with them.[114]

Once a nurse built that trust, "They say everything. They don't hold any secrets," Thoto explained. "And they even when they are really used to you, they'll call you by your clan name. They will not say Mrs. Thoto or Sister Thoto. They will say MaRadebe."[115] Rulashe similarly felt that in working in Nompumelelo and Keiskammahoek clinics, the key to community education was "to establish good relationships, relations with the people you work with," because "if they understand you, you've got no problem." She summed up the approach many took, carefully working with *amagqirha*, one-on-one with patients, and in community health education when she said, "You can't just shake them off their beliefs and traditions. The important thing is to make people understand. And as long as you take your time, you accept the people, and then you . . . give them information—you won't have that much trouble."[116]

The Struggles of Gendered Health Care

Female nurses made up the overwhelming majority of nurses in the Ciskei. While they did not encounter resistance in helping women with childbirth as much as others have elsewhere, they found that treating ailments specific to Xhosa men required careful negotiation and cultivation of trust. Before biomedicine changed Xhosa birthing practices, women usually gave birth in the woman's parents' home with the help of older women (especially if it was her first child). These older women could be considered traditional birth attendants—women with experience and special knowledge to help in childbirth. In the Xhosa understanding, these women had experience in this natural physical process but could also be seen as unpolluted if they were no longer menstruating.[117] The Xhosa viewed pregnancy, childbirth, and the immediate postnatal period as vulnerable times for women and newly born babies. As Ngubane described it in relation to the Zulu, birth was a process "associated with the other world." As a mother brought a child into "this world," she was in a "marginal state between life and death" and could be easily contaminated.[118] As menstruation was considered impure, women who were no longer menstruating could safely attend a woman giving birth. The new mother was also considered to be more protected when giving birth in her natal home. Even before the birth, certain protective restrictions were placed on pregnant women about what they could eat, where they could travel, and who they could associate with. After the birth, the mother and child were secluded for a number of days, and some procedures were performed to help strengthen and protect the child and its mother.[119] For example, the afterbirth or placenta would be buried in a secret place to prevent anyone from using it for malevolent purposes, and the baby may have had protective medicines rubbed into its skin.

Maternal and infant health services have been significant parts of the extension and contestation of biomedicine throughout Africa. However, although nurses sought to entice women to give birth at the clinics and engaged women about certain conventions related to pregnancy, childbirth, and infant care in the Ciskei at this time, they did not clash much with traditional birth attendants or highlight birthing practices and beliefs as major obstacles to their work. Midwifery district services began quite early in South Africa. Mashaba cited forms of midwifery training beginning in the early nineteenth century, and McCord's Zulu Hospital was recognized as a center for training African midwives in 1924.[120] In mission hospitals and district services, childbirth and maternal care were extended to Africans because significant health problems were linked to infant and maternal mortality rates; maternity care was less challenging to traditional practices; missions thought they could make the most effective change by targeting women; and missions believed that district nurses would be the most effective in converting people to the clinic and hospital.[121] By the 1960s, fully qualified nurses who worked in the clinics had midwifery training, and it was not uncommon for those with only single qualifications to be registered midwives (rather than qualifying in other grades of general nursing). Scholars have pointed to the widespread acceptance of biomedical midwives in South Africa, with Digby arguing that district nurses and birth attendants developed good relations in a number of places, and Burns estimating that by the end of the twentieth century, 84 percent of South African mothers used nurses or midwives while they were in labor and 90 percent gave birth in medical facilities.[122] Indeed, for most of the nurses I interviewed, traditional birth attendants played a minor role, if they saw them at all. Those who talked about encountering them (about five) worked in times and places when biomedical clinics and nurses were scarce or talked about educating them to refer women to nurses, clinics, and hospitals.

Problems with biomedical practitioners becoming involved in childbirth came more so in the early years, when young, single nurses and midwives lacked credibility among communities for helping with births and when nurses found some practices surrounding birth and taking care of infants as detrimental.[123] Some Xhosa practices and beliefs persisted, especially those more associated with the unpredictable aspects of conceiving and giving birth. Expectant mothers could easily have a nurse help them through the physical process of giving birth but have other Xhosa procedures done for extra protection. Four nurses I interviewed talked about the continuance of Xhosa beliefs and practices. Some they sought to change. Others they worked with or merely acknowledged. For example, some talked about women taking Xhosa medicine to ease the labor or open the cervix.[124] On the other hand, Victoria Hospital and clinic nurse Mavuso talked about the prevalent idea that young girls should not eat eggs because it would make them like boys too much.[125] Nurses tried to change this idea when teaching the community about nutrition. Thoto talked about how since the Rabula clinic did not have an incinerator, they allowed the women to take the placenta home to either burn it or do their "traditional things" with it.[126] This practice was related to more spiritual beliefs that did not interfere with the birthing process. Digby also described the patient pluralism of mothers who would call a Xhosa practitioner to come and perform "formalities" to initiate and strengthen the babies after the nurse performed her work.[127] On the other end of things, Mcako talked about women going to *amagqirha* for help conceiving. Many advertisements for medicines in *Izimvo Zabantsundu* included those for enhancing fertility, suggesting a demand from women for those medicines. Yet for the most part, these sorts of practices did not seem to be a big concern for nurses. Rather, they focused on the importance of the antenatal and well-baby clinics in spreading health education and getting women to the clinic and hospital to give birth. Evidence from the nurses and the high number of women using biomedical services for childbirth by the end of the twentieth century indicates then that Xhosa women largely made the transition from relying on birth attendants to nurses and midwives for the natural process of childbirth.

When dealing with Xhosa men, nurses had to negotiate more carefully. Some male patients resisted female-delivered health care in situations that prohibited female involvement, such as with ailments related to male sexual organs or male circumcision, a major part of Xhosa society. This posed a particular problem

Engaging Xhosa Beliefs and Practices

for younger female nurses. Mount Coke and Bhisho Hospital nurse Memane remarked, "You need males [in nursing] very much. Because there are people who still adhere to the old culture that 'you can't touch me being a female—I'm a man,' you know?"[128] At a health education course sponsored by the Transkei and Ciskei Association of Mission Hospitals in 1969, David Bosch, a radical missionary with the Dutch Reformed Church in the Transkei who spoke Xhosa, gave a talk on the role of the Christian nurse in the hospital, wherein he gave insights into how Xhosa men may have felt about being cared for by the female nurses. Bosch particularly highlighted the problems elderly men encountered when being nursed by young women. He emphasized, "Taken from his or her own familiar surroundings, the first experience in a hospital can be a traumatic experience for the patient." This was particularly difficult for "elderly Xhosa men, who are nursed by 'mere children,'" who could unintentionally "take away his dignity entirely" by "having all his clothes taken off by the nurse" and by having to wear "short pyjama trousers, and so on."[129] Indeed, nurses commented on men not wanting to be given an injection by a female nurse or shaved or washed by a female nurse. Hewana remembered a man coming to the Debe Nek clinic and demanding an injection without explaining what his problem was. It turned out he was "sexually . . . not okay," and so the nurses tried to persuade him to come back when the doctor visited the clinic.[130] Mount Coke and St. Matthew's Hospital and clinic nurse Hilary K. Mnyanda related the stories of two men with hydrocele (swelling in the scrotum) who wore coats even when it was hot so as to hide their ailment instead of going to the nurses for treatment.[131] Other nurses talked about the difficulties of dealing with male initiates (*abakwetha*) who were circumcised and, according to Xhosa customs, not allowed to interact with women until they finished their initiation into manhood. Botched circumcisions at times, however, demanded immediate, professional care.

Necessity drove men and boys to accept the care of a female nurse. At other times, nurses and patients found ways around these obstacles by going through a wife, seeing an initiate in secret, simply reasoning with patients, or calling upon male nurses (if available). Mhlambiso found that she could work through a wife or other female villagers "since I was a woman here [at the Amathole Basin] and knowing the community, working, staying with the community." As she explained, "It was easier for me for the wife to come, *esithi*, 'MaDlamini I've got this problem.' Privately. So . . . I used to have the way out to get to the husband."[132] In the case of the two men with hydrocele, Mnyanda talked with a wife and brother to arrange for the men to come see a doctor at the clinic. Like other nurses, Ann Shaw and Middledrift district nurse Sodlulashe described how she treated initiates in secret, sometimes at

142   Engaging Xhosa Beliefs and Practices

night. Sneaking to the clinic, they would send a signal or send someone in to whisper to the nurse.

> Then they didn't want a female to interfere with *abakwethas*, but somebody would come during the day and tell you that they have a problem there. Then, you ask that somebody to bring that somebody at night; early evening, they bring that somebody and sometimes they call you from the veldt [open grassland] side of the clinic. Then you say it's safe, they come, now they come. Sometimes they don't want the *umkwetha* to come through the gate where the other people come. Then you make them climb the fence because you want to help this somebody. Then you'll know that every evening he's going to come for the treatment the same way.[133]

Concerned peers or family members also got involved, especially mothers. Sodlulashe told of another initiate who sent word to his mother to tell the nurses he needed care. One can imagine the worried mother rushing to the clinic after receiving the news. Tshatshu clinic nurse Mkwelo told of another mother who broke the rules of initiate isolation from females and carried her son on her back to the clinic.[134] When male patients were forced to receive care from nurses in hospitals or clinics, nurses adapted to their concerns. Mavuso talked about finding a way to talk to male patients when she was going to wash them. She would explain to them what she needed to do and that she would allow them to take care of their private parts and cover themselves so she would not see.[135] Working in clinics in the Ciskei and in the now Gauteng Province, Janjties similarly found she had to talk to her older male patients carefully: "And you don't talk as a nurse to them because what they know, they are men. You are a woman. You sit down and say, '*Tata*, just sit down and listen, I'm going to tell you. Then you'll decide.'"[136] Unfortunately, male nurses were very rare in rural clinics, so nurses had to make adjustments and work with, rather than against, their male patients to ensure they received care.

Conclusion

Some scholars have argued that indigenous nurses are more effective in delivering biomedical community health care because they understand local beliefs and thus have a greater ability to translate biomedical terms linguistically and conceptually.[137] The experiences of nurses in the Ciskei support this assessment. However, these nurses did more than translate terms and concepts. Ciskei nurses succeeded not only in delivering biomedicine but also in shaping the way patients drew on various healing systems. Xhosa nurses, exercising their agency while working closely with individual patients and communities, contributed to the continued coexistence and adaptation of Xhosa healing systems and biomedicine, even as Xhosa methods and beliefs changed, perhaps more than biomedicine. While not all Xhosa nurses respected or believed in Xhosa therapies, many of them did, and they learned that the best way to reach their patients was by respecting their beliefs. In attempts to motivate patients to continue to draw on biomedicine, they encouraged patients to use Xhosa therapies along with biomedicine to increase the chances of healing. When a divergence between the two healing systems was irreconcilable—such as with treatments for gastroenteritis, TB, and psychiatric cases—nurses turned to individual consultation and community education and sought the cooperation of local authorities and *amagqirha* to change beliefs and practices. Nurses also worked around the limitations of gender roles that affected the care they could deliver by treating male patients through male practitioners, female relatives, in secret, or with more understanding and coaxing. Employing these strategies helped nurses succeed as they brought new ideas and practices into the communities they served. New gender roles in families emerging in the 1960s through the 1980s demanded as much negotiating as well.

CHAPTER FIVE

Negotiating Marriage and Family Relations

WHEN TUNYISWA, HEWANA, AND VUYO MDLEDLE recited the nurse's pledge at the end of their training, they felt that they had committed themselves to putting the patient before self.[1] The promise to "pledge myself to the service of humanity" and make the health of patients "my first consideration" was an important part of the professional ethos of nursing of their time.[2] Nurses were expected to sacrifice themselves and follow orders with strict obedience, regardless of their own personal circumstances or political views. The historical record mirrors this subordination of a nurse's personal life to her work. Surprisingly, many secondary sources as well as reports, studies, and newspaper articles from the 1960s through the 1980s rarely address Black South African nurses' family relations or off-duty activities in depth, seemingly seeing nurses only as nurses at work.[3] Even memoirs written by nurses have paid little attention to their private lives, and women I interviewed initially offered very little about their marriages and families.[4] The health care systems in the Ciskei also made little accommodation for the family considerations of nurses. Hospitals and clinics made considerable demands on a nurse's time and physical resources. Nurses worked up to twelve-hour shifts in hospitals (especially when on night duty) and would be stationed at rural clinics for all but two weekends during a month, where they would also be on call after hours. Many found great difficulty in obtaining jobs near their families or accommodating their children in those circumstances. Marriage and pregnancy during training were discouraged, with some training programs restricting entrance to single trainees, requiring all student nurses to live in the nurses' quarters and threatening student nurses who fell pregnant with expulsion. Inadequate or nonexistent maternity leave for full-time nurses working in the Ciskei added further stress to nurses struggling to provide childcare for their own families while they attended to patients at the hospital or clinic.

Negotiating Marriage and Family Relations

The labor supply and the large number of African women applying for training meant that for the most part, the system was not forced to adjust to accommodate the family considerations of the nurses.

Despite the silences in the historical record and an unsympathetic system, these women clearly had considerable lives outside their work. They married, had children, continued relationships with their own parents, siblings, and in-laws. Throughout all this, their careers and family lives intersected in significant ways. A nurse's family members impacted her career by encouraging her to obtain education or training, influencing her to change jobs to be geographically closer to family, or halting her training and work for different lengths of time. In turn, a nurse's career had an important impact on her marriage and family life, with varying consequences. Examining the intersection of their work and family lives reveals the dynamics of changing marriage and family roles and expectations for professional women at a time of growing opportunities for women.

The interviews I conducted demonstrate that while marriage choices for these women moved toward a preference for companionate marriage, this change was uneven and nonlinear as it occurred among a wide group of women from different socioeconomic backgrounds. Nurses, their spouses, parents, and in-laws all had to negotiate the changes brought by women's new economic and social roles. The way all of them accepted or rejected these changing roles and expectations in family relations became a significant factor in how nurses fared when attempting to balance their work and family lives. Some women experienced marital tensions related to their professional status and the adjustments their careers demanded. Others had more supportive family members, especially husbands, which made it easier for them to balance all their responsibilities. Almost all of them shared the fact that they continued to shoulder the greater part of the burden of childcare and home management even as they took on demanding careers. The extant sources allow for more confident conclusions about the impact the nurses' careers had on their family lives than vice versa; however, some evidence suggests that these family considerations may have in turn influenced the delivery of health care in the Ciskei by affecting staffing and the quality of care individual nurses offered. The stories of three women in particular vividly illustrate the range of issues and outcomes these women experienced.

A Variety of Experiences
Lulu Msutu Zuma

Lulu Msutu Zuma was the youngest daughter of a chief of the Tyefu village. Her father's political position and commitment to her education helped her obtain the training she achieved. She graduated from high school and passed the matriculation exam; then in the mid-1950s, she trained as a nurse and a midwife. Even though her father thought her personality was too quiet for a profession that required one to interact closely with people, Zuma remembered that above all, he wanted a daughter to become a nurse. Thus, when marriage interrupted her older sister's plans to go to nursing school, he said Zuma must go. Zuma explained that at that time, they still followed what she termed the "old culture." This meant that when her sister got married, she had to devote herself to her new family—her husband, children, and father- and mother-in-law. Xhosa marriage negotiations, ceremonies, and expectations had changed over time, particularly with the arrival of Christianity. Still, when Zuma was training in the 1950s, marriage was seen as a contract between two families—known as *lobola* in Xhosa. Put simply, when a woman married a man, the man's family gave the woman's family a number of cattle in return, the number of which was determined in a series of negotiations. The two families exchanged gifts at different phases in the process. In the end, the bride, or *umakoti*, was taken to the groom's family and viewed as a new, junior member of the family and given a new name. She retained her own clan name, but her children would belong to the clan and family she married into. In the first few years of her marriage, she was expected to prove her worth and serve the family, not just her husband.[5] In Zuma's words, "If you were married, you were married. You just stayed and that's that—and look after your family. And that was the criteria of being a successful married woman, that you were able to look after your family and you cannot go and leave your family and go and study. You must concentrate on the family." Zuma further explained that the *makoti*'s new family, particularly her mother- and father-in-law, had "a lot to say about what you do and what you don't do."

Once Zuma started her training to become a nurse, her father wanted to see to it that she finished. Part way through her general nursing program, she got engaged, but her father said, "No," not before she finished her certificate. Apparently, he was afraid she might not finish her training, given the expectations for young married women at the time. According to Zuma, her father wanted to be sure she would have a profession to support herself if something happened to her marriage. The marriage was postponed and then eventually called off. In the end, Zuma said she herself decided against the marriage because there was no one at home to take care of her own parents. While Xhosa marriage expectations for women would allow *umakoti* to attend to her own family, Zuma wanted to make sure that she would be freely available.

Zuma eventually did get married, years after her first proposal. When she first mentioned her marriage in our interview, she talked about it in relation to her troubles having children. Zuma attributed her problems sustaining a pregnancy to her age—she was in her mid-thirties. She only had one daughter, who died at the age of five. After describing her difficulties in having children, Zuma then turned her attention to the political and economic situation in South Africa. She had been politically involved herself, but apartheid laws restricting the movement of Black people also disrupted her married life. She and her husband ended up moving to the Transkei to avoid dealing with pass laws.

It was only later in the interview that Zuma came back to her marriage when I asked her about challenges she experienced at a particular hospital. It was then in her career that her "social life" became her biggest challenge. Her husband began to say that he did not want her to work as a nurse. She speculated that he felt "his ego was challenged" because when she asked him what she would do, he said, "You just stay at home and listen to me, I will tell you what to do." They often had relatives staying with them whom she had to look after at home, and he apparently now wanted to have her do this under his instruction. But giving up her career was unacceptable for her: "And of course straight away I said, 'There's no such thing that is going to happen with me. I'm not going to stay at home.'"

Things came to a head with both stress at work and at home one day when a new, demanding doctor asked Zuma to write out instructions at the end of her shift. This made her late coming out of work. Her husband was outside waiting in the car and was angry with her for coming late. When he demanded to know why she was late, she could not tell him because she had to respect the confidentiality of her patients. As he drove home, she started to cry, which frustrated and angered him even more. "And he said to me," she remembered, "if you don't tell me what you are crying for you are not going to work tomorrow. I'm not going to have a wife who is crying all over the place and not telling me why." For her, this was the beginning of the end: "Then from that day, I had a challenge—it was either my husband or my work." During this time, she experienced what she later counted as her greatest professional accomplishments. She worked as a matron in the Mthatha Hospital and oversaw disaster management for the region. This often took her away from home and earned her praise from top politicians. Zuma lamented that she could not tell her husband about the successes that she had at work. When politicians praised her in public, it made her husband "mad."

While work was going well, Zuma's husband began physically abusing her and having girlfriends who even came to the hospital where she worked to harass her. Then, he gave her an ultimatum: she had to stop nursing, stop studying (she was working on a nursing administration degree), and stop going to church.

She replied, "I am not stopping anything. So if you say if I want this marriage to be successful, I must stop those things, we might as well go straight for a divorce because I'm stopping none of them." They divorced in 1989. Later in the interview, Zuma shared one thing that consoled her. Even though she divorced her husband, he always said she was the best housekeeper (and even asked her to come back twenty years later). She always made sure that even when she was at work, family members who stayed with them did not feel "there was something missing at home. . . . I designed all the meals at home, . . . even when I was not there, what people were going to have for breakfast, for dinner . . . for lunch, every day. Even if I wasn't going to be there, I designed the meals." She also made sure relatives had the necessary school fees and took care of her husband's son from his first marriage. Thus, although she lost her only child and divorced her husband, she took pride in the fact that she had reached one of the measures of success in Xhosa marriage that she pointed to at the beginning of the interview—to look after her family.[6]

Theresa Nonceba Ntonga

Theresa Nonceba Ntonga was brought up primarily by her mother in Duncan Village in East London. Unlike Zuma, Ntonga did not come from the political elite. Her parents had been part of a rising middle class of people with post-secondary education. Her father was a policeman and her mother was a teacher until she got married (during the 1940s and 1950s, female teachers were not allowed to be married). By the time Ntonga came along, her father had passed away, and to make a living, her mother had obtained work as a domestic worker in the nearby Frere Hospital. She earned enough to send her daughter to school. After finishing high school, Ntonga trained as a nurse and midwife. She met her husband as they both visited relatives in Zwelitsha.

In the first few years of her career in the early 1970s, Ntonga worked in three different clinics and then a hospital. Being stationed out in rural clinics was challenging—in the Mgwali clinic near Port Alfred, for example, she had to do all the clinic work, including cleaning the building. But she was committed to her work. She also had family responsibilities. She was married and had two children (born in 1976 and 1978). When I asked how she balanced her work and being a mother, she acknowledged her difficulties, saying, "Well, at that time, you find that we had some helpers, somebody who'll help you at home, keep your children. Otherwise, it's not easy. It's not easy being a mother and a nurse at the same time." When I asked what her children thought of her career, she said she thought they liked that she was a nurse. She noticed that her children liked to tell other people that their mother was a nurse, indicating to her that they were proud of her profession. Furthermore, Ntonga speculated that her daughter did not have a problem with her mother being a nurse because it was her nursing career that supported the family financially. Yet her daughter would never take up nursing as a profession for herself. She explained, "I used to come back tired and then shout at them and she [her daughter] said, 'Nursing, hm-m, I can't take nursing.'"

Ntonga said she found it easier to take care of her children when she worked at the Bhisho Hospital in the early 1990s, because unlike working in a rural village, "everything was there," including her husband. She and her husband stayed together in their marriage "right through" until he died. His jobs allowed him to live with his wife and children even as his wife moved around to different hospitals and clinics. He first did window dressing and then had a career in consulting municipal governments. When asked what her husband thought of her career, Ntonga asked, "You mean assisting?" then broke into laughter. "I'm sorry," she said. "He was useless." Then she laughingly told me I must not get married. When she became more serious, she said, "I wouldn't be struggling like this if . . . I really struggled, I don't want to lie." Her main problem was that her husband did not contribute much financially. Her children adored their father, especially her daughter; but Ntonga apparently had to be the primary breadwinner for her family. When her own salary was not enough to pay for her children's school fees, she even had what she described as "sideline jobs," such as selling chickens. She remarked, "If I wasn't a hard worker, I wouldn't have anything now." Unlike Zuma, she denied that her career caused any tension in their marriage. It was just that her husband was irresponsible. She explained, "They see that you can work hard, then they lean on you." She concluded that she was able to survive because God gave her strength. She did give her husband credit for helping in the house—"because he was good, even in cooking at times," she explained, laughing. He knew how to cook certain dishes that she did not. He also helped with cleaning when they did not have money to hire someone, and he helped slaughter the chickens. "If he wasn't there, it would be so hard for me," she said in a follow-up visit in 2018. But in the end, he did not leave her any money.[7]

Thando Lucas

Thando Lucas was born in 1945 in Port Elizabeth, the eldest of eleven children in her family. She described her parents as "hard working." Unlike Zuma and Ntonga's parents, they had little formal education. Her father worked in garages with cars and her mother was a domestic worker. "During the olden days," she narrated, "it was not easy to educate such a lot of siblings," so her maternal grandmother offered to ensure she got an education. Lucas speculated that her parents and grandparents could see that she had a future because of how well she was doing in school. She studied up through high school, when she met her (now) husband. He was already working and was "in too much of a hurry to get married."[8] Her parents could not afford a church wedding, so they only got married the "traditional way," with *lobola* and all the expectations that could come with a "traditional" marriage.

After offering this simple narrative, Lucas then talked about how her parents initially did not want her to get married at that time. Apparently, like Zuma's father, they feared marriage would halt their daughter's education, an education that family members had carefully invested in and within which she showed promise. When Lucas's husband promised to ensure she would receive further education, her parents agreed to their marriage. Lucas recounted, "He promised them that whatever was to be done by me, being the one being educated in the family, he is going to do that." And "that he did." He paid for her education and everything that "he could do for me and my family." He even supported her through all her degrees and certificates beyond her general nursing training. Incidentally, I interviewed Lucas shortly after she and her husband celebrated their fiftieth wedding anniversary with a big party.

Lucas's husband's support did not mean that her career did not take certain turns because of her marriage and children. When they moved to Port Elizabeth for his job, Lucas started training at Livingstone Hospital. To do so, she was required to live in the nurses' quarters. Unhappy with this arrangement, her husband asked her to cut her training short so she could live with him. Thus she only trained to be an auxiliary nurse then. However, Lucas's husband's support was crucial later in her further training. When they moved to the King William's Town area, she wanted to train at Mount Coke. Initially, she was turned down because she was married and the hospital only accepted single trainees. "There I come, with my husband, without knowing that," Lucas said. "And the matron [who] was there, Mrs. Tolmay, told us that 'you are not supposed to be trained here because she is a married somebody, married to you.' Then my husband argued [out] that day," pointing out that they both wanted to be educated and did not have children with them, that the matron should regard them as her own children wanting to be educated, and furthermore, that she could not be 100 percent sure that all of her trainees were single. The matron was persuaded. According to Lucas, she was the first known married person to be admitted into the training program. Like Livingstone Hospital, the trainees had to live in the nurses' quarters and abide by curfew rules. While this living arrangement was not acceptable for her husband earlier, it was okay at Mount Coke after he had struggled to secure her admission. Luckily, during her last year she had a matron who "understood family life" and allowed her to stay with her husband. But for two years, she and her husband barely

Negotiating Marriage and Family Relations   151

saw each other as they passed each other on their way to and from work and school.

Lucas had her first child early on in her career, but then had trouble getting pregnant. After ten years, she had what she calls her miracle baby—a daughter. Her daughter was followed by another son seven years after that. When asked how she balanced her work and raising her children, she exclaimed, "Man! I would never know, but it happened. We *had* to." As was common in Xhosa culture, she took her first child to be cared for by her in-laws as it was believed that a man's parents should raise the first-born child since they had more experience raising children than the new parents. With the second child, her husband decided "not to take any child to anybody—'Let's stay with our children.'" Lucas was training for a certificate in midwifery at the time. When she left for work in the morning, she would leave the baby with her husband and the "auntie" they hired to work for them. Because the hospital was an hour by bus from where she and her husband stayed, she sometimes slept at the hospital overnight and her husband would care for the baby alone. When she had her third baby, she was working at the Zwelitsha clinic, in the township where they lived, and was able to keep the baby in a cot at the clinic and breastfeed him during the day when needed.[9]

Changing Nature of Marriage and Family Expectations

The nurses I interviewed trained, married, and had children anywhere from the mid-1950s through the 1980s. As in other African societies, changing economic and social opportunities for women in the twentieth century had a great impact on the nature of marriage relationships in the Ciskei. In earlier decades, many female nurses came from, and married men within, the Black Christian elite who had adopted European Christian ideas of marriage (even as they mixed these ideals with African ones).[10] As nursing training for Black women grew in leaps and bounds in the mid-1950s and 1960s, nurses came from more varied socioeconomic backgrounds, as exemplified by Zuma, Ntonga, and Lucas. Thirty-three of the nurses I interviewed told me that their parents had little formal education or engaged in agricultural and menial work, while nineteen told me their parents had education beyond primary school. Forty-one were born in rural areas versus twenty-six in urban. Xhosa women had long found ways to be economically independent, particularly in urban areas that offered them opportunities to gain economic power and social independence.[11] Yet the 1950s and 1960s saw a growing number of educated professional women who had salaries and prestigious careers like nursing, often rivaling that of men at the time. Thus more people in both the new and older generations had to face the implications of the widening roles for women.[12]

Debates among writers and readers of *Imvo Zabantsundu*, the local Xhosa-language newspaper, show that new ideas and roles for women challenged relationships between men and women and their parents in the 1960s through the 1970s among the Xhosa in the Eastern Cape. An article about Witness K. Tamsanqa's 1958 play *Buzani Kubawo*, wherein a young man rebels against his father's choice of marriage, pointed out how the play addressed changing customs and intergenerational struggles, especially as children migrated to urban areas for work.[13] Articles addressing the African woman's position in the early 1960s questioned if women had a place outside the home.[14] Throughout the 1960s and into the early 1970s, some men and women wrote scathing critiques of women's liberation coming from "the West" or boldly claimed that women held inferior intelligence or devious desires.[15] These passionate writings suggest that the authors felt threatened by the new challenges to male authority or to a system they had invested in as women. Some women defended themselves in the paper, critiquing men as well as asserting women's innate abilities. These authors were not always as progressive as contemporary feminists may have wished. Some just wanted recognition for the work that women did in the homes, reaffirmed women's power with her husband and children, or said that marriage was a partnership, but the woman was the junior partner.[16] As the 1970s progressed, more articles highlighting women's accomplishments and the need to recognize women's oppression appeared along with articles reporting on the various roles open to women. Some wrote about women using professions traditionally accepted as female as springboards to careers in business or highlighted female politicians, medical professionals, and judges.[17] Depicting the Ciskei as a potentially progressive option for women at a National Council of African Women meeting in Queenstown in 1971, L. S. Mtoba, an executive councilor from the Ciskei Department of Justice, said that while "Bantu law and culture" needed to be respected, Xhosa society also needed to "keep pace with social changes." Recognizing the different roles women played, he continued, "We cannot be so orthodox as to accept no change. . . . Today we have Bantu women who are University graduates, lecturers, principles of schools, presidents of national organisations, hospital sisters, medical practitioners, lawyers, etc." Mtoba mentioned famous Port Elizabeth nurse and politician Dora Nginza as a specific example and asked why women should be perpetual minors.[18]

Women, men, and their parents negotiated these new economic and professional roles for women in different ways depending on their backgrounds, personalities, and career options. Historians of Africa have charted how colonialism, urbanization, and religious conversion changed the institution of marriage. Generally, their work creates a sense of men and women across the

Negotiating Marriage and Family Relations

continent in the late nineteenth and twentieth centuries tending toward individual choices about marriage and management of family life less tied to kin structures (or what others would term the extended family).[19] Along with these changes, scholars have analyzed the rise of what is often termed companionate marriage—a marriage wherein a husband and wife have romantic love for one another, are expected to have more egalitarian roles within the marriage, and have more autonomy as a couple.[20] For historical subjects and scholars, this kind of marriage has often been termed a "modern" marriage. But as other scholars have noted, the ideal did not always match reality, and changes have come unevenly.[21] Men and women have held on to different ideals. What was once considered traditional was not wholly replaced by a new Christian and European form of marriage.[22] As studies on recent marriage trends in South Africa and Senegal have shown, marriage relations and expectations have also not always moved in a linear direction toward companionate marriage.[23]

Moreover, ties to extended family and women's responsibility for childcare and household management have persisted over time. Even if African marriages trended toward couples freely choosing their future spouses and exercising more independence in making decisions about their own households, husbands and wives were still closely connected to their broader kinship networks. Sharon Stitcher theorized that as Kenyan middle-class families made the transition to a more Western nuclear unit, with the husband and wife both working outside the home, more egalitarian gender relationships should emerge. However, her research found that "customary" marriage still had a presence in society, that members of the extended family often lived with the immediate family, that men and women worked for different reasons, and that women still had primary responsibility over domestic work but not a greater share in decision-making.[24] This blending of old and new family and marriage relations could be found in South Africa in the 1960s through the 1980s, with wives particularly beholden to their in-laws. As Zuma described, looking after "your family" for *umakoti* included performing domestic chores such as cooking and cleaning for *umakoti*'s husband, her father- and mother-in-law, her husband's siblings and their children, and other extended family members in the home. *Umakoti* was also expected to serve as the primary caregiver for her own children. As in Lucas's case, a husband's parents would often take a leading role in raising the first-born child since they had more experience raising children than the new parents.[25] However, women in general performed most of the duties of taking care of their children's physical needs and managing their households.

The discrepancies between husbands and wives regarding changing marriage expectations is evident in the history of the Eastern Cape in the 1960s through the 1980s. In addition to the three telling examples given at the beginning of this chapter, a study done in a township just west of the Ciskei in the mid-1970s provides vocabulary and data for further analysis. The study highlighted the way that women and men negotiated changes in expectations in marriage using what they termed "traditional" and "modern" ideas of marriage. Virginia van der Vliet found that younger, educated women in a Grahamstown township were more likely to desire what Vliet termed a closed joint monogamous marriage, where husband and wife performed duties together or interchangeably or spent leisure time together, even if they segregated their domestic duties. Men, on the other hand, were more likely to want what they called traditional marriage because they believed it gave them patriarchal privileges, offered them social and sexual freedom, meant they did not have to do chores, and granted them acceptance by their male peers who shared their beliefs. Vliet found that younger, educated women struggled with husbands asserting superiority.[26]

Discussions about marriage, love, and dating that were common in *Imvo Zabantsundu* in the 1960s through the 1970s similarly reveal shifts in ideas and practices toward more equality and companionship in marriage but expose resistance to those changes as well. Starting in 1968, the paper would periodically publish articles explaining the legal rights of married women. Authors and activists felt it important to explain that women married under Xhosa customary law were considered legal minors who could not inherit property or conduct business without their husband, but that women could request a different arrangement at the time of marriage, including one where the husband and wife shared property.[27] In the mid-1970s, one article encouraged women to exercise newfound agency in dating, while another argued that a husband had no right to his wife's paycheck and asked questions such as: "Must [the woman] not have things and real rights that are hers exclusively? Must the woman be a glorified slave?"[28] Articles about the importance of choosing a good partner, marriage partners working as a team, expectations about romance, watching out for the influence of in-laws, and the desire that wives be treated as they were during courtship demonstrate that a number of people believed love to be an important element of marriage and that many women expected marriage to have companionship and affection.[29] They also indicate that some men and in-laws resisted more companionate marriage or *umakoti* independence. One 1975 article in particular reinforces van der Vliet's findings, claiming research showed that companionship in marriage was better for one's mental health, but that men complained about the sexual limitations and economic responsibilities the arrangement imposed on them.[30] A couple of other articles addressed the differences in expectations of people with an urban versus rural outlook, or as the article implied, those looking to reinforce traditional roles versus those more open to new kinds of relations. Writing somewhat disparagingly of Xhosa marriage practices, the author claimed that "people who live in urban areas believe that relations between two people cannot be built by cows only. A loving relationship is a prerequisite between the two people who are going to build a life together and bring about a union between two families."[31] In 1976 the paper reported that a nurse's husband filed for divorce when she left her husband's home to finish her nursing training after only three days of staying with her in-laws after their wedding.[32] A few articles sought to balance Western versus Xhosa or African values among these changes and to show that men, women, and their parents held different views for different reasons.[33] For example, in 1979 *Imvo Zabantsundu* staff writers questioned what was going to happen to *lobola*. They reported that single men found it to be a system of financial exploitation, whereas married women and parents wanted to keep it to hold men and women to their responsibilities and maintain ties between families.[34]

The tensions and negotiations the nurses I interviewed had to engage in with both their husbands and in-laws show that their marriage relations were undergoing a similar, uneven change. While all the nurses I interviewed had to balance the demands of child-rearing and marriage with the demands of their profession, their responses regarding negotiating marriage relationships varied. Like Zuma, the experiences of some of the women I interviewed reflected the tension between women in skilled and economically profitable careers and men desiring the more "traditional" marriage that Vliet highlighted.[35] On the other hand, while some women found that their nursing careers exacerbated marital problems, others like Lucas had supportive husbands and extended family members who helped them balance family and professional work. Evidently, the ability of a nurse to balance both her profession and family life had less to do with her profession and more to do with the family relationships she had. Similar to Elizabeth Hull's application of Belinda Bozzoli's concept of "domestic struggles" then, the history of these nurses demonstrates the need to take into account the "variability of domestic situations" when assessing the relationship between a woman's profession and her marriage and family life.[36]

Marital Tensions

Although few women I interviewed talked about it directly, there is evidence that some nurses' careers indeed exacerbated marital tensions. Of the sixty-seven I interviewed, seven had never married, forty-seven reported remaining married (or widowed), and at least eleven were divorced (about 16 percent). Most of the divorced women attributed the breakup of their marriage to infidelity and abuse. Only one, Zuma, reported that her career was a direct source of contention in her marriage. However, the details she related were telling. When she and her husband lived in the Transkei, Zuma speculated that her husband felt "his ego was challenged" because she worked as a matron, traveled for work, and gained public recognition. In other words, he felt threatened by her achievements and reacted by demanding that she submit to his wishes and commands. He also started having girlfriends and physically abusing her. The infidelity and abuse reported by other nurses may have been linked to a husband feeling threatened or neglected as well. Perhaps men in troubled marriages were just irresponsible and unfaithful, or perhaps they did not know how to adjust to this new situation—what others have referred to as a crisis of masculinity.[37] As a social worker writing in the local newspaper cautioned, her advice about improving marriage relations would not work "where a husband is too unsure of his masculinity to cope with an independent wife."[38] At the same time, there very well could have been reasons that the nurses did not want to discuss their divorce with me. Zuma said that she did not hear others having the same problems she did, but she herself did not tell others at work about her marital struggles—she hardly even told her sister. Perhaps just as Zuma kept her troubles to herself, some women refrained from telling me, a stranger, very personal and even painful details of their marriages. On the other hand, in the meeting I had with retired nurses about this book, a few talked about how nurses endured "unbearable" things in marriage because they were trained to be empathetic and endure difficult circumstances. This led them to believe that they suffered through more abuse than other women.[39]

Still, when asked to talk about other nurses' marriages, other interviewees indicated that more than just Zuma's divorce was linked to the threat a husband may have felt by his wife's status and training. Just like Zuma and professional women in East Africa, a 1973 article in the *Imvo Zabantsundu*'s women's page, edited by Lulama Jijana, addressed the tensions that could arise if the husband felt the woman was encroaching on what he felt were his manly duties.[40] "Another problem, although not so very common," the article read, "arises if a wife's income is very close to or equals, or even exceeds, that of her husband. He will tend to resent any inroads into the dominant male role of economic responsibility for the family unit."[41] Some nurses I interviewed similarly observed that husbands could have felt a sense of competition or felt threatened by their wives' achievements. For example, Baleni admitted that friction can come when marriage partners have different levels of "sophistication."[42] Mount Coke and Twecu clinic nurse Kwatsha said that because her husband had a college degree, he was not threatened by her career (he was a teacher by profession). She explained, "Now there's that competition, yeah, and you see that, okay this person is better than myself, maybe. But I don't think it's a problem when the person is learned like my husband."[43] Although I did not obtain as much information about nurses' husbands' backgrounds as I did about the nurses themselves, it is revealing that many of the nurses' spouses had education beyond secondary school (at least thirty-five), indicating that nurses often married someone with a similar level of education. This could reflect the desirability of nurses as spouses for those with more education, the nurses' choice to marry more educated men, or the likelihood of choosing a spouse from a peer in urban or rural centers of training and education. Yet husbands who did not support their wives or expressed discontent with their jobs had a range of occupations and education levels, showing that while professional competition affected some marriages, there were other factors at play as well.

Other marital tensions came from complaints about a nurse's work schedule and absence from the home.[44] Those who trained in earlier years found it especially difficult to work while married since their husbands and in-laws were more likely to require they stay at home full-time. Penelope Ntshona, for instance, completed her training in 1951 and was married in 1952 to a young medical doctor. Because her husband wanted her to focus on taking care of their children, he did not allow her to find a full-time job until the children were grown.[45] In the 1980s, the nature of nursing employment in the Ciskei meant that a nurse could spend a significant amount of time away from home. Nurses could move many times to obtain posts or seek further training. Since the majority of the nurses I interviewed had worked in clinics in rural villages at one point in their career, many of them had to live away from their families for long periods of time. If a nurse did not live in the village where she was stationed, she had to stay in the nurses' quarters in the village. Nurses would have only two weekends off per month. The other weekends, the nurse would be on call and expected to be available for after-hours emergencies. At least sixteen of the nurses I interviewed lived away from their husbands at one point in their careers. At least eight reported that their husbands did not like the fact that their work schedules kept them away from their families. Some of these men wanted their wives to stay at home with the children, while others were either afraid they would be lonely or feared their wives would have relationships with other men while they were outside the home.[46] On the other hand, at least two nurses believed that their absence from the home facilitated their husband's infidelity, especially if they had to work the night shift.

In addition to negotiating relationships with their husbands, women had to deal with the expectations of their parents and in-laws. Few interviewees faced opposition from their own parents to their nursing training. Whether educated or not, these parents valued education, if only because it ensured their daughters' future economic security.[47] As with Zuma, some nurses' parents discouraged them from marriage while they were training, fearing that the demands of marriage would prevent them from finishing their educations and limit their economic prospects. A decade later, Lucas's parents had a similar reaction, showing the enduring or growing desire by parents to see their daughters trained and the fear that nursing training would be incompatible with their marriage arrangements. Gaining nursing training was especially important for those in lower economic statuses like Lucas, whose family counted on her academic success to help secure her economic future and possibly the economic future of the family. At least thirteen women said they chose to train as a nurse for primarily economic reasons—they could get paid while training and needed a quick way to start bringing an income into their natal family. At least seven mentioned that they continued to help their parents and siblings throughout their careers, with cash assistance, building houses, or providing care for ailing family members.[48]

While the woman's natal family may have supported her education, a woman's husband's family may have had different expectations. Even if wives and husbands shared the same vision of the kind of roles they would play in their marriage, the in-laws may have demanded or expected otherwise. A social worker in the region, Pumla Sangotsha, wrote in 1973 that women wanted to be married and yet were finding it "harder and harder to accept their subordinate role, . . . sacrifice their fulfillment to that of their hubbies, . . . live second-hand lives." She reminded her female readers to remember the culture their husbands grew up in. Even though their courtship may have taken place in a different context, his expectations for his wife—and I would add his parents' expectations—would be heavily influenced by what he saw growing up.[49] One nurse I interviewed, Hilary Mnyanda, struggled with negotiating her position as a professional woman who worked outside the home with her husband and father-in-law's more "traditional" demands—tensions she also cast as arising from marrying into a "rural area." Her husband always expected her to cook for her, even if she was at work all day. Her father-in-law challenged her abilities to cook and serve food and questioned her decisions about her children's education and travel. As this woman portrayed it, her husband seemingly did not get involved in these struggles, leaving his wife to argue with her father-in-law on her own until she decided to leave the family's homestead to go live with her husband where he was stationed as a teacher.[50] Fortunately for her, she could leave the homestead and still stay with her husband. Others, like the woman divorced for leaving her husband's family to finish her nursing training, may not have had that option. Yet others may have found that their careers gave them more negotiating power.

Negotiating Economic Power

A number of other husbands of the nurses I interviewed accepted their wives' careers because they saw the economic benefits of their work. A nurse's salary could help her family become part of this expanding Black middle class of new professionals in the Ciskei, people with economic power to accumulate property and gain higher levels of education, despite the racial restrictions in South Africa.[51] Like urban areas in the South African Republic, more educational and economic opportunities in the 1960s through the 1980s resulted in an increase in salaried men, traders, entrepreneurs, and more female teachers and nurses (and more professional politicians rather than the educated elite who dominated politics in earlier times). This brought the hope of new social mobility, especially in "homelands" where promised political and business opportunities and a large public service sector provided "substantial material benefits."[52] While ten nurses complained about the inadequate pay they received for the amount of work they did, nurses still earned a significant salary compared with the impoverished of the Ciskei.[53] Single, divorced, and widowed nurses supported themselves, their children, parents, or other extended family members with their earnings. For husbands and wives running an independent household during this time, that extra income could make the difference in the kind of education their children received. At least five women reported that their husbands accepted their careers merely because of the financial contributions to their families' living expenses. The other eight who reported that their husbands enjoyed their careers did not highlight the nurses' salaries as the reason, although this could have contributed to their husbands' acceptance.

At least three nurses voiced the feeling that their husbands took advantage of their incomes, raising questions about the men's complacency in accepting the women's greater earning power. For example, one woman complained that her husband treated the money she earned as belonging to him. He did not even ask her for it but expected her to give it to him. Another woman grumbled about how her husband left it up to her to secure and pay for post-secondary education for their children, remarking that he cared more about other people than those inside his own house.[54] Ntonga described her husband as faithful to their monogamous marriage but "useless" when it came to providing a living. His jobs allowed him to live with his wife and children even as his wife moved around to different hospitals and clinics. Yet her main problem was that her husband did not contribute to the family's financial security. Articles in *Imvo Zabantsundu* support the idea that some men took advantage of professional women's financial assets throughout this time. In what appears to be a letter to the editor in *Imvo Zabantsundu* in August 1964, the unnamed author indicated that men were indeed viewing professional women as bringing in economic benefits. In addition to the nurse's training being a potential help to her family, the article read, "Nowadays, men prefer to marry nurses for purely logical good reasons. On account of the high cost of living standards, a professional wife is an asset to the home."[55] Over a decade later, authors took a more cynical view. A 1977 article indicated that some men married professional women like nurses because "men want people who will be able to support themselves" so they could spend their own money on what they wanted and still have the status of being married. "They want the title and not its responsibilities," the author wrote.[56] Another woman reportedly said in 1980, "Men of today like comfort for which they are not prepared to pay, they expect women to do that."[57] Had the tables turned by the 1980s as far as who was expected to financially support the family? Did men find that their wives' incomes allowed them more freedom outside the marriage or family responsibilities? Or were men perhaps more desperate after the economically difficult decade of the 1970s, whereas nurses had more secure careers? It is possible that Ntonga's husband shirked some of what society deemed were his financial responsibilities for supporting the family because of his wife's earning power. As Ntonga described it, once her husband saw that she could work hard, he depended on her income. Husbands like Ntonga's may have also struggled to know what their roles were as the role of women in marriage was changing during this time of women's increased education and economic power. In any case, whereas some men saw their wives' achievements as a threat and reacted by asserting their masculinity, others may have passively or gladly accepted a reversal in traditionally accepted economic roles.

Some of the women also struggled to accept new roles for both women and men as women's economic power increased. Even when married couples had established a more nuclear family unit and had more characteristics of a companionate marriage, this did not mean that the women I interviewed had entirely changed their expectations of the role of women and men in the family. As Hull argued, even though men and women may have been taking on a variety of roles, the women she interviewed still used "fixed representations of gender roles" as they spoke about their lives.[58] In addition to her disappointment that her husband did not fulfill his role in supporting the family financially, Ntonga laughed when she talked about his cooking, presumably because it was considered a woman's role to cook. Although Magodla similarly complained about her husband not fulfilling his expected financial responsibilities by not paying for their children's education, she also expressed frustration that he would not change some of his expectations of her duties. She pointed out the unhappy situation of a nurse who was working full time but also expected to perform the role of a wife once she is home if she wanted to keep her marriage.

Two o'clock I must be on duty and come back at seven o'clock. Seven o'clock I was to see that my *umngqusho* [samp and beans] was all right, see that my ironing *yabantwana* [children's ironing]—I mean, it was too much?! It was too much. But we survive. . . . Whether we are educated or we are working, you have to do your *ii-chores*, *ii-chores zomfazi ne* [the wife's chores, no]? You have to cook for your husband, your husband will come home from work, he'll sit there with a newspaper, and see that you will give him a cup of coffee, and then you prepare *i-supper* and all that, *ne*? And tomorrow morning you both, one's going the other side, you're also going but when you come back we are going to play *i-nantsika yabomama*, the wife's role, *ne*?

Although she saw the injustice of expecting the woman to perform all the domestic duties on top of her full-time work without any help from the man, she also said that those who endured had lasting marriages.[59] Despite her marriage breakdown, Zuma longed for children and gained satisfaction in fulfilling what she saw as the role of *umakoti* in her husband's family by taking care of extended family members and running the household well.[60] Nompumelelo and Ciskei medical council nurse Maniwe Catherine Mvubu speculated, "You treat them [husbands] nicely then they like your profession."[61] Figlan, a Nompumelelo nurse who also worked closely with VHWs, insinuated that nurses themselves caused problems at home when they tried to change gender roles, stating that because they were in charge at work, they wanted to be in charge at home too.[62] Two *Imvo Zabantsundu* articles two decades apart expressed similar ideas, demonstrating that this view was held by more people. A 1973 article reported that some wives "exert altogether too much of their personalities in the home at the expense of their husbands' self-respect."[63] In 1991 an article warned working women who had managerial positions at work against trying to be a manager at home as well.[64] "But a working wife must always remember that her husband, family and home have priority over everything," a 1973 article affirmed.[65] All these comments indicate that while some practices changed, some nurses held on to more traditional expectations of men acting as the heads of their families and providing the main economic resources and wives focusing more on performing domestic duties in service of their husbands and children.

Supportive Husbands

Of course, not all nurses experienced friction in their family relations as a direct result of their careers. The interviews I conducted also indicate that a number of men saw themselves as part of joint monogamous or companionate marriages and supported their wives by encouraging their personal aspirations, providing extra assistance in their work, or taking a greater part in childcare and housekeeping chores. Lucas's husband, for example, not only promised her parents that he would ensure she finished her training. At one point, he even convinced a matron to admit his wife to the nursing school. Other husbands expressed pride and satisfaction in their wives' careers. Eight women said that their husbands in fact enjoyed their careers (as opposed to others who tolerated their careers for economic reasons). These husbands actively facilitated their wives' work by supporting their aspirations for further training, helping them cope with their schedules, and even assisting with patients.[66] In addition to long workdays in hospitals or weeks in clinics, some nurses moved from home for weeks or months to gain further training. Some husbands reportedly helped their families through times when their wives were absent by maintaining stable home bases. Frere Hospital nurse Nombasa B. Dubula remarked, "I was fortunate because my family, my children [grew up] knowing that I'm going to be out, in and out; but my husband kept the family together." Like other husbands, he also supported her by taking her to and from work.[67] Fort Beaufort Hospital nurse Ethel Nonkululeko Gwayi's husband similarly provided transportation to make sure she could be home immediately after her shift to share the evening meal with her children.[68] Mhlambiso's husband drove from Amathole Basin to Cecilia Makiwane Hospital every Friday while she was doing a community health course there so that she could spend the weekend with her family.[69] Mbombo's husband helped transport patients with his own car when she was based at a rural clinic.[70] In addition to helping their wives manage their time and transportation, husbands might also help their wives by providing companionship. Janjties mentioned that just discussing cases that worried her with her husband could help her cope. She remarked, "There are times when you go home with this thing and then you feel okay after discussing it with your husband and you tell him how I treated this person or . . ."[71]

A number of interviewees talked about their husbands taking on household chores seen as traditional women's duties. For example, Hewana's husband took care of their baby when she was on night duty instead of hiring a nanny to work through the night.[72] Kwatsha's husband changed the baby's nappies, and Ntonga's husband sometimes cooked.[73] Lucas told how her husband took care of their second baby at night when at times during her midwifery training she stayed at the hospital overnight. They could have asked the nanny to stay, but her husband wanted to care for the baby himself.

There were certainly various factors that determined why a husband helped in this way. The information provided in the interviews gives some insight into the role of education and family relations. Many of these husbands had service-oriented jobs in nursing's peer sectors. Like Kwatsha's husband, most of the husbands whom nurses reported supported them in their professions were teachers.[74] Other supportive husbands were employed by the government in an office or service delivery position such as a policeman. A couple of others were political activists, some had wage-earning jobs, and others had family members who had been nurses. Gwayi's husband, for example, came from a family where all his sisters were nurses. He even persuaded her to change from teaching to nursing.[75]

Having a supportive husband and other family members did not mean that the nurses I interviewed did not make sacrifices or changes in their career for family reasons. At least twenty nurses I interviewed moved to different cities or regions because their husbands got jobs there or because their children or parents needed them. Nine nurses mentioned that getting married or having children interrupted their training or jobs, especially when hospitals or clinics did not offer maternity leave. Yet women with supportive husbands tended to work more in partnership with them. In these families, husbands and wives compromised to make things work so that these women found it easier to cope with their demanding jobs and family responsibilities.

Child-Rearing

One of the most prominent familial roles the nurses shared was that of motherhood. Almost all the women I interviewed shared the experience of raising children while also working as a nurse. Even if a woman was not married, having children gave her a more respected status in Xhosa society.[76] Of the sixty-seven women I interviewed, seven never married and only two never had any of their own children (although at least one of those two helped raise children of a family member at some point). Raising children while working full time as a nurse was challenging. The difficulties these women faced included maintaining employment through pregnancy and childbirth, spending adequate time with children at home, and arranging childcare. The health care systems within which they worked did not do much to facilitate their motherhood. At times, they were at the mercy of the matrons. If a matron understood family life, such as the one Lucas had at Mount Coke, a nurse could make provisions to balance her different responsibilities.[77] If not, the matron could make life harder, such as when a matron denied Kwatsha's request to be reassigned from the Twecu clinic back to Mount Coke Hospital so she could stay with her children.[78]

The majority of the women I interviewed (thirty-nine) had three to four children, fourteen reported having one or two children, and nine had five or more. Although my evidence does not indicate precisely how a nurse's profession influenced the number of children she had, certainly factors such as staying separately from one's husband for work or training, physically taxing jobs, and an emphasis on family planning in the health profession could all have influenced nurses to have fewer children. Others who waited to marry or have children until they had finished training, like Zuma, similarly may have naturally reduced the number of children they had, although the age at which they gave birth and its relation to their time of training varied among the nurses I interviewed.

For those who had children while training or working for government or mission hospitals, the difficulties started as soon as they fell pregnant. Nine of the women I interviewed told of how getting married or bearing children either led to a job resignation or a postponement of their training. Training programs, especially those run by mission hospitals, viewed pregnancy as a problem and grounds for expulsion if the nurse was not married. The hospitals expected nurses to serve as examples of their definition of civilized, Christian ladies, after all. One woman told how she fell pregnant outside marriage during her first year of training at Baragwanath Hospital in the mid-1960s. She was required to go back home to the Eastern Cape to give birth to the baby, but she also went because, as she put it, "You had to feel that there is something wrong that you have done."[79] The same moral expectations applied to full-time employees, although maternity leave could be an option instead of expulsion. As a template for contracts with nurses in the 1960s and 1970s stated: "The nurse must at all times be an example to the people to whom she ministers. This must be reflected in her personal neatness and appearance, her attitude to her work, the handling of her patients, and in her moral standard and general living habits. An unmarried nurse who has illegitimate children is hardly an example of a high moral code."[80]

Maternity leave policies for those working full time varied depending on the time and the location where a nurse worked but seem to have generally caused women stress, as they found the leave inadequate or nonexistent. Judith Nolde described how the Wiehahn Commission in the late 1970s recommended longer maternity leaves. Union and political groups advocated for it at the same time. Still, Nolde argued that maternity leave was not protected well in general in South Africa during this time.[81] Indeed, three nurses who worked in Cape Provincial hospitals in the 1960s to the early 1970s (including Victoria and Grey Hospitals), talked about having to resign and reapply when they fell pregnant.[82] The Ciskei Territorial Authority granted four months', mostly unpaid, leave in the 1960s and 1970s for district or clinic nurses. Contracts stipulated that a pregnant nurse should be released from work starting two months prior to the birth of her child until two months after the birth. The nurse could use her annual paid leave as part of this four months, but otherwise her

Negotiating Marriage and Family Relations

time away was counted as unpaid leave and she would not be granted any more leave during the rest of the year. If she lived in the nurses' accommodations at a rural clinic, she was expected to take all her personal belongings with her to make room for a relief nurse.[83] It is unclear from archival records whether this same contract carried over into the independent Ciskei; however, the interviews suggest that the contracts were at least similar. Some nurses I interviewed said there was no maternity leave in the independent Ciskei, while others affirmed that they were granted a short amount of unpaid time off. The unpaid aspect of the leave may have led some nurses to declare there was no maternity leave. They also may have had a shorter amount of time than under the territorial authority. Nompumelelo and Mount Coke Hospital and clinic nurse Tyileka Malo remembered having six weeks, and Mbie said they had to save their annual leaves to make up for a lack of maternity leave.[84] Overall, for women working full time as nurses, pregnancy and childbirth had the potential to significantly disrupt their job security and income.

As soon as a nurse returned to work after giving birth, she would struggle to give enough time to her children, especially if she lived in nurses' quarters that had no provision for children. Nonkululeko Vena said she really only saw her children on weekends, even when she lived at home near Victoria Hospital, because she left early in the morning and came home late at night.[85] Similarly, Magodla said, "Most of the time you are in the hospital. You have got no time to look after your family."[86] As Gwayi explained, "You have to leave the children very early in the morning, most of them are still asleep, especially the young ones. And then you come back, . . . you reach home 'round about past eight. Either you find the children asleep or they have had supper already."[87] Night duty was especially taxing on children because their mothers would be gone as they settled down for the night and got ready for the next day. Others said their children did not like it when their mothers had to work far away at rural clinics or when they had to work on holidays. Tunyiswa thought her children "had a bad experience" with nursing "because mama was always busy." She remembered one Christmas when she was supposed to go home, but then a maternity case came. "I had to stay and deliver that mother," she said. "Then I couldn't go for Christmas at home. I had to go late in the evening because when you deliver a woman you had to stay with her for about three hours."[88] Similarly, Vakalisa said, "So, my children are not interested in nursing at all because they had a rough time because I used to work even on Christmas Day. '*Yho!* Mama, we'll never be nurses. When you work even on public days and Christmas Day?!'"[89] Magodla even wondered if she had been home one Friday, maybe her son would not have left home and later been caught in a fight that led to his death.[90] "But," as one nurse said,

166 Negotiating Marriage and Family Relations

"you survive, because others survived. You have to survive. . . . It's part of the package."[91]

As households moved toward a more nuclear family living situation, especially when jobs took couples away from family homesteads, arranging for childcare when both parents worked outside the home was difficult. Although it was an accepted practice for their own mothers and mothers-in-law to help raise children, the nurses I interviewed still held the primary responsibility for childcare and upkeep of the home, even when marriages looked more like companionate marriages. As with marriage, kinship networks continued to play an important role in child-rearing even as expectations and family structures changed. Almost half the women I interviewed received help from a family member at one point or another to raise their children. Around ten said their mother-in-law (or in-laws in general) helped, and at least fifteen said their own mothers looked after their children. Family help also included relatives who came to work as nannies and husbands who stepped in to carry part of the load. Eleven of the women I interviewed reported that their husbands helped with childcare at home in some way.

Yet even if women preferred to recruit help from among their relatives, this was not always an option, especially if they lived far from other family members because their jobs or their husbands' jobs took them away. At least twenty-seven hired aunties or nannies at one point or another. Many expressed that this option could be risky if they did not find a trustworthy person. Vena remarked that she had to undo some of what the nanny taught her children during the week.[92] Ciskei and Transkei hospital nurse Nozipho Tom arrived at home one day just in time to stop the nanny from giving her child an enema, a practice she preached against as a nurse.[93] Others complained of unreliable nannies who made them late for work. As Figlan said, "You are fortunate if you can get somebody whom you say is reliable. . . . Sometimes you are fortunate to get somebody whom you can trust with your kids. But unfortunately, the one whom you can trust will only stay for a short time and leave. So we are always gambling." She remembered a particularly difficult time when she was left with no one to stay with her children: "I just had to take my kids straight home [to my mother in Port Elizabeth] because the person who was looking after my children said, 'I'm going, now,' and I was doing night duty and I had to be on duty."[94] Another alternative was to find some arrangement that allowed the nurse to bring her children closer to her place of work. A few of the women I interviewed did this. For example, when Lucas had her third baby, she brought the baby to the clinic to breastfeed him during the day.[95] Christina Njamela managed to arrange for her children to live with her in mission housing when she worked at the St. Matthew's Hospital.[96] Some women also

Negotiating Marriage and Family Relations

said it was easier to have their children staying with them in the villages if they were stationed at a rural clinic.[97] However, women who lived in nurses' quarters at rural clinics or hospitals often did not have that option and had to find other ways to ensure their children were cared for. Overall, as has been observed, in the late twentieth century, African women who gained more gender equality in their professional opportunities and their economic power did not see corresponding changes in their home responsibilities. Instead, they just handled added responsibilities.

The longer-term effects of a nurse's career on her children as reported by the nurses were mixed. Some highlighted the positive benefits of their careers for their children. Economically, nurses gave their children more stability and opportunities, particularly when it came to education. The majority who talked about their children's careers said they had received university educations or had skilled and secure employment. Some also noted that their careers gave their children a desire to work in their communities. On the other hand, most children of nurses did not want to become nurses or go into the medical field. This was largely because their children saw how much their mothers worked and did not want such demanding jobs. As Ntonga explained, her daughter would not take up nursing because her mother would come home tired and irritable. A few other comments also indicated that the stresses and demands of a nurse's work could make for a cranky mother. For example, Mbombo discussed how terrible it was when she was working at a rural clinic with a newborn baby. While she was grateful to be allowed to have her baby with her in the village so she could breastfeed her, at the same time, "it was tough because you had to work day and night and you are having a baby at the same time. You didn't have much rest yourself. You were so tired and irritable." On top of that, it was expensive because she had to pay for a nanny to help her in the village in addition to the expenses at her permanent home.[98] Janjties remarked that she often took her worries and thoughts about challenging cases at work home with her, which would affect her mood and even her sleep. This, she admitted, affected her family at times because "you won't have time for them."[99] Thus, at the same time that children could appreciate the work their mothers performed in the communities, they also missed their mothers or felt they had irritable mothers at times because of their work. Nurses relied on various kinds of help to cope, and those with family help did better at keeping the family together and performing well at work at the same time.

Impact on Health Care Delivery

Indeed, what happened at home and with a nurse's family relationships had an impact on her work. Coming to accurate conclusions about the exact cause and effect on the health care system requires the correlation of sources and a different set of measurements unobtainable in the historical record. However, some secondary sources and the extant archival and oral history evidence do point to some possible ways health care in the Ciskei was shaped by nurses' family relations. Family considerations influenced where nurses were willing to work and train and interrupted careers. This affected the staffing of hospitals and clinics and led to some difficulty in securing staff at rural clinics, a high turnover rate in some places, or career-long posts for nurses in other places. On the personal level, experience giving birth and having nurturing family relations themselves gave nurses greater understanding and at times sympathy for their patients, whereas stresses at home may have negatively affected the quality of care offered by other nurses.

The number of women I interviewed who reported changing jobs for family reasons indicate that nurses' family situations could have had a significant impact on staffing clinics and hospitals in the Ciskei. Again, at least twenty of the nurses I interviewed talked about changing jobs to move closer to family members, with almost all of those moving to stay with their husbands and children. Nurses explained that they did so to provide stability for the family and to keep the family together. Several had initially obtained jobs far away from their family and then sought posts to work in the same city or townships as their husbands, while others moved with their husband as soon as he obtained work elsewhere and sought a nursing position after the move. Two said that they moved specifically to obtain a position that allowed them to better care for their children, and two others changed jobs to care for a parent or sibling. After her father passed away, one nurse transferred from Baragwanath Hospital to Nessie Knight Hospital to be closer to her mother. Another two remarked that they never considered working internationally because they would miss their children.[100]

The location and demands of working at rural clinics had a more significant impact on personnel availability and staff changes than hospitals. It could be difficult to entice nurses to accept posts at rural clinics where nurses would be stationed for all but one or two weekends per month or where their children may have had difficulty accessing a good school. When asked what would bring someone to quit nursing, three interviewees cited family reasons—nurses would change professions or resign from a rural clinic to live near their families. Some Ciskeian politicians recognized these struggles. A few Ciskei legislative members voiced concern about the difficulties nurses faced in accommodating their families when moving to rural areas. For example, R. B. D. R. Myataza from the Hewu district urged the minister of health and welfare in 1982 to handle nurses' transfers better, stating, "Those who have the authority to effect

Negotiating Marriage and Family Relations

the transfers should remember this one thing, namely that an individual has a family." He pointed out that difficult and untimely transfers sometimes forced nurses to leave their children at home alone.[101] However, the testimonies of nurses and the written record indicate that authorities were not willing to accommodate nurses' families.[102] On the other hand, a few nurses requested posts at particular rural clinics so that they could live near family, either their natal family or their spouse's family. For example, Mfengqe worked at the Perksdale clinic for most of her career because she grew up in that community, her own family lived there, and her children were living there with relatives while she worked elsewhere. She requested to be allocated to the clinic so she could live with her family. She worked there for the rest of her career. At least three other women I interviewed chose to do the same.[103]

However, just because numerous nurses changed and sought jobs in the Ciskei, frequent transfers did not lead to systemwide changes, especially if the heads of the system did not see it as a problem. Up until the mid-1980s, if a number of nurses resigned or were fired for reasons linked to family considerations, matrons could easily fill the positions, regardless of the difficult working conditions. The St. Matthew's matron reported to the hospital board in 1962 that she had four hundred applications for six vacancies.[104] A decade later, the matron at Mount Coke emphasized the high incidence of unemployment among nurses in the area and reported in 1975 that she continued to receive numerous applications to work at the hospital from nurses of all grades.[105] Perhaps this oversupply caused the Ciskei minister of health and welfare in the mid-1970s to explain why he did not see a need to modify the system, commenting in the legislative debates that assembly members should not worry about the frequent transfer of nurses because it was just the nature of the profession.[106] Even when the Ciskei health care system started facing a shortage of nurses in the mid to late 1980s, authorities did not see family considerations as part of the cause. Instead, they explained that nurses left the Ciskei because they could receive better pay in the Republic of South Africa or in the expanding private hospital sector. They recognized it was difficult to retain nurses because rural clinics were less attractive but did not give specific reasons why this was the case in the official documents.[107] The government sought to address the shortage of nurses by increasing their pay and making additional provisions in 1988; but for the most part, there is little evidence that the authorities saw family considerations as a major reason to make changes.[108] Thus the system did not change explicitly because of nurses' family situations.

Pregnancy and childbirth also had a mixed impact, with the potential influence on the broader system again minimized by the labor supply. Pregnancy affected staffing in hospitals with training programs and in the broader system when women had to resign or take maternity leave. Numerous pregnancies among student nurses had the potential to affect changes in some training programs. For example, while St. Matthew's Hospital board reports do not detail the number of nurses who fell pregnant every year, from time to time the matron would report the need for greater discipline when too many student nurses had to leave because of pregnancy. Although she did not specify if the nurses were married or not, in 1969 the matron reported that she dismissed three nurses of a total of around thirty for pregnancy, and three more left pregnant at the end of their training. In the same meeting, the hospital board agreed to remove the clause in the student applications that required women to report if they had been pregnant prior to the application, presumably because doing so could help prevent a "wastage of staff."[109] At the same time, resignation because of pregnancy or maternity leaves opened up positions for those looking for temporary posts, either because their own family situation would not allow them to work full time or because jobs were scarce.[110] And if Lucas's experience is any indication, more married women seeking training eventually led training programs to change the marital status entrance requirements. Oftentimes, however, women managed to continue with their training while pregnant by keeping their marital status or pregnancies secret as long as possible. For example, Gamase Mtyeku related how she kept her pregnancy secret from Frere Hospital when she earned a study leave to complete a course in nursing education in Natal. She did not want to give up the opportunity she had worked hard to obtain. She did not even let giving birth stop her from writing an important elimination exam. On the morning of the exam, she woke up in labor. After a quick external checkup, she decided to write the exam, with the invigilator "watching me like a hawk!" She sweated through the three-hour exam and then frantically found a car and a driver to take her to the hospital, where she gave birth to her daughter after a difficult labor.[111]

Marital tensions, childbirth, the demands of child-rearing, and other family responsibilities most certainly affected the way nurses treated their own patients to some degree or another. The evidence of just how and how much is sparse. There is research yet to be done to determine any correlation between family-related stress and the way some nurses abuse patients. The scant literature on the popular view that South African public health nurses are cruel does not shed light on the influence of domestic situations. Rather, it focuses on the effect of working conditions, ideology, and insecurity as main contributing factors.[112] Daphne Murray's master's thesis on the effects of divorce on the work performance of twelve nurses in the early twenty-first century demonstrated that when the emotional, mental, and physical health of a nurse was affected by divorce, the quality of care the nurse delivered was also affected

Negotiating Marriage and Family Relations 171

negatively, as stress and exhaustion could make them irritable and less focused. At the same time, Murray also pointed out that some nurses found solace in their work, which made them more focused and caring with their patients.[113] Although her sample size was small, Murray's findings are reasonable and correspond with some of the experiences of the nurses I interviewed. For example, her finding that one of the biggest stressors after divorce was arranging for childcare certainly echoes the concerns of nurses who worked in earlier decades. Yet more research on this issue would help deliver firm conclusions about the actual correlation between stress at home and the treatment of patients.

The interviews I conducted suggest more conclusively that a nurse's own experiences with childbirth could make her more sympathetic and effective in helping women through the process. As Thoto said, "Because when you didn't have children, you don't really understand. But when . . . you've experienced it yourself, then you are more understanding."[114] Four others made similar comments. Mtyeku in particular talked about how she gained more patience for first-time mothers after having gone through the experience herself. She explained: "There may be, what, three patients in the labor ward and you're looking after these three, and this one has no control—she's in labor, they're all in labor—but they have no control if the baby will come at such-and-such time and so on, so you are bound to be impatient and jump around. But once you've delivered yourself, you summon more sympathy and more understanding."[115]

Comments by other nurses about how one is supposed to treat patients as if they were their own family members may also be an indication that good family relations made nurses more sympathetic and caring. For example, Gwayi talked about how she delighted in the social intimacy she felt with her patients. She explained that she cultivated this by greeting them as if they were her own children. For her, this was a way she could help them feel as if they were at home.[116] Kwatsha felt that whether or not a nurse treated her patients rudely had a lot to do with her own upbringing. Thinking of her patients as her own family helped her treat her patients with care. She commented, "I don't remember ever scolding a patient or being nasty to a patient because I always thought about my own relative."[117] However, as with the other issues addressed here, without more aggregate data or contemporary surveys dissecting these issues directly, it is difficult to come to firm conclusions.

Conclusion

Political, social, and economic changes led to the growth in Black nursing in South Africa, especially in "homelands" such as the Ciskei. Yet the health care system did not generally accommodate nurses' family considerations. Pregnancy and childbirth necessarily interrupted or delayed career advancement, and many nurses relocated or resigned to live near their families. As these women obtained new professional roles, they and their family members from various socioeconomic backgrounds responded differently to changing demands on the women's time and resources and the possibilities for new kinds of relationships. The testimonies of the nurses I interviewed about the challenges they faced in balancing their careers and family responsibilities attest to the uneven nature of changes in marriage and family expectations for professional African women in the 1960s through the 1980s. And yet, as they moved into demanding, prestigious careers and may have hoped for a "modern" companionate marriage, the expectation that women took primary responsibility for childcare and household management persisted. Some had a more difficult time than others negotiating responsibilities and expectations with a spouse and in-laws as they all held to different beliefs about what marriage and family life should look like.

Ultimately, the work of these nurses and the sacrifices they made were the key to the provision of rural biomedical health care in the Ciskei in the 1960s through the 1980s. As they looked back on their careers, most of the women I interviewed expressed satisfaction and joy in the role they played in delivering that health care, despite the challenges they faced in doing so. "I don't have regrets when I look back," Gqomfa concluded. "I feel that I have worked for the community. I have done what I had to do, I've imparted my knowledge to them and to my fellow workers."[118] Mhlambiso, who was stationed at the Amathole Basin clinic and later served as a government official, said, "I used to love my profession. . . . In fact, I felt satisfied. . . . Now I can see I've got old men [who I] delivered by myself. I've got ladies who are working at better places. I delivered them here. So at least I'm recognized in my area *kakhulu*. They love MaDlamini *kakhulu*. I did my best for my people."[119] Indeed, many of these nurses did their best for their people as they managed to nurture both their communities and their families.

Conclusion

WHEN I FIRST CONCEIVED OF THIS BOOK, I imagined I would conclude with an epilogue that chronicled the evolution of the health care system from the final years of the Ciskei through the transition from apartheid to the ANC-led government. I quickly realized that to do so adequately would require a book on its own. The ANC government was faced with an enormous, complex, and difficult task in reorganizing and expanding the public health sector. There have been challenges and disappointments along the way. What I offer here is a brief narrative of the final years of the Ciskei homeland and a discussion of how the retired nurses I interviewed talked about the transition to democracy's impact on the nursing profession. This provides insight into how senior nurses experienced the transition and how those experiences influenced the way they framed the past. I also present messages the nurses I interviewed had for nurses currently working in South Africa. These messages further reflect the influence of the past and present on the nurses' interpretations of their history while also offering wisdom for the future.

The unraveling of the Ciskei began even as the South African government granted it independence in 1981. As indicated in chapter 3, the 1980s were turbulent for Lennox Sebe and the Ciskei, with economic and political challenges exposing the tenuous basis of the republic. Corruption and political opposition from within and without undermined the Ciskei homeland system and Sebe's power into the early 1990s. As Jeff Peires, Cecil Manona, and Luvuyo Wotshela have described, a "wave of popular resistance" swelled in rural locations and Ciskei townships in the final years of the 1980s, resulting in widespread rejection of Ciskei National Independence Party membership cards within the Ciskei and growing resistance led by resident associations and other liberation movements in the broader region. Sebe and his associates attempted to quell this opposition. Sebe declared a state of emergency in the

174   Conclusion

face of widespread strikes on February 2, 1990, the same day F. W. de Klerk announced the unbanning of the ANC (and a little over a week before Nelson Mandela's release from prison).[1] By this time, the South African government knew the homeland system in general was failing but still attempted to have a hand in homeland politics. On March 4, 1990, South African Defense Force Brigadier Oupa Gqozo took over the Ciskei government while Sebe was visiting Hong Kong. Although the coup was peaceful, violence and looting followed in the Ciskei's biggest township of Mdantsane.

Immediately after he took over the Ciskeian government, Gqozo seemed to open up the political process in the Ciskei. He declared the Ciskei a "people's government" at his inauguration, an event attended by the United Democratic Front and graced by an ANC banner. He expressed support for residents' associations and forced all headmen to resign (as they were implicated in the apartheid system).[2] As Peires noted, he also abolished the death penalty, started investigating corruption during Sebe's time, and in some cases negotiated with workers.[3] In the meantime, a number of different nongovernmental groups increasingly worked to negotiate local economic and political development.[4] It did not take long, however, for Gqozo to show that he was more interested in upholding the system and maintaining his power rather than working for the greater good. The South African government and Ciskei leaders like Gqozo held on to the homelands as long as possible. Gqozo brought in his own security forces, supported other homeland leaders' refusal to relinquish their power (Gatsha Buthelezi in KwaZulu and Lucas Mangope in Bophuthatswana), established his own political party (the African Democratic Movement), and turned against the Ciskean people by restoring the headmen system and banning residents' associations.[5] In January 1991 Gqozo demonstrated his ruthlessness with the brazen, brutal murders of Charles Sebe (former Ciskeian chief central intelligence officer) and Onward Guzana (former Ciskei Defense Force colonel and Gqozo military council member).[6] All this behavior led to an attempted coup by the Ciskeian Defense Force in February 1991.

In an effort to salvage the situation, the South African government moved in to take over parts of the government, such as the military and Ministries of Justice and Finance. The struggle over control in the Ciskei climaxed the following year. The South African Civic Organization (SANCO) was formed in 1992 as an umbrella organization for several local movements. This strengthened civic resistance and liberation movement ties in the Ciskei. As part of the ANC's mass action campaign for the Nationalist Party to negotiate in good faith in 1992, an estimated eighty thousand protestors marched on Bhisho on September 7 to demand the reintegration of the Ciskei into South Africa and the end to military rule. The Ciskei Defense Force opened fire on the marchers, killing

Conclusion   175

twenty-eight and wounding more than two hundred.[7] Violence and resistance in various localities continued into 1993, while other local municipalities brokered their own transitions. A "caretaker" administration under the leadership of Rev. Bongani Finca (of the Border Council of Churches) was appointed to oversee the Ciskei in the month leading to the first fully democratic elections in 1994, after which the Ciskei was reincorporated into South Africa.[8]

Officials and nurses working in the Ciskei health care system generally continued to press forward with their apolitical work even as the Ciskei government was falling apart until conditions became too unbearable in the early 1990s. Some nurses had already voted with their feet, so to speak, by turning to the private sector for employment, causing staff shortages in the late 1980s. Tensions erupted with deteriorating conditions and maladministration under Gqozo. According to Mbie, this is when it started to be "a bit chaotic."[9] The military government brought in a new minister of health, welfare and pensions in April 1990, a Dr. Henk Kayser, president of the Medical Association of South Africa.[10] Six days later, nurses at Cecilia Makiwane Hospital closed the hospital to new admissions to demand better pay and working conditions. General workers had striked for similar reasons the previous month. Gqozo condemned the strikers and the National Education Health and Allied Workers' Union (Nehawu) for attempting to destabilize the government (although the union was not responsible for the strike). The strike lasted for two days, and six hundred nurses were arrested before Gqozo's military council agreed to hear their demands.[11] The following year, a civil servants' strike throughout the Ciskei stripped the hospitals of their clerical and domestic staff, leaving them in crisis.[12] Signs of further problems within the Ciskei health administration continued to surface: a director general was mysteriously suspended in 1992, Kayser was replaced by a retired teacher with no health experience, and an inexperienced director general was appointed in 1993 amid simultaneous allegations of community program funding corruption.[13] Moreover, health care workers were "faced with difficulties in delivering health care, while being associated with an unpopular regime."[14] In March 1993 Cecilia Makiwane Hospital workers declared the health system at "the point of complete collapse," in large part because of incompetent and unconcerned government officials. They lacked vital supplies and infrastructure, while the Bhisho Hospital was built in a convenient location for Ciskei politicians. Dedicated individuals sustained hospital operations.[15] Yet in March 1994 Ciskei nurses gave the director general, Dr. G. Weissinger, and his deputy an ultimatum to resign or they would "destabilize" health services. They were fed up with the behavior of these top officials as well as the mismanagement of resources. They complained that Weissinger had no interest in restructuring health services, had not been attending meetings, and dealt with staff with a sarcastic attitude. What's more, they accused some senior nurses and other officials of not representing their interests. The hospitals were dirty and the infrastructure was in "shambles," yet "huge sums of money [were] being spent every month."[16] Those working in clinics were not as affected by the hospital strikes of this period but were still no doubt influenced by the broader context.

Soon after the March 1994 threats by the nurses, the transitional administration took over in the Ciskei, and in April 1994 South Africa held elections. Subsequently, the newly formed Eastern Cape province inherited a Ciskei health care system in desperate need of new leadership and resources. The new provincial government faced the difficult task of integrating previously segregated state systems and addressing major health challenges, poverty, and underdevelopment. While the Ciskei had made progress in extending primary health care, the overall system was plagued by the "injustices and irrationality of apartheid, with grossly fragmented maldistribution of health care by 14 different health departments [ten in homelands] which emphasized curative medicine instead of placing preventative medicine first."[17] As Roger Southall and Zosa De Sas Kropiwnicki wrote, "Combining the Transkei and Ciskei bantustans with a large segment of the former (white) Cape, Eastern Province had to deal with highly uneven development, desperate poverty in the former homelands, rampant unemployment, and miserable levels of service delivery in historically Black areas."[18] In some instances, the government had to start from scratch; in others, it pieced existing structures together. As the government created new provincial and local structures in the Eastern Cape, it faced the challenges of administering a new public health care system that grappled with rising health care costs, the effects of poor living conditions, malnutrition, and illnesses such as TB, measles, diarrhea, and a new, mushrooming HIV/AIDS epidemic.[19] Wotshela further outlined how the new province had to deal with people rushing to settle on previously restricted land, seeking housing and economic opportunities.[20] This created new sanitation and infrastructure needs even as the rest of the rural and urban areas required electricity, sanitation, water, and paved roads.

The ANC devised a unified health care system to address these issues and reach the needs of all people (although some of the complaints of Ciskei nurses in March 1994 ring eerily familiar today). Starting in 1991 the South African government began to integrate its public health system, and the ANC began holding a series of meetings with the South African government, homeland officials, medical councils, and international consultants.[21] The ANC's guiding principle was that, as opposed to apartheid, everyone should have access to health care regardless of their socioeconomic situation or race. The basic

Conclusion 177

idea put forth from the beginning was to establish a "unitary national health service" administered through four levels: national, regional, district, and community. Drawing on visons of primary health care as well as community health centers of previous times, district nurses would still play a significant role in this new system.[22] There was also more openness to African medicine.[23] These meetings resulted in the adoption of a three-tiered system wherein nine new provinces oversaw smaller districts. The districts took the main administrative role, overseeing hospitals and clinics until 2004 when the provinces streamlined the system more under their control. Under the Reconstruction and Development Program adopted by the South African government in 1994, the government promised free primary health care along with upgraded housing and improved infrastructure for many people, administered through the districts. In the first decade or so after 1994, the government built 1,345 new clinics and upgraded 263 more. It also increased mass immunization.[24] In doing so, it implemented some aspects of primary health care the homelands had attempted previously. However, implementation of the new health care plan was hampered by ironing out the jurisdiction of geographic regions, stringent funding, poor management, a lack of human resources, and the HIV/AIDS crisis.[25]

Some nurses in management positions talked about the difficulties of the integration process in the Eastern Cape. Beauty Nongauza remembered many symposia held to work out the changes, and Nomali Bangani talked about how difficult it was to standardize practices when they met with nurses from the former Transkei, who did things differently like charging patients money for family planning services.[26] Ntombentsha Figlan worked in the head office overseeing VHWs. She remarked, "With the takeover, there's so much that was transitioned, there was so much that was changed, so much that was changed."[27] Others had difficulty transferring their pensions to the new system.[28] Many of the nurses I interviewed retired soon after the transition from apartheid to democratic South Africa so had little experience with the new system. Yet most of them certainly had opinions about its results. Of the forty-seven who talked about the transition, all but three talked about the changes they observed. Although a fair number commented on the better pay, greater attention to HIV/AIDS, racial integration, and better working hours of the new era, many talked about the decline in infrastructure, equipment, and supplies in both the clinics and hospitals after 1994. Six said they had shortages of medicines, while five talked about the decline in the upkeep and cleanliness of facilities. Four said the number of vehicles or the ambulance service declined. Seven lamented the waning of outreach programs such as the end of VHWs, the dropping of special mobile teams, and fewer home visits paid to patients. Although the

178 Conclusion

dreaded on-call system was discontinued and some VHWs were absorbed as paid and better-trained practitioners, those who noted the lack of community outreach were saddened by the decline in what they felt was a virtue of clinic work—taking health care to the community members, one by one. Eight nurses complained of problems with the management of the new era—too much bureaucracy and not enough accountability, putting people in upper management based on political loyalties and not merit, and the lack of funding for public health care.

The strongest theme in the responses about the changes brought on by the transition to a new South Africa was the negative effect that it had on the competency and behavior of nurses. A few made comments about the system itself, with one saying the government did not care, others commenting on the lack of practical education, and a few others saying that the government should hire retired nurses to help them fix the system. Five complained that the four-year university nursing course did not equip nurses with enough practical training. Ten interviewees talked about the presence of unions or the prevalence of strikes (legal for nurses from 1992). Some said nurses earned better pay because unions and strikes were now allowed while others felt strikers neglected patients.[29] The majority, however, talked about the deteriorating respect and discipline of junior nurses. Many did so in response to a question about what advice they would give to current or future nurses. The more grievous charge was bad nursing behavior that led to the reputation of public nurses as cruel and lazy.[30] Baleni stated curtly, "Have respect for human life. That's the message: Have respect for human life. Because nurses these days, they have no respect for human life. They do whatever."[31] Three others said current nurses did not listen to patients or their superiors, and one said they did not put patients first. This led nine to remark that current nurses cared more about money than the patients. A number compared the standard of contemporary nurses to that of their day. "The standards of nursing must go back to what we had," Mdledle argued. "But they won't listen. They've got rights."[32] Similarly, Njamela stated, "Hey! You see, when you compare them with the old stock I would say they are not that dedicated to their work, yeah. . . . The respect, their attitude towards people, you see they are not like those nurses of the olden days, yeah."[33]

Like the nurses Hull interviewed at Bethesda Hospital in KwaZulu-Natal, six nurses I interviewed directly associated this behavior with democracy. In some places, "it was a real confusion," according to Mhlambiso, "because immediately there was a change, everybody thought she was free to do anything, because it's democracy." She felt nurses even put people's health in danger at clinics when they postponed seeing a sick patient so they could take their tea

Conclusion

179

or lunch break. She continued, "We used never to have things like that. We used to get our tea time when we've finished our clients."[34] Virginia M. Mkosana called it "madness" that "people lost their respect for adults, for seniors." Clerks would come and read the newspaper the whole day because "you dare not say anything because people have their own right."[35] Even cleaners would not follow orders at times.[36] When I presented my book to retired nurses in 2018, other nurses remarked that whereas patients had respect and a feeling of *ubuntu* toward nurses before, even patients became unruly in the new era. This led Nontsikelelo Biko to conclude that democracy had "destroyed the whole system" because all "these rights" clashed with one another.[37]

The problem was not with having democracy, but the way people interpreted it. As Biko's comment indicates, for these nurses, there was a misunderstanding about what rights meant in public health care and in relation to other rights. Although Gqomfa acknowledged the unforgiving hierarchy of prior times, stating that "there was no democracy of a nurse, proper democracy in the nursing field" before, others said that younger nurses interpreted democracy to mean that anyone could do what she wanted despite the needs of the patients, that she could take chances with coming late or neglecting those in need of care.[38] Similarly, Mbombo remarked: "And at least nurses had rights now. Yeah. They could challenge some of the bad practices towards them. At least *ke* it was good in that. But the bad thing is that now there's such a lot of challenges like staff shortages, medicines are short. . . . And since people have rights now their discipline is . . . not there anymore."[39] As Ncukana put it, "You know people took democracy in a different way because though it is said everybody has a right, but each and every one saw to his or her own rights."[40] For Nkani, those who interpreted democracy in that way did not know what democracy meant. For her, it did not mean one could do what one liked but that one was self-disciplined.[41]

For nurses trained to follow a strictly hierarchical system or for those who had obtained a superior position, this challenge to authority and seeming self-interested behavior was difficult to deal with. They had been taught to put the patient first, that politics should not mix with nursing. They expected currently employed nurses to sacrifice and serve the patients regardless of the circumstances under which they worked, just as they had done. The disorder and the poor reputation of public nurses of the present sharpened the contrast they drew between the present and the positive memories of nursing in their past. Even if they acknowledged the problems of the Ciskei and the older nursing profession, some longed for the days when there was more order. As Jacob Dlamini has argued, these kinds of nostalgic expressions are not just about yearning for the good old days but also constitute wishes for the present that reveal a sense of loss. The system had changed, with a new political and professional context to which nurses had to adjust. As Dlamini wrote, systems did not change for everyone "in the way often imagined."[42] As they felt the loss of their status and struggled with junior nurses and patients in a new system, retired nurses who made these comments likely felt what they had worked so hard to attain and maintain was slipping away.

Indeed, the transitional period for health professionals in public institutions was marked by uncertainty and tension, as they had to navigate different relationships with the state, the public, patients, and other employees. As Hull has argued, comments about the problems democracy brought signal that a "new moral terrain of citizenship [was] dislodging the previous, taken-for-granted hierarchies that the nurses enjoyed as professionals."[43] Hull interviewed more midlevel and early career nurses than I did. This allowed her to discuss the tension between those asserting their citizenship or rights in a profession where they may have felt threatened by old hierarchies and new accountability structures versus those wanting to maintain control and a particular professional ethos. Hull described nurses fearing the loss of their jobs because managerial authority threatened their citizenship in the profession. Retired nurses I interviewed, on the other hand, talked more about the individual demands of junior nurses and general workers based in claims about democratic rights. Hull also analyzed comments that nurses of today are only in the profession for money. As Hull pointed out, money was an incentive for nurses entering the profession in the past and a major concern for them today, so monetary considerations are not new. However, these comments expressed a perceived individual selfish behavior on the part of a new generation of nurses, either when they voiced demands for better working conditions or perpetuated the reputation of public nurses as cruel. Perhaps the younger nurses had gone too far in asserting an entitlement. Yet Hull points to a generational tension with nurses from different age groups all fearing a loss of status, job, or appreciation.[44] This all contributed to the uncertainty and tensions of the post-apartheid period in public nursing.

Focusing on just the uncertainty and loss of the transition would leave out the legacy the nurses left. In over half the interviews I conducted, I concluded the interview by asking the nurses what advice they had for current nurses or nurses just starting their careers. The answers I received reflected not only their reaction to current trends but also nurses' individual personalities and commitments that drove their work and led to their success. The most common and fervent message the nurses I interviewed had for the next generation was that nurses should love, understand, and treat their patients with care and respect. This message came in various ways. For example, seven talked about

Conclusion

181

the importance of caring for patients. As Macaula put it, "I must tell them that . . . wherever they work and whenever they work, . . . they must care for the patients. They must love their patients and their job."[45] Likewise, Ngqokwe said, "You must love the people that you are dealing with, you see? Have your heart with them. You must do that, so that at least you know—you know them. And you know what they need, their needs nicely. Then you can't go wrong." She continued, "Medical field, it's quite nice, Les, if you really understand people. You must have the understanding of the people."[46] Like Ngqokwe, six others encouraged nurses to be understanding and empathetic. Mjikeliso, for instance, would counsel younger nurses to recognize that their patients have problems beyond just their physical health and to offer advice. As she put it, she would encourage nurses "to show interest in whatever they do, to know that people need them, to be patient with the people and tolerant with them, and to be good counselors."[47] In Francine Zani's words, they must "listen to their problems. Listen to their problems."[48] Another common phrase given: "They must be patient with the patients." In other words, nurses must not be offended easily or must not be rude, even if the patients are. Others framed this in terms of being "kind," "meek and gentle," or doing "good to the patient."[49] Rulashe used the Christian adage "do unto others as you would them unto you."[50] Indeed for some, this approach was tied up in their religious beliefs, with Dubula and Vakalisa also talking about the importance of being a Christian and drawing on God's help in nursing.[51] The need for kindness and respect for patients likely also came from their training, especially if they trained in mission hospitals. Overall, the main message was that for them, successful nursing included respect, understanding, love, and caring for patients as fellow human beings. Health care and healing was not just about the physical mechanics of the body but about human connection as well.

The other main messages the nurses I interviewed had for contemporary nurses had to do more with the character of the nursing profession, including sacrifice and selfless service. Eight nurses talked about the importance of putting the patients first, while seven talked about the need to view nursing as a calling and not merely a job. Mtyeku thought hard about what advice she would give. "*Yho!* What is that going to be?" she wondered. She finally settled on, "Don't forget that the most important person in the *whole* nursing enterprise is the patient."[52] Others made remarks such as, "Patients come first. They come first," "Patients should be their first consideration," and "They must put people first—*batho pele*."[53] This was part of the nurses' pledge and the motto of public service in the new era (*batho pele*—Sotho for "people first"). It was also tied to the notion that nursing was a calling that required courage, personal sacrifice, and a commitment to one's community or nation. As Ntonga advised, "I think a person must come to nursing because she liked it, because you want to help people, because you want to assist them, to be a relief or a helper to a person who is not well." She continued, "They must not go there for money in nursing. . . . Nursing needs somebody with a call."[54] Monetary compensation could not fully reward working in the sluice room, emptying bedpans, dealing with death, suffering, accidents, long hours, negotiating community relations, constant health education, and high-stress maternity cases. Seeing a patient walk away healthy or relieving pain had to be a reward for this kind of work as well. This was a sentiment taught and reinforced by their training, with its Christian roots.[55] Thus Majiza said, "I would think I would tell them that nursing is not a job. It's a calling. Because we have to endure so much."[56] This was the understanding that the nurses who worked in earlier times had of what was required of them, what made nursing a noble profession. They held to this professional ethos and wanted to see those in the next generation adhere to this as well.

The work of Black African nurses stationed in the Ciskei in the 1960s through the 1980s ought to be commended. Exploring apartheid homeland history with all its complexity allows us to recognize their work and achievements as a part of a problematic broader context as well as a product of varied and individual forces. The system that evolved with different political configurations during the Ciskei's lifetime relied heavily on these highly skilled practitioners to deliver preventive, primary, and curative biomedicine to an increasing number of people through clinics and hospitals. A greater understanding of the shortfalls as well as the achievements of the preceding system and its actors can lead to solutions for present or future problems. The system fell short of reaching all it had promised to reach. The broader socioeconomic context meant nurses fought a losing battle against diseases linked to malnutrition and poverty, and corrupt politics crippled the delivery of health care. However, the Ciskei did extend health care to many more people than it had before and curbed the effects of some diseases, in large part because of the nurses' training, acknowledgment of Xhosa medical beliefs and practices, and the nurses' commitment—at times at the sacrifice of attention to their own families.

South Africa continues to deal with the legacy of apartheid and the inequities of the past. Health care suffers from uneven development between geographic regions, between the urban and rural, and between private and public sectors. The poor still struggle to gain adequate access to care, and the inequities in broader society lead to great inequities in the health of individuals. There is a shortage of health workers and poor management and leadership in many places.[57] The Eastern Cape has been hit especially hard with these challenges,

Conclusion 183

becoming a "by-word for inefficiency and mismanagement," making some express nostalgia for homeland leaders in the face of inadequate service delivery today.[58] This history has shown that having adequate funding and staff can support the diffusion of health care through community clinics that can reach more people in remote locations in dire need of health care. It also demonstrates that nurses' demands for better pay and greater attention to their working conditions are valid and need to be balanced with expectations of caring and respectful nursing. Adequate practical, theoretical, and ethical training for nurses who are committed to their work is key—but should also be accompanied by appropriate renumeration and working conditions that accommodate family life. It was the hope of nurses who openly shared their personal stories of marital tensions and difficulties raising their children that other women would learn from their experiences to be more resilient and self-respecting. Continued openness to and cooperation with African medicine could also improve people's health and access to care, especially when there is mutual respect and a desire to find points of commonality. All these lessons are important as South Africa and other nations work to provide health care to more of their people and nurses continue to play a key role in delivering care and shaping the health of their people.

Notes

Introduction

1. For example, African nurses working in all the homelands combined numbered 10,725 in 1973 whereas the total number was 20,000 in 1978. See Shula Marks, *Divided Sisterhood: Race, Class, and Gender in the South African Nursing Profession* (New York: St. Martin's, 1994), 170; South African Institute of Race Relations, *A Survey of Race Relations in South Africa 1973* (Johannesburg: South African Institute of Race Relations, 1974), 351.

2. Joan Van Dyk, "Why Covid Likely Won't Change the Plight of Community Health Workers," *Mail and Guardian*, November 2, 2020.

3. Mafika Pascal Gwala, ed., *Black Review 1973* (Durban: Black Community Programmes, 1974), 14. For more on the effects of apartheid on South African health and the health care system, see Director General, World Health Organization, "Health Implications of Apartheid in South Africa," Notes and Documents/Unit on Apartheid; no. 5/75 (United Nations, Dept. of Political and Security Council Affairs, 1975); Saldru Community Health Project, *Health and Health Services in the Ciskei*, Saldru Working Papers, no. 54 (Cape Town: Saldru, 1983); Cedric de Beer, *The South African Disease: Apartheid Health and Health Services* (Trenton, NJ: Africa World, 1986); Randall M. Packard, *White Plague, Black Labor: Tuberculosis and the Political Economy of Health and Disease in South Africa* (Berkeley: University of California Press, 1989); Steven Feierman and John M. Janzen, eds., *The Social Basis of Health and Healing in Africa* (Berkeley: University of California Press, 1992); Diana Wylie, *Starving on a Full Stomach: Hunger and the Triumph of Cultural Racism in Modern South Africa* (Charlottesville: University Press of Virginia, 2001); Stephens Ntsoakae Phatlane, "Poverty, Health and Disease in the Era of High Apartheid: South Africa, 1948–1976" (PhD diss., University of South Africa, 2009). For more on the history of South African health care and medicine, see Anne Digby, "The Medical History of South Africa: An Overview," *History Compass* 6, no. 5 (2008): 1194–1210; Julie Parle and Vanessa Noble, "New Directions and Challenges in Histories of Health, Healing and Medicine in South Africa," *Medical History* 58, no. 2 (April 2014): 147–65.

4. The scattered "homelands" included the Ciskei, Transkei, KwaZulu, QwaQwa, Bophuthatswana, KwaNdebele, KaNgwana, Lebowa, Gazankulu, and Venda. The

process of reorganizing governments and local services into these supposed new nations started in 1959 with the Promotion of Bantu Self-Government Act, and homelands persisted into the early 1990s (though only four gained official independence). Instead of using the term "homeland," some have used the term "Bantustan" as a derogatory term to indicate the governments were a political stunt (Bantustan being related to the term "Bantu" used by the apartheid government to classify people). I use the term "homeland" or "apartheid homeland" because most local South Africans I interviewed used that term, and it is now widely recognized that the homelands were not true reflections of the land these ethnic groups had occupied prior to European colonization.

5. Jeff Peires, "The Implosion of Transkei and Ciskei," *African Affairs* 91, no. 364 (1992): 365–87; Bernard Magubane et al., "Resistance and Repression in the Bantustans," in *The Road to Democracy in South Africa*, vol. 2, ed. South African Democracy Education Trust (SADET) (Pretoria: Unisa Press, 2006), 749–802; Timothy Gibbs, *Mandela's Kinsmen: Nationalist Elites and Apartheid's First Bantustan* (Melton, Woodbridge, UK: James Currey, 2014); Luvuyo Wotshela, "The Fate of Ciskei and Adjacent Border Towns: Political Transition in a Democratic South Africa, 1985–1995," in *Road to Democracy in South Africa*, vol. 4, pt. 3 (Ibadan, Nigeria: Pan-African University Press, 2019), 1855–99.

6. Marks, *Divided Sisterhood*. Racial restrictions were formally introduced into the South African Nursing Association in the late 1950s.

7. Charlotte Searle, *The History of the Development of Nursing in South Africa, 1652–1960* (Cape Town: Struik, 1965); Charlotte Searle, *Towards Excellence: The Centenary of State Registration for Nurses and Midwives in South Africa, 1891–1991* (Durban: Butterworths, 1991); Idalia Loots and Molly Vermaak, *Pioneers of Professional Nursing in South Africa* (Bloemfontein, South Africa: P. J. de Villiers, 1975); Eugéne Potgieter, *Professional Nursing Education 1860–1991* (Pretoria: Academica, 1992); Grace Mashaba, *Rising to the Challenge of Change: A History of Black Nursing in South Africa* (Kenwyn, South Africa: Juta, 1995); Martina Egli and Denise Krayer, *"Mothers and Daughters": The Training of African Nurses by Missionary Nurses of the Swiss Mission in South Africa*, Histoire et Héritages—Approche Pluridisciplinaire 4 (Lausanne, Switzerland: Le Fait missionnaire, 1997); Simonne Horwitz, "'Black Nurses in White': Exploring Young Women's Entry into the Nursing Profession at Baragwanath Hospital, Soweto, 1948–1980," *Social History of Medicine* 20, no. 1 (2007): 131–46.

8. Ntsoaki Senokoanyane, *Their Light, Love and Life: A Black Nurse's Story* (Cape Town: Kwela Books, 1995); Mashaba, *Rising to the Challenge of Change*; Mazo Sybil T. MaDlamini Buthelezi, *African Nurse Pioneers in KwaZulu/Natal, 1920–2000* (Victoria, BC: Trafford, 2004); Doreen Merle Foster, *Lahlekile: A Twentieth Century Chronicle of Nursing in South Africa* (Brentwood, UK: Chipmukapublishing, 2007); Thokozani Mhlongo, "Profiling Black South African Nurse Pioneers: Promoting the Black Biography," *Nursing Times Research* 9, no. 65 (2004): 65–72; Horwitz, "'Black Nurses in White'"; Elizabeth Hull, *Contingent Citizens: Professional Aspiration in a South African Hospital* (New York: Bloomsbury Academic, 2017).

9. Anne Digby, "'The Bandwagon of Golden Opportunities'? Health Care in South Africa's Bantustan Periphery," *South African Historical Journal* 64, no. 4 (2012): 827–85; Hull, *Contingent Citizens*; Elizabeth Hull, "International Migration, 'Domestic

Struggles' and Status Aspiration among Nurses in South Africa," *Journal of Southern African Studies* 36, no. 4 (December 2010): 851–67.

10. Anne Digby and Howard Phillips, *At the Heart of Healing: Groote Schuur Hospital, 1938–2008* (Auckland Park, South Africa: Jacana Media, 2008); Simonne Horwitz, *Baragwanath Hospital, Soweto: A History of Medical Care, 1941–1990* (Johannesburg: Wits University Press, 2013); Hull, *Contingent Citizens*.

11. Horwitz, *Baragwanath Hospital*; Hull, *Contingent Citizens*.

12. Pat Holden and Jenny Littlewood, eds., *Anthropology and Nursing* (New York: Routledge, 1991).

13. Digby, "Bandwagon," 832, 849. Lack of resources hindered implementation in most homelands, but Digby points out that the Ciskei and Bophuthatswana were best endowed as far as financial resources went, with two or three times the per capita expenditures of KwaNdebele and Lebowa. Digby writes that this may have been in part due to Ciskei's more widespread urbanization and Bophuthatswana's mines. Salaries made up the bulk of the budget in the Ciskei.

14. Les Switzer, *Power and Resistance in an African Society: The Ciskei Xhosa and the Making of South Africa* (Madison: University of Wisconsin Press, 1993); Peires, "The Implosion of Transkei and Ciskei"; Luvuyo Wotshela, "Homeland Consolidation, Resettlement and Local Politics in the Border and the Ciskei Region of the Eastern Cape, South Africa, 1960–1996" (PhD diss., Oxford University, 2001); Luvuyo Wotshela, "Territorial Manipulation in Apartheid South Africa: Resettlement, Tribal Politics, and the Making of the Northern Ciskei, 1975–1990," *Journal of Southern African Studies* 30, no. 2 (June 2004): 317–37.

15. Peires, "The Implosion of Transkei and Ciskei," 382.

16. Saldru Community Health Project, *Health and Health Services in the Ciskei*; Switzer, *Power and Resistance in an African Society*. The population almost doubled between 1973 and 1983, from about 350,000 to 630,000 (Saldru, *Health and Health Services in the Ciskei*, 6). As Switzer pointed out, although the Ciskei had increased the number of beds in hospitals and clinics in the 1970s, the proportion of those beds to the population virtually stayed the same, increasing from 2.1 per 1,000 in 1946 to only 2.3 in 1980 (Switzer, *Power and Resistance in an African Society*, 339).

17. Jeffrey Butler, Robert I. Rotberg, and John Adams, *The Black Homelands of South Africa: The Political and Economic Development of Bophuthatswana and KwaZulu* (Berkeley: University of California Press, 1977), 241; South African Institute of Race Relations, *A Survey of Race Relations in South Africa*, 1960–83; Saldru Community Health Project, *Health and Health Services in the Ciskei*, 35; Switzer, *Power and Resistance in an African Society*, 340.

18. De Beer, *The South African Disease*. De Beer's chapter 4 on Bantustan health and health care paints a dismal picture of overcrowded, poverty-stricken areas and failing health systems.

19. Switzer, *Power and Resistance in an African Society*, 213 and 339.

20. "East Cape Head of BPC Denies Plan to Kill Homeland Leaders," May 13, 1975, *Daily Dispatch*. See also Magubane et al., "Resistance and Repression in the Bantustans," 774.

21. Wotshela, "Homeland Consolidation, Resettlement and Local Politics"; Luvuyo Wotshela, "Insurrection and Locally Negotiated Transition in Stutterheim, Eastern

Cape, 1980–1994," in *From Apartheid to Democracy: Localities and Liberation*, ed. Christopher Saunders (Cape Town: Department of Historical Studies, University of Cape Town, 2007), 49–68; Wotshela, "The Fate of Ciskei."

22. Meghan Healy-Clancy, "The Everyday Politics of Being a Student in South Africa: A History," *History Compass* 15, no. 3 (2017): 5, https://doi.org/10.1111/hic3.12375; Daniel Magaziner, *The Art of Life in South Africa* (Athens: Ohio University Press, 2016), 8–9, n. 25.

23. William Beinart, "Beyond 'Homelands': Some Ideas about the History of African Rural Areas in South Africa," *South African Historical Journal* 64, no. 1 (2012): 5.

24. Steffen Jensen and Olaf Zenker, "Homelands as Frontiers: Apartheid's Loose Ends—An Introduction," *Journal of Southern African Studies* 41, no. 5 (2015): 939.

25. Beinart, "Beyond 'Homelands.'" Beinart's article was the publication of a talk he gave at a conference held at Wits University in 2011 that resulted in a special journal issue titled "Let's Talk about Bantustans." For discussions of the Ciskei and homeland health care in this issue, see Laura Evans, "South Africa's Homelands and the Dynamics of 'Decolonization': Reflections on Writing Histories of the Homelands," *South African Historical Journal* 64, no. 1 (2012): 117–37; and Elizabeth Hull, "The Renewal of Community Health under the KwaZulu 'Homeland' Government," *South African Historical Journal* 64, no. 1 (2012): 22–40.

26. Retired nurses' dialogue with author, November 7, 2018, Ginsberg.

27. Lulu Msutu Zuma, interview by the author, May 30 and 31, 2012, Jubisa.

28. Hull, *Contingent Citizens*, 94.

29. Digby, "Bandwagon," 835–36.

30. Horwitz, *Baragwanath Hospital*; Jacob Dlamini, *Native Nostalgia* (Auckland Park, South Africa: Jacana Media, 2009). See also Mwelela Cele, "Even Apartheid Couldn't Kill TV's Splendor," New Frame, August 20, 2018, www.newframe.com.

31. For a prominent example, see Feierman and Janzen, *The Social Basis of Health and Healing in Africa*.

32. Jean Comaroff and John Comaroff, *Of Revelation and Revolution: Christianity, Colonialism, and Consciousness in South Africa*, vol. 1 (Chicago: University of Chicago Press, 1991).

33. Anne Digby and Helen Sweet, "Nurses as Culture Brokers in Twentieth-Century South Africa," in *Plural Medicine, Tradition and Modernity, 1800–2000*, ed. Waltraud Ernst (New York: Routledge, 2002), 113–29; Anne Digby, *Diversity and Division in Medicine: Health Care in South Africa from the 1800s* (Oxford: Peter Lang, 2006); Barbra Mann Wall, *Into Africa: A Transnational History of Catholic Medical Missions and Social Change* (New Brunswick, NJ: Rutgers University Press, 2015); Karen E. Flint, *Healing Traditions: African Medicine, Cultural Exchange, and Competition in South Africa, 1820–1948* (Athens: Ohio University Press, 2008); Ruth J. Prince and Rebecca Marsland, eds., *Making and Unmaking Public Health in Africa: Ethnographic and Historical Perspectives*, Cambridge Center of African Studies Series (Athens: Ohio University Press, 2014); David Baranov, *The African Transformation of Western Medicine and the Dynamics of Global Cultural Exchange* (Philadelphia: Temple University Press, 2008); David Gordon, "A Sword of Empire? Medicine and Colonialism at King William's Town, Xhosaland, 1856–91," in *Medicine and Colonial Identity*, ed. Mary P. Sutphen and Bridie Andrews (New York: Routledge, 2003), 41–60; Parle and Noble, "New Directions."

Notes to Pages 11–14   189

34. Gordon, "A Sword of Empire"; Flint, *Healing Traditions*.

35. Wall, *Into Africa*, 24; Nancy Rose Hunt, *A Colonial Lexicon: Of Birth Ritual, Medicalization, and Mobility in the Congo* (Durham, NC: Duke University Press, 1999).

36. Baranov, *The African Transformation*.

37. For quote see Baranov, *The African Transformation*, 18.

38. Digby, *Diversity and Division*. See also Flint's discussion of "tradition" in *Healing Traditions*.

39. Baranov, *The African Transformation*, 19.

40. Digby and Sweet, "Nurses as Culture Brokers"; Digby, *Diversity and Division*; Wall, *Into Africa*, 24; Hunt, *A Colonial Lexicon*.

41. Pat Holden, "Nursing Sisters in Nigeria, Uganda, Tanganyika, 1929–1978," Oxford Development Records Project (Oxford: Rhodes House Library, 1984); A. Mangay Maglacas and John Simons, eds., *The Potential of the Traditional Birth Attendant* (Geneva: World Health Organization, 1986); Karin A. Shapiro, "Doctors or Medical Aids—The Debate over the Training of Black Medical Personnel for the Rural Black Population in South Africa in the 1920s and 1930s," *Journal of Southern African Studies* 13, no. 2 (January 1987): 234–55; Pearl T. Robinson, "Fatimata Traore, Nurse-Midwife: Combining a Successful Family Planning Program with Community Development," *Sage* 7, no. 1 (1990): 55–56; Hunt, *A Colonial Lexicon*; Chishamiso Rowley, "Challenges to Effective Maternal Health Care Delivery: The Case of Traditional and Certified Nurse Midwives in Zimbabwe," *Journal of Asian and African Studies* 35, no. 2 (2000): 251–64.

42. Mechthild Reh and Gudrun Ludwar-Ene, eds., *Gender and Identity in Africa* (Munster: Lit, 1995); Jean Allman, Susan Geiger, and Nakanyike Musisi, eds., *Women in African Colonial Histories* (Bloomington: Indiana University Press, 2002); Tabitha Kanogo, *African Womanhood in Colonial Kenya: 1900–1950* (Athens: Ohio University Press, 2005); Iris Berger, *Women in Twentieth-Century Africa* (Cambridge: Cambridge University Press, 2016); Kathleen Sheldon, *African Women: Early History to the 21st Century* (Bloomington: Indiana University Press, 2017).

43. Ifi Amadiume, *Daughters of the Goddess, Daughters of Imperialism: African Women, Culture, Power, and Democracy* (New York: Zed Books, 2000); Corrie Decker, *Mobilizing Zanzibari Women: The Struggle for Respectability and Self-Reliance in Colonial East Africa* (New York: Palgrave Macmillan, 2014); Liz Walker, "'They Heal in the Spirit of the Mother': Gender, Race and Professionalisation of South African Women," *African Studies* 62, no. 1 (2003): 99–123.

44. Other historians have analyzed the mission-educated elite or marriage during the colonial period, including Kristin Mann, *Marrying Well: Marriage, Status and Social Change among the Educated Elite in Colonial Lagos* (New York: Cambridge University Press, 1985); Jane L. Parpart, "'Where Is Your Mother?': Gender, Urban Marriage, and Colonial Discourse on the Zambian Copperbelt, 1924–1945," *International Journal of African Historical Studies* 27, no. 2 (1994): 241–71; Allman, Geiger, and Musisi, *Women in African Colonial Histories*; Jean Comaroff and John Comaroff, "Homemade Hegemony," in *Ethnography and the Historical Imagination: Selected Essays*, ed. Jean Comaroff and John Comaroff (Boulder, CO: Westview, 1992); Meghan Healy-Clancy, "The Politics of New African Marriage in Segregationist South Africa," *African Studies Review* 57, no. 2 (September 2014): 7–28; Meghan Healy-Clancy, "Introduction: ASR

Notes to Page 14

Forum: The Politics of Marriage in South Africa," *African Studies Review* 57, no. 2 (September 2014): 1–5; Monica Wilson, "Xhosa Marriage in Historical Perspective," in *Essays on African Marriage in Southern Africa*, ed. Eileen Jensen Krige and John Comaroff (Cape Town: Juta, 1981), 133–47. An exception would be Wilson, "Xhosa Marriage in Historical Perspective," 133–47.

45. Christine Oppong's book on the conjugal and maternal roles of Accra nurses, Daphne Murray's study on divorce among nurses, and Elizabeth Hull's article on the domestic struggles that influenced nurses' employment decisions stand out as exceptions yet are not written as histories. See Christine Oppong, "Nursing Mothers: Aspects of the Conjugal and Maternal Roles of Nurses in Accra" (Canadian African Studies Association Meeting, Toronto, 1975); Daphne Murray, "The Impact of Divorce on Work Performance of Professional Nurses in Tertiary Hospitals of the Buffalo City Municipality" (master's thesis, University of Fort Hare, 2012); Hull, "International Migration." Works on marriage and motherhood mostly focus on the political or public aspect of these categories: Lynn M. Thomas, *Politics of the Womb: Women, Reproduction, and the State in Kenya* (Berkeley: University of California Press, 2003); Emily Osborn, *Our New Husbands Are Here: Households, Gender, and Politics in a West African State from the Slave Trade to Colonial Rule* (Athens: Ohio University Press, 2011); Rhiannon Stephens, *A History of African Motherhood: The Case of Uganda, 700–1900* (New York: Cambridge University Press, 2013); Emily Burrill, *States of Marriage: Gender, Justice and Rights in Colonial Mali* (Athens: Ohio University Press, 2015); Rachel Jean-Baptiste and Emily Burrill, "Love, Marriage, and Families in Africa," in *Holding the World Together: African Women in Changing Perspective*, edited by Nwando Achebe and Claire Robertson (Madison: University of Wisconsin Press, 2019), 275–93.

46. Meghan Healy-Clancy, "Women and the Problem of Family in Early African Nationalist History and Historiography," *South African Historical Journal* 64, no. 3 (2012): 450–71; Healy-Clancy, "The Politics of Marriage in South Africa"; Healy-Clancy, "The Politics of New African Marriage"; Zubeida Jaffer, *Beauty of the Heart: The Life and Times of Charlotte Mannya Maxeke* (Bloemfontein, South Africa: SUN, 2016); Iris Berger, "An African American 'Mother of the Nation': Madie Hall Xuma in South Africa, 1940–1963," *Journal of Southern African Studies* 27, no. 3 (2001): 547–66; Lynn M. Thomas and Jennifer Cole, eds., *Love in Africa* (Chicago: University of Chicago Press, 2009); Cherryl Walker, ed., *Women and Gender in Southern Africa to 1945* (Cape Town: David Philip and James Currey, 1990); Cherryl Walker, *Women and Resistance in South Africa* (New York: Monthly Review Press, 1991); Cherryl Walker, "Conceptualising Motherhood in Twentieth Century South Africa," *Journal of Southern African Studies* 21, no. 3 (September 1995): 417–37; Julia C. Wells, *We Now Demand! The History of Women's Resistance to Pass Laws in South Africa* (Johannesburg: Wits University Press, 1993); Deborah May, *You Have Struck a Rock!*, DVD (California News Reel, 1981); Nomboniso Gasa, ed., *Women in South African History* (Cape Town: Human Science Research Council Press, 2007); Zine Magubane, "Attitudes Towards Feminism Among Women in the ANC, 1950–1990: A Theoretical Re-Interpretation," in *The Road to Democracy in South Africa*, vol. 4, *1980–1990* (Pretoria: Unisa Press, 2010), 975–1034; Daniel Magaziner, "Pieces of a (Wo)Man: Feminism, Gender, and Adulthood in Black Consciousness, 1968–1977," *Journal of Southern African Studies* 37, no. 1 (2011): 45–61; Shireen Hassim, *Women's Organizations and Democracy in South Africa: Contesting*

Authority (Madison: University of Wisconsin Press, 2006); Shireen Hassim, *The ANC Women's League: Sex, Gender and Politics*, Ohio Short Histories of Africa (Athens: Ohio University Press, 2014); Arianna Lissoni and Maria Suriano, "Married to the ANC: Tanzanian Women's Entanglement in South Africa's Liberation Struggle," *Journal of Southern African Studies* 40, no. 1 (2014): 129–50.

47. Hospital reports for Mount Coke and St. Matthew's proved very helpful in gauging changes in health care approaches, clinical work, diseases, and obtaining a glimpse into the conditions nurses trained and worked under. Records for the Victoria Hospital were scattered in various archives and did not include many documents from the late 1960s and 1970s. The Nompumelelo Hospital in Peddie, founded in 1964 by a Dutch Reformed Church mission, had no mission records in public collections.

48. Les Switzer, *Media and Dependency in South Africa*, Africa Series 47 (Athens: Ohio University Monographs in International Studies, 1985).

49. "The Ciskeian Nursing Council: Report of the Second Council, Term of Office, 1 August 1987 to 31 July 1992," 26, in author's possession.

50. Joe Lunn, *Memoirs of the Maelstrom: A Senegalese Oral History of the First World War* (Portsmouth, NH: Heinemann, 1999), 5.

51. The number of retired nurses interviewed who worked in each major hospital catchment area include (some worked in multiple areas, so may be counted multiple times): twenty-seven in Mount Coke Hospital and clinics and its successor, Bhisho Hospital; twenty-five in St. Matthews Hospital and clinics and its successor, S. S. Gida Hospital; twelve in Victoria Hospital and clinics (which had many fewer clinics); and eleven in Nompumelelo Hospital and clinics (which also had fewer clinics and a shorter life span). I interviewed two who worked in the northern areas (Thornhill and Sada, newly built in the Ciskei) and nine who worked at Cecilia Makiwane Hospital (which became the main referral hospital that focused on urban clinics).

52. For those in retired nurses' associations, I provided a list of general, open-ended questions in advance to give them time to think about the questions and understand the purpose of the interview. This could have restricted the women's process of remembering, yet some paid attention to these questions and others did not.

53. Sherna Berger Gluck and Daphne Patai, eds., *Women's Words: The Feminist Practice of Oral History* (New York: Routledge, 1991); Sherna Berger Gluck, "Women's Oral History: Is It So Special?," in *Handbook of Oral History*, ed. Thomas Charlton, Lois E. Myers, and Rebecca Sharpless (Lanham, MO: AltaMira, 2006), 357–83; David William Cohen, "Doing Social History from Pim's Doorway," in *Reliving the Past: The Worlds of Social History*, ed. Olivier Zunz (Chapel Hill: University of North Carolina Press, 2014), 191–235. See also life history work noted below.

54. For discussions of life histories of African women and oral history, see Edward Alpers, "The Story of Swema: Female Vulnerability in Nineteenth-Century East Africa," in *Women and Slavery in Africa*, ed. Claire Robertson and Martin Klein (Madison: University of Wisconsin Press, 1983); Sarah Mirza and Margaret Strobel, *Three Swahili Women: Studies in Social and Economic Change* (Bloomington: Indiana University Press, 1989); Belinda Bozzoli, *Women of Phokeng: Consciousness, Life Strategy, and Migrancy in South Africa, 1900–1983* (Portsmouth, NH: Heinemann, 1991); Marcia Wright, *Strategies of Slaves & Women: Life-Stories from East/Central Africa* (New York: Lilian Barber Press, 1993); Heidi Gengenbach, "Truth-Telling and the Life Narrrative of African

Women: A Reply to Kirk Hoppe," *International Journal of African Historical Studies* 26, no. 3 (1993): 619–27; Nwando Achebe, *Farmers, Traders, Warriors, and Kings: Female Power and Authority in Northern Igboland, 1900–1960* (Portsmouth, NH: Heinemann, 2005), 7–8.

55. Leslie Anne Hadfield, "Can We Believe the Stories about Biko? Oral Sources, Meaning, and Emotion in South African Struggle History," *History in Africa* 42, no. 1 (2015): 239–63.

56. Alecia Phiwo Dubula, interview by the author, May 4, 2012, Bhisho; Penolope Ntshona, interview by the author, October 21, 2013, Alice; Lumka Someketha, interview by the author, May 29, 2012, King William's Town. The challenge of clearly separating chronology in one's memory may have also made for exaggerations of improvements made in the Ciskei independent period, but they are a natural reflection of how the changes in homelands occurred over time, with actual independence acting as an artificial break from the past.

Chapter 1. Medical Systems and the Rise of African Nursing

1. Thandiswa Florence Makiwane also married Xhosa intellectual D. D. T. Jabavu and helped found the Zenzele Women's Self-Help organization. More on Florence Jabavu can be found in Catharine Higgs, "Helping Ourselves: Black Women and Grassroots Activism in Segregated South Africa, 1922–1952," in *Stepping Forward: Black Women in Africa and the Americas*, ed. Catharine Higgs, Barbara A. Moss, and Earline Rae Ferguson (Athens: Ohio University Press, 2002), 59–72.

2. Flint, *Healing Traditions*.

3. Digby, *Diversity and Division*, 302.

4. Baranov, *The African Transformation*, chap. 4.

5. Digby, *Diversity and Division*, 279.

6. Elizabeth van Heyningen, "Medical Practice in the Eastern Cape," in *The Cape Doctor in the Nineteenth Century: A Social History*, ed. Harriet Deacon, Howard Phillips, and Elizabeth van Heyningen (Amsterdam: Rodopi, 2004), 169–94. Van Heyningen argues that the work of anthropologists in two different decades demonstrates the continuities in Xhosa healing, but this chapter will also highlight major changes.

7. Harriet Ngubane categorizes Zulu recognized causes of ill-health as natural causes, sorcery, pollution and the withdrawing of protection of ancestors. See Harriet Ngubane, *Body and Mind in Zulu Medicine: An Ethnography of Health and Disease in Nyuswa-Zulu Thought and Practice* (New York: Academic, 1977). Hammond-Tooke also emphasized that pollution caused by natural forces was one of the recognized causes of illness or misfortune among Nguni people. W. D. Hammond-Tooke, "The Uniqueness of Nguni Mediumistic Divination in Southern Africa," *Africa* 72, no. 2 (2002): 279.

8. Flint, *Healing Traditions*, 46–56. See also Ngubane, *Body and Mind*, chap. 2.

9. Jeff B. Peires, *The Dead Will Arise: Nongqawuse and the Great Xhosa Cattle-Killing Movement of 1856–7* (Bloomington: Indiana University Press, 1989), 71.

10. Dr. A. B. Xuma, "The African Concept of Disease," address delivered at Study Course in African Culture and Its Relation to the Training of African Nurses conference of 1954, Jane McLarty Papers, B.1.4, Historical Papers, William Cullen Library, University of the Witwatersrand (hereafter HP).

Notes to Pages 23–26

11. Baranov, *The African Transformation*, 181.

12. Jeff Peires, *The House of Phalo: A History of the Xhosa People in the Days of their Independence* (Johannesburg: Jonathan Ball, 2003), 75.

13. See in particular, Ngubane's discussion in Ngubane, *Body and Mind*, chap. 4.

14. Gordon, "A Sword of Empire," 43.

15. Manton Hirst, "Dreams and Medicines: The Perspective of Xhosa Diviners and Novices in the Eastern Cape, South Africa," *Indo-Pacific Journal of Phenomenology* 5, no. 2 (December 2005): 2.

16. Hirst, "Dreams and Medicines," 3–4. Hirst argued that there is no real distinction between witches and sorcerers among the Xhosa.

17. John Henderson Soga, *The Ama-Xhosa: Life and Customs* (Lovedale, South Africa: Lovedale, 1932), 213, 215, 298.

18. Philip Mayer and Iona Mayer, *Townsmen or Tribesmen: Conservatism and the Process of Urbanization in a South African City*, 2nd ed. (New York: Oxford University Press, 1971), 162. See also Hirst, "Dreams and Medicines," 4. This description of being kicked by the bird to describe TB likely arose with the spread of TB in South Africa in the late nineteenth and early twentieth centuries, although Packard argues that TB was also likely present among African populations before European contact, even if at low levels. Packard, *White Plague, Black Labor*, 25.

19. Hirst, "Dreams and Medicines," 12–13.

20. Xuma, "The African Concept of Disease," Jane McLarty Papers, HP.

21. See Peires, *The Dead Will Arise*.

22. Soga, *The Ama-Xhosa*, 178.

23. Gordon, "A Sword of Empire," 43.

24. Soga, *The Ama-Xhosa*, 178.

25. Soga, *The Ama-Xhosa*, 156.

26. Digby, *Diversity and Division*, 294.

27. Manton Hirst, "The Healer's Art: Cape Nguni Diviners in the Townships of Grahamstown, Eastern Cape, South Africa," *Curare* 16, no. 2 (1990): 111, n. 3; Soga, *The Ama-Xhosa*, 167–68, 173, 175. See also Xuma, "The African Concept of Disease," Jane McLarty Papers, HP. Hammond-Tooke lists various types of diviners, found in Southern African groups that were at one point found among the Xhosa as well, in W. D. Hammond-Tooke, *The Bantu-Speaking Peoples of Southern Africa* (London: Routledge and Kegan Paul, 1980), 349.

28. Flint has shown in *Healing Traditions* that in the course of the nineteenth and twentieth centuries, because of the interaction with British colonialism in Natal, the roles of various Zulu healers were simplified. Whereas before there were doctors for specific purposes with specific skills, the different categories all fell into one larger category of *isangoma* (a term now also used by the Xhosa). The same has apparently happened with Xhosa terms for healers, although the experience with colonialism in the Eastern Cape differed from that in the Natal colony. Both Soga and Hirst also noted the decline in the first half of the twentieth century of *imilozi*, *amagqirha* who could give voice to ancestors, who would speak through them (Soga, *The Ama-Xhosa*, 163, 169; Hirst "The Healer's Art," 97).

29. Gordon, "A Sword of Empire," 44; Hirst, "Dreams and Medicines," 6; Soga, *The Ama-Xosa*, 160.

194 Notes to Pages 26–32

30. Hirst, "Dreams and Medicines," 7; Gordon, "A Sword of Empire," 44.

31. Soga, *The Ama-Xhosa*, 165.

32. Soga, *The Ama-Xhosa*, 5.

33. Hirst, "The Healer's Art," 100.

34. Hammond-Tooke, "The Uniqueness of Nguni Mediumistic Divination."

35. Hirst, "Dreams and Medicines," 7. See also Catherine Burns, "Louisa Mvemve: A Woman's Advice to the Public on the Cure of Various Diseases," *Kronos* 23 (November 1996): 108–34.

36. Flint, *Healing Traditions*. Flint also argues that the gender makeup of Zulu healers changed because of the way the colonial law licensed herbalists as opposed to *isangoma*.

37. Hammond-Tooke, "The Uniqueness of Nguni Mediumistic Divination," 278.

38. Gordon, "A Sword of Empire," 44.

39. Gordon, "A Sword of Empire," 43.

40. Hirst, "Dreams and Medicines," 6. In this article, Hirst demonstrated how *amagqirha* draw on dreams to discover upcoming clients or certain medicines or receive communication from ancestors. Soga also emphasized the importance of dreams in *The Ama-Xosa*, 156–58. By the 1930s Soga described shillings replacing the assegai or spear as an initial form of payment to *amagqirha* (Soga, *The Ama-Xosa*, 158, 160, 170–73).

41. Hirst, "Dreams and Medicines," 14; Baranov, *The African Transformation*, 19.

42. Peires, *The House of Phalo*, 15 and 11, respectively.

43. Peires, *The House of Phalo*, 11.

44. Hirst, "Dreams and Medicines," 4.

45. Rankin wrote that environmentalism was especially employed by practitioners in tropical environments in Africa (John Rankin, *Healing the African Body: British Medicine in West Africa, 1800–1860* [Columbia: University of Missouri Press, 2015]). Gordon described how Fitzgerald at Grey Hospital designed the hospital to protect patients from atmospheric pollution according to the miasmatic theories of medicine (Gordon, "A Sword of Empire," 49).

46. Rankin, *Healing the African Body*, especially 30–38. See also Jonathan Roberts, "Western Medicine in Africa to 1900, Part 1: North, West and Central Africa," *History Compass* 15, no. e12400 (2017): 1–8, https://doi.org/10.1111/hic3.12400; Jonathan Roberts, "Western Medicine in Africa, Part 2: Ethiopia, East and Southern Africa to 1900," *History Compass*, 15, no. e12393 (2017): 1–8, https://doi.org/10.1111/hic3.12393.

47. Peires, *The Dead Will Arise*, 59. See also Gordon, "A Sword of Empire."

48. Gordon, "A Sword of Empire." 45.

49. Peires, *The Dead Will Arise*, 60.

50. Mashaba, *Rising to the Challenge*, 2.

51. Peires, *The Dead Will Arise*, 12.

52. Peires, *The Dead Will Arise*, 319.

53. Searle, *History of the Development of Nursing in South Africa*, 130.

54. Mashaba, *Rising to the Challenge*, 3.

55. Searle, *History of the Development of Nursing in South Africa*, 131–33.

56. Catherine Burns, "'A Man Is a Clumsy Thing Who Does Not Know How to Handle a Sick Person': Aspects of the History of Masculinity and Race in the Shaping of Male Nursing in South Africa, 1900–1950," *Journal of Southern African Studies* 24,

no. 4 (December 1998): 695–717; Shula Marks, "'We Were Men Nursing Men': Male Nursing on the Mines in Twentieth-Century South Africa," in *Deep hiStories: Gender and Colonialism in Southern Africa*, edited by Wendy Woodward, Patricia Hayes, and Gary Minkley (Amsterdam: Rodopi, 2002), 177–204.

57. Holden and Littlewood, *Anthropology and Nursing*; Marks, *Divided Sisterhood*.

58. Marks, *Divided Sisterhood*, 85–87.

59. Peires, *The Dead Will Arise*, 60; Flint, *Healing Traditions*; Rankin, *Healing the African Body*.

60. Marks, *Divided Sisterhood*, 79; Peires, *The Dead Will Arise*, 60; Gordon, "A Sword of Empire," 47.

61. Peires, *The Dead Will Arise*, 60.

62. Gordon, "A Sword of Empire," 42, 48. Similarly, Marks pointed out that "African healers and patients were adept at adopting and adapting those aspects of western medicine that worked without allowing this to undermine belief in the efficacy of their remedies and belief system" (Marks, *Divided Sisterhood*, 80).

63. A prominent example was the Xhosa prophet and war doctor (*igqirha*) Nxele Makana. Nxele led the Xhosa against the British in a battle near Grahamstown in 1819 and taught a mixture of Christian and Xhosa cosmology.

64. Gordon, "A Sword of Empire," 53–54.

65. Steven Feierman, "Struggles for Control: The Social Roots of Health and Healing in Modern Africa," *African Studies Review* 28, nos. 2/3 (September 1985): 119.

66. See also Flint, *Healing Traditions*; Kirsten Rüther, "Claims on Africanisation: Healers' Exercises in Professionalisation," *Journal for the Study of Religion* 15, no. 2 (2002): 39–63.

67. Allan M. Brandt and Martha Gardner, "The Golden Age of Medicine?," in *Medicine in the Twentieth Century*, ed. Roger Cooter and John Pickstone (Amsterdam: Harwood Academic, 2000), 22.

68. Brandt and Gardner, "The Golden Age of Medicine?," 28–29.

69. Megan Vaughan, *Curing Their Ills: Colonial Power and African Illness* (Stanford, CA: Stanford University Press, 1991).

70. Baranov, *The African Transformation*; Vaughan, *Curing Their Ills*; Feierman and Janzen, *The Social Basis of Health and Healing in Africa*.

71. Baranov, *The African Transformation*, 34–35. Baranov further writes, "As such, biomedicine today is unmistakably identified with a range of scientific-material forms (from syringes to CAT scans) that mediate the relationship between physician and disease, between physician as active investigator and patient as passive object, and between the patient (a full person) and his or her body (a mass of biochemical functions and reactions)."

72. Michael Gelfand, *Christian Doctor and Nurse: The History of Medical Missions in South Africa from 1799–1976* (Sandton, South Africa: Aitken Family and Friends, 1984); Comaroff and Comaroff, *Of Revelation and Revolution*; Welcome Siphamandla Zondi, "Medical Missions and African Demand in KwaZulu-Natal, 1836–1918" (PhD diss., University of Cambridge, 2000); Norman Etherington, *Missions and Empire* (Oxford: Oxford University Press, 2005); Digby, *Diversity and Division*; Martin J. Lunde, "An Approach to Medical Missions: Dr. Neil Macvicar and the Victoria Hospital, Lovedale, South Africa, circa 1900–1950," (PhD diss., University of Edinburgh, 2009);

Radikobo P. Ntsimane, "Amandla Awekho Emuthini, Asenyangeni: A Critical History of the Lutheran Medical Missions in Southern Africa with Special Emphases on Four Mission Hospitals, 1930s–1978" (PhD diss., University of KwaZulu-Natal, 2010).

73. Comaroff and Comaroff, *Of Revelation and Revolution*, chap. 7, "The Medicine of God's Word: Saving the Soul by Tending the Flesh," 323–65.

74. Lunde, "An Approach to Medical Missions," 178.

75. Lunde, "An Approach to Medical Missions," 134.

76. McCord Zulu Hospital soon followed suit, training African nurses by 1910 and offering the full professional course in 1924.

77. Martin J. Lunde, "North Meets South in Medical Missionary Work: Dr Neil Macvicar, African Belief, and Western Reaction," *South African Historical Journal* 61, no. 2 (2009): 336–56.

78. Pat Holden, "Colonial Sisters: Nurses in Uganda," in *Anthropology and Nursing*, ed. Pat Holden and Jenny Littlewood (New York: Routledge, 1991), 67–83; Digby and Sweet, "Nurses as Culture Brokers"; Egli and Krayer, *"Mothers and Daughters"*; Isa Schuster, "Perspectives in Development: The Problem of Nurses and Nursing in Zambia," in *African Women in the Development Process*, ed. Nici Nelson (London: Frank Cass, 1981), 77–97; Marks, *Divided Sisterhood*; Meghan Healy-Clancy, *A World of Their Own: A History of South African Women's Education* (Charlottesville: University of Virginia Press, 2014); Agnes Rennick, "Mission Nurses in Nyasaland: 1890–1916," in *Twentieth Century Malawi: Perspectives on History and Culture*, ed. John McCracken, Timothy J. Lovering, and Fiona Johnson Chalamanda (Stirling, UK: University of Stirling, Center of Commonwealth Studies, 2001), 21–37; Lunde, "North Meets South in Medical Missionary Work," 347–48.

79. Marks, *Divided Sisterhood*, 83. Lunde cites Nokose Matade as the second graduate of nurse training at Lovedale (Lunde, "North Meets South in Medical Missionary Work," 346, n. 50). It is possible that Matade started training after Makiwane and Colani but graduated before Colani.

80. Digby, *Diversity and Division*, 240; Marks, *Divided Sisterhood*, 81.

81. Marks, *Divided Sisterhood*, 84–86.

82. Marks, *Divided Sisterhood*, 87–88.

83. Unfortunately, her career was cut short by an unspecified illness that led to her death in 1919.

84. Digby, *Diversity and Division*, 241.

85. Foster, *Lahlekile*.

86. Digby, *Diversity and Division*, 244; Mashaba, *The Challenge of Change*, 24–25.

87. On witchcraft and superstitions, see Mashaba, *The Challenge of Change*, 15; Searle, *History of the Development of Nursing in South Africa*, 125; and also Macvicar's comments quoted in Marks, *Divided Sisterhood*, 81. On preparing the ground for professional nursing, see Mashaba, *The Challenge of Change*, 5. Marks highlights that African nurses were advertised as acting as "harbingers of modernity to their own people, 'evangelists for western medicine,' often with painful results" (*Divided Sisterhood*, 82).

88. Marks, *Divided Sisterhood*, chap. 3.

89. Catherine Burns, "A Long Conversation: The Calling of Katie Makanya," *Agenda* 54 (2002): 134. Burns estimated that 50 percent of patients from all of South Africa had shifted from home-based childbirth to hospitalized childbirth by 1950.

90. Letter from Lovedale Hospital Superintendent to Acting Native Commissioner, Alice, August 8, 1941, Box 224, vol. 2, Archives and Records Services, Eastern Cape Department of Sport, Recreation, Arts, and Culture, King William's Town (hereafter Eastern Cape Archives and Records).

91. Letter from Herbert M. Bennett to Native Commissioner, Lady Frere, Regarding Native Mission Hospitals: Finances and Statistics, June 27, 1947, Box 224, Hospitals: General, KWT, vol. 2, Eastern Cape Archives and Records.

92. On October 15, 1945, the superintendent reported to the Secretary of Native Affairs that the hospital had eleven maternity cases (even though it only had four maternity beds), with four waiting to enter at any time (letter from Herbert M. Bennett to Mr. Mears, Secretary for Native Affairs, October 15, 1945, Box 226, Mount Coke Hospital File, Eastern Cape Archives and Records). In a previous year's report, it noted that it dealt with a total of ninety-six maternity cases (Mount Coke Hospital Annual Report for the year ended 30 June 1944, Box 226, Mount Coke Hospital File, Eastern Cape Archives and Records).

93. Mount Coke Hospital Board Report 1957, Box 226, Mount Coke Hospital 1958, Eastern Cape Archives and Records.

94. St. Matthew's Hospital Board Meeting Minutes, March 30, 1954, and Hospital Report, March 7, 1957, AB1354, vol. 1, HP. By 1946 the number of inpatients had risen to 675 (excluding over 100 maternity cases) and outpatients, to 2,067.

95. Letter from Dr. R. A. Spaulding (Medical Superintendent) to "friends" of the hospital giving a report of 1955, February 1956, Minute Books, AB1354, vol. 1, HP.

96. Box 563, St. Matthews Mission Farm, File 2, Eastern Cape Archives and Records; The 15th meeting, June 26, 1945, AB1354, Minute Books, CPSA Diocese of Grahamstown, St. Matthew's Hospital, Keiskammahoek, vol. 1: 1939–1955, HP.

97. "Memorandum on Hospitalisation," May 26, 1958, Box 224, Hospitals: General, KWT, vol. 1, Eastern Cape Archives and Records.

98. Packard, *White Plague, Black Labor*.

99. In practice, the Department of Health would calculate the cost of treatment on a per diem basis per patient for those suffering from infectious diseases in areas where there was no statutory local authorities and often refunded local authorities from 50 to 100 percent of the costs. Hospitals could apply to provincial governments and the Native Affairs Department or the Ciskei General Council for the other costs of running the hospital.

100. For more on the concern over labor and debates about training more African doctors versus medical aides, see Shapiro, "Doctors or Medical Aids," 234–55.

101. Ciskeian Missionary Hospital—Minutes of Meetings, 1925–1949, AD1715, 9.6, HP.

102. Searle, *History of the Development of Nursing in South Africa*, 353.

103. The hallmarks of this movement were the 1942–44 Gluckman Commission and the community health center experiments that recognized the impact of social and economic conditions on health and sought to establish integrative curative, preventive, and promotive (education) health care services. See, for example, Shula Marks, "South Africa's Early Experiment in Social Medicine: Its Pioneers and Politics," *American Journal of Public Health* 87, no. 3 (March 1997): 452–59; Alan Jeeves, "Health, Surveillance and Community: South Africa's Experiment with Medical Reform in the

1940s and 1950s," *South African Historical Journal* 43, no. 1 (November 2000): 244–66; Alan Jeeves, "Delivering Primary Health Care in Impoverished Urban and Rural Communities: The Institute of Family and Community Health in the 1940s," in *South Africa's 1940s: Worlds of Possibilities*, ed. Saul Dubow and Alan Jeeves (Cape Town: Double Storey Books, 2005), 87–107; Howard Phillips, "The Grassy Park Health Centre: A Peri-Urban Pholela?," in *South Africa's 1940s: Worlds of Possibilities*, ed. Saul Dubow and Alan Jeeves (Cape Town: Double Storey Books, 2005), 108–28; Vanessa Noble, "A Medical Education with a Difference: A History of the Training of Black Student Doctors in Social, Preventive and Community-Oriented Primary Health Care at the University of Natal Medical School, 1940s–1960," *South African Historical Journal* 61, no. 3 (September 2009): 550–74; Steve Tollman and Derek Yach, "Public Health Initiatives in South Africa in the 1940s and 1950s: Lessons for a Post-Apartheid Era," *American Journal of Public Health* 83, no. 7 (July 1993): 1043–50; Neil Andersson and Shula Marks, "Industrialization, Rural Health, and the 1944 National Health Services Commission in South Africa," in *The Social Basis of Health and Healing in Africa*, ed. Steven Feierman and John M. Janzen (Berkeley: University of California Press, 1992), 131–61.

104. For example, in some cases the Department of Health paid one-third while the Ciskei General Council paid two-thirds, whereas in other cases, the Department of Health paid seven-eighths of the salary and the Ciskei General Council paid one-eighth. Local communities, the Ciskei General Council, or other sources may have paid for uniform and living allowances or accommodation.

105. The government encountered difficulty persuading nurses to work in the rural clinics. Some sought jobs in hospitals and others left the profession when they got married. The commissioner suggested increasing the salaries and providing a bigger uniform allowance to entice more nurses to work in the clinics (letter from A. G. Walker, Chief Native Commissioner, King, to Secretary for Native Affairs, Pretoria, August 17, 1944, Box 224, vol. 2, Eastern Cape Archives and Records).

106. Annual Report of Native Affairs Department 1948–1949, October 21, 1949, Box 55, Eastern Cape Archives and Records.

107. Letter from Chief Native Commissioner, A. G. Walker, to Secretary for Native Affairs, Cape Town, June 7, 1945, Box 224, Hospitals, vol. 2, Eastern Cape Archives and Records.

108. The Victoria Hospital reported in 1940 that it had temporarily opened two clinics, sent a district nurse to Kwezana and held clinics at Ngwenya and Sityi ("Victoria Hospital Board, Lovedale, Report for the Year 1940," Box 226, Victoria Hospital, Alice File, Eastern Cape Archives and Records). St. Matthews started establishing its first clinics in 1941 and had four within a decade (Rabula started and stopped in 1941–43, but then the hospital established clinics at Burnshill [circa 1943], Cata-Emnyameni [1946], Gxulu [1948], and Gwili Gwili [circa 1948]).

109. "A Memorandum on Public Health to be submitted to the National Health Services Commission," Box 549, Eastern Cape Archives and Records.

110. "Mount Coke Hospital Annual Report, 1941," Box 226, Mount Coke Hospital File, Eastern Cape Archives and Records.

111. Mount Coke Hospital Report 1958, Mount Coke Hospital Reports, Newsletters Quarterly Reports, Methodist Papers, Folder 1, Cory Library for Historical Research, Rhodes University (hereafter Cory Library).

Notes to Pages 41–43

112. "Mount Coke Hospital Report 1956," Mount Coke Hospital Reports, Newsletters Quarterly Reports, Methodist Papers, Folder 1, Cory Library.

113. 1958 and 1959 Mount Coke Hospital Reports, Mount Coke Hospital Reports, Newsletters Quarterly Reports, Methodist Papers, Folder 1, Cory Library.

114. "Mount Coke Hospital, The Methodist Church of South Africa, Reports and Statements for the Year 1947," Box 226, Mount Coke Hospital File 1958, Eastern Cape Archives and Records.

115. "Memorandum on Hospitalisation," May 26, 1958, Box 224, Hospitals: General, KWT, vol. 1, Eastern Cape Archives and Records.

116. Digby, *Diversity and Division*, 243.

117. Its graduates worked in hospitals, at mission stations, and in district nursing services. Fourteen had married and not resumed work, but many found an informal role in their communities (Digby, *Diversity and Division*, 244). By 1941 Lovedale had trained, in total, ninety registered nurses and six midwives (letter from Lovedale Hospital Superintendent, A. F. G. Guiness, to Acting Native Commissioner, Alice, August 8, 1941, Box 224, Hospitals: General, KWT, vol. 2, Eastern Cape Archives and Records).

118. Mount Coke Hospital Board Report 1957, Box 226, Mount Coke Hospital 1958, Eastern Cape Archives and Records; Pamphlet, "The Door Is Ever Open But—," Pamphlet Box 193, Cory Library.

119. "St. Matthew's College, Annual Report 1946," Box 563, St. Matthews Mission Farm, File 2, Eastern Cape Archives and Records.

120. In 1933 three hospitals trained African nurses in the whole of South Africa—Victoria Hospital, Elliot Hospital in Mthatha, and the American Board Hospital, Ridge Road, in Durban. St. Monica's Home in Cape Town, Bridgman Hospital in Johannesburg, and the American Board Hospital offered training in midwifery to Africans (Records of the South African Institute of Race Relations, Part 2 AD 843/RJ, Kb24 Nursing 1933–1950, HP). By 1942 forty-seven hospitals, thirty-seven municipalities and councils, and twenty-six missions (apart from mission hospitals) and welfare committees employed Black nurses of all racial origins (Marks, *Divided Sisterhood*, 89). Mashaba listed the following hospitals that were established or that started to have Black sections in the 1930s and 1940s: St. Mary's Roman Catholic Mission (Marianhill), King Edward VIII Provincial Hospital in Durban, Umlali Hospital in the Cape, Frere Hospital in East London, and Pretoria Hospital (Mashaba, *Rising to the Challenge*, 22). The Non-European Hospital in Johannesburg started to train Black nurses in 1940 and was transferred to Baragwanath in 1948, which became the largest training school in Transvaal and country (see Horwitz, *Baragwanath Hospital*). In 1941 the Native Affairs Department reported that the following hospitals were training African nurses in the Eastern Cape: Frere Hospital (public, East London), Mount Coke, Frontier (public, Queenstown), Umlamli (mission, Herschel/Sterkspruit), Victoria, and St. Matthew's (letter from Native Affairs Department to Mr. Rose-Innes, December 4, 1941, Hospitals: General, KWT, vol. 2, Eastern Cape Archives and Records).

121. A number of problems hindered an increase in the training: inadequate prior education, overcrowded training facilities, a lack of tutors, long hours, the prejudice of trainers, and heavy-handed matrons (Mashaba, *Rising to the Challenge*, chap. 3). A study conducted by the South African Institute of Race Relations also found that

200   Notes to Pages 43–44

African women viewed other professions such as teaching and factory work as more attractive because of the better pay and teaching's higher status and flexibility (89.1.5 Report on the Shortage of Nurses in South Africa, Records of the South African Institute of Race Relations, Part 1 AD 843/B, HP).

122. Pamphlet, "School of Nursing for Native and Coloured Nurses. The Victoria Hospital, Lovedale," circa 1930, Box 226, Victoria Hospital, Alice File, Eastern Cape Archives and Records. The St. Matthew's Hospital board noted in 1957 that one nurse was sent away because she was pregnant, but that this was the first case in more than eighteen months. It is unclear from the record if this nurse was married, but the tone of satisfaction that this was not a common occurrence indicates that the hospital expected its trainees to remain separate from regular life and live as examples of Christian virtue. See St. Matthew's Hospital Board Meeting Minutes, May 9, 1957, AB1354, Minute Books, CPSA Diocese of Grahamstown, St. Matthew's Hospital, Keiskammahoek, vol. 2: 1956–1969, HP.

123. Victoria Hospital, "Report for the Year 1937," Box 226, Victoria Hospital, Alice File, Eastern Cape Archives and Records. See also Lunde, "An Approach to Medical Missions."

124. This religious orientation showed up in the hospital's reports (often penned by Bennett). Every year, the reports included comments about the "spiritual aspects" of the hospital, such as declarations that the spiritual needs of the patients were the most important or that "nothing can overcome superstition, heathen beliefs and practices, with their damaging effects on body and mind, like a vital religious experience." See Mount Coke Hospital Report 1956, Mount Coke Hospital Reports, Newsletters Quarterly Reports, Methodist Papers, Folder 1, Cory Library; Mount Coke Hospital Board, the Methodist Church of South Africa, "Report and Statement for the year 1953," Box 226, Mount Coke Hospital File, Eastern Cape Archives and Records.

125. Victoria Hospital Report, Lovedale, 1932, Box 226, Victoria Hospital, Alice File, Eastern Cape Archives and Records.

126. Mount Coke Hospital Board Report 1955, Box 226, Mount Coke Hospital File, Eastern Cape Archives and Records.

127. Hill's outpatient's department apparently saw a decline in patients, while others traveled over thirty miles (fifty kilometers) to see Murray (Digby, *Diversity and Division*, 338).

128. Digby's description of Macvicar's teaching at Lovedale gives us a glimpse of how he hoped to convert his students to science. Macvicar reportedly would give "two-hour lectures to the nurses in a classroom equipped for practical work with microscopes, a bacteriological incubator and anatomical aides." Digby quotes Mager in, *Diversity and Division*, 272. See also Lunde, "North Meets South in Medical Missionary Work."

129. Mount Coke Native Hospital, Annual Report 1940, and Mount Coke Hospital Annual Report for the year ended 30 June 1944, both in Box 226, Mount Coke Hospital File, Eastern Cape Archives and Records. In the Mount Coke Hospital Board Report 1957 report in the same archive and file, the hospital reported that mothers of children admitted to the hospital sometimes brought medicines from the *amagqirha* or tried to take over the care, and so they decided to house mothers in a separate building and control their visiting hours.

130. Lunde, "An Approach to Medical Missions," 208, n. 558.

131. Mount Coke Native Hospital, Annual Report 1940, and Mount Coke Hospital Annual Report for the year ended 30 June 1944, both in Box 226, Mount Coke Hospital File, Eastern Cape Archives and Records.

132. Rüther, "Claims on Africanisation"; Flint, *Healing Traditions*.

133. "Magic and Witchcraft in the Hospital Ward," Mr. E. C. Jali and "The African Concept of Disease" by Dr. A. B. Xuma, Jane McLarty Papers, B.1.4, HP.

134. Marks, *Divided Sisterhood*, chap. 5.

135. Anne Mager, *Gender and the Making of a South African Bantustan: A Social History of the Ciskei, 1945–1959* (Portsmouth, NH: Heinemann, 1999), 204.

136. Annual Report of Native Affairs Department—1948–1949—dated October 21, 1949, Box 55, Eastern Cape Archives and Records.

137. Mager, *Gender and the Making of a South African Bantustan*, 204–5; Digby, *Diversity and Division*, 251. A similar incident threatened to occur at the Nessie Knight Hospital in the same year, and Baragwanath and Pretoria General also had strikes in the 1940s and 1950s. Both Lovedale hospitals had already started negotiations with the provincial government to come under direct government control to relieve the financial worries of the hospital. This change officially took place January 1, 1950, further cementing the state's influence on the institution (although the hospitals maintained that they kept their Christian character). See *Lovedale Missionary Institution Report for 1949* (Lovedale: Lovedale Press, 1950), 30–31, Lovedale Annual Reports, Cory Library.

138. Horwitz, *Baragwanath Hospital*, chap. 5.

139. Digby, *Diversity and Division*, 247–49.

140. Discussion Following the Lecture "African Attitudes to Sex," V. Habedi, Study Course in African Culture and Its Relation to the Training of African Nurses conference of 1954, Jane McLarty Papers, B.1.4, HP.

141. Digby, *Diversity and Division*, 252.

142. In 1957 the Mount Coke Hospital related that it received applications for training every week (Mount Coke Hospital Board Report 1957, Box 226, Mount Coke Hospital 1958, Eastern Cape Archives and Records). In 1959 St. Matthew's reported that the hospital had received 524 applications for training for only fourteen vacancies. That year, the hospital had three fully trained African sisters permanently employed, evidence that the hospital was increasing its African staff at the same time that its graduates obtained employment elsewhere (St. Matthew's Hospital Board Meeting Minutes, December 10, 1959, AB1354, Minute Books, CPSA Diocese of Grahamstown, St. Matthew's Hospital, Keiskammahoek, vol. 2: 1956–1969, HP). Similarly, the Victoria Hospital reported in 1960 that it could only accept one out of every one hundred applications (Lovedale Hospital Board, Report for the Year 1960, Pamphlet Box 5, Cory Library).

Chapter 2. The Politics of Ciskei Homeland Health Care

1. Marks, *Divided Sisterhood*, 170; South African Institute of Race Relations, *Race Relations Survey 1984* (Johannesburg: South African Institute of Race Relations, 1985), 713. This number included all those registered with the South African Nursing Association, which would have included those living in the Ciskei at the time, since the Ciskei Nursing Association was only officially established in 1984, after Ciskeian independence in 1981. The *Daily Dispatch* reported that in 1966, for every African vacancy

Notes to Pages 49–51

at East London's Frere Hospital, there were 70–80 applications, but 79 of the 250 positions for white student nurses were vacant ("79 Nurses Wanted at Hospital," October 7, 1966, *Daily Dispatch*).

2. South African Institute of Race Relations, *A Survey of Race Relations in South Africa 1973*, 351. This would have been an ideal number if all of them worked in the Ciskei, with its population in 1973 estimated at 350,000 (for a ratio of 1:33); however, these nurses worked in ten different rural areas.

3. These numbers come from "The Ciskeian Nursing Council: Report of the First Council, Term of Office, 1st August 1984 to 31st July 1987," 11, and "The Ciskeian Nursing Council: Report of the Second Council, Term of Office, 1 August 1987 to 31 July 1992," 26, Leslie Hadfield Collection, NAHECS.

4. In the colonial era, local councils (made up of three members) fed into district councils. Each district was to have a council of twelve members, six chosen by the governor general and six chosen by the local councils. The Native Affairs Act of 1920 refined the council system under the direction of Native Affairs Commissioners and provided for the establishment of general councils—broader, regionally based councils such as the Ciskei General Council that covered seven districts: Middledrift, Tamacha (or King William's Town), Peddie, Victoria East, Keiskammahoek, Herschel, East London. Glen Grey was also, at times, part of the Ciskei General Council. D. M. Groenewald, "The Administrative System in the Ciskei," in *Ciskei: Economics and Politics of Dependence in a South African Homeland*, ed. Nancy Charton (London: Croom Helm, 1980); Peires, *The House of Phalo*; Switzer, *Power and Resistance in an African Society*; Roger Southall and Zosa De Sas Kropiwnicki, "Containing the Chiefs: The ANC and Traditional Leaders in the Eastern Cape, South Africa," *Canadian Journal of African Studies* 37, no. 1 (2003): 48–82. See also Mager, *Gender and the Making of a South African Bantustan*.

5. Effectively, the creation of tribal authorities brought more people into the government (especially as the government appointed more chiefs), yet with limited power. It centralized political power in the hands of appointed chiefs and white (now-called) Bantu commissioners at the exclusion of educated Africans with no "traditional" authority claims, and the local authorities did not have power to change South African law. Switzer, *Power and Resistance*, 305; Southall and Kropiwnicki, "Containing the Chiefs"; Laura Evans, "Resettlement and the Making of the Ciskei Bantustan, South Africa, c. 1960–1976," *Journal of Southern African Studies* 40, no. 1 (2014): 21–40.

6. "Mount Coke Hospital Report, 1963," Mount Coke Hospital Reports, Newsletters Quarterly Reports, Folder 1, Cory Library.

7. Letter to the Bantu Affairs Commissioner, Whittlesea, Re: Erection of Clinics: Ciskei Bantu Authorities, March 10, 1967, Hewu District Box 78, National Archives and Records of South Africa, Cape Town Archives Repository (hereafter Cape Town Archives Repository).

8. "Notes on the Establishment of District Nursing Services," Hewu District, Box 78, Cape Town Archives Repository.

9. Application for Clinic Site, Keiskammahoek Region, Ref D49/1319/7/1 1968, National Archives Repository, Pretoria (hereafter National Archives), SAB BAO1/2199.

10. Hewu District Box 78, Cape Town Archives Repository. This included clinics at Lahlangubo and Lower Didimana, which were later built.

Notes to Pages 51–53

11. "Mount Coke Hospital, 1968 Report," Mount Coke Hospital Reports, Newsletters Quarterly Reports, Folder 2, Cory Library. The Mtombe clinic was closed after land reform put it in a bad position to serve a larger number of people ("Mount Coke Hospital, 1964 Report"), and the Tshabo clinic closed in 1967 because there was another clinic very nearby. The Tamara and Ander's Mission clinics were taken over by the Ndlambe Regional Authority in August 1969. "Mount Coke Hospital Report, 1969," Mount Coke Hospital Reports, Newsletters Quarterly Reports, Folder 1, Cory Library.

12. Magubane et al., "Resistance and Repression in the Bantustans," 749–802; Southall and Kropiwnicki, "Containing the Chiefs"; Luvuyo Wotshela, "Territorial Manipulation in Apartheid South Africa: Resettlement, Tribal Politics, and the Making of the Northern Ciskei, 1975–1990," *Journal of Southern African Studies* 30, no. 2 (June 2004): 317–37; Wotshela, "Insurrection and Locally Negotiated Transition,"; Mager, *Gender and the Making of a South African Bantustan.*

13. Mager, *Gender and the Making of a South African Bantustan,* 112–14. Proapartheid white government officials justified the separation of the Ciskei and Transkei leadership by claiming that Sandile came from the Right Hand House of the Xhosa.

14. Groenewald, "The Administrative System in the Ciskei"; Southall and Kropiwnicki, "Containing the Chiefs"; Switzer, *Power and Resistance*; Jeff Peires, "Ethnicity and Pseudo-Ethnicity in the Ciskei," in *Segregation and Apartheid in Twentieth-Century South Africa,* ed. William Beinart and Saul Dubow (London: Routledge, 1995), 256–84.

15. Magubane, "Resistance and Repression in the Bantustans," 770; Wotshela, "Territorial Manipulation"; Laura Evans, "Resettlement and the Making of the Ciskei Bantustan, South Africa, c. 1960–1976"; Anne Mager and Phiko Velelo, *House of Tshatshu: Power, Politics and Chiefs North-West of the Great Kei River c 1818–2018* (Cape Town: UCT Press, 2018), 155–57.

16. Switzer, *Power and Resistance,* 336.

17. Digby, "The Bandwagon," 829.

18. Digby, "The Bandwagon"; Mtobeli Mxotwa, "Preventive care—Key Role in Ciskei Health," *Daily Dispatch,* June 4, 1988.

19. "Minister Wants Lots of Hospitals in Homelands," *Daily Dispatch,* May 12, 1969. In this article, it was reported that "nearly R7-million has been spent by the Dept of Bantu Administration and Development on hospitals in the African homelands during the past year and indications are that this amount will be greatly exceeded during the current year."

20. "Utilization of Nursing Personnel in Health Services in the Transkei and Ciskei," by Miss P. M. Burton, MS 17 211, Folder 5, Cory Library; Report on Clinics, July 5, 1974, MS 17 205, Folder 18, Cory Library; "A statement of policy objectives: 1979 Department of Health and Welfare," January 22, 1979, Ciskei Commission, MS 16 581, Cory Library; "Memorandum on Development of Hospital and Health Services," December 4, 1978, Ciskei Commission, MS 16 581, D.B.31, Cory Library, 7; St. Matthew's Hospital Board Meeting Minutes, July 26, 1972, AB1354, vol. 3: 1970–1977, HP. In recognition of the role nurses played in directing and delivering care to populations lacking access to doctors, the Republic of South Africa would pass a law in 1981 allowing nurses to carry out certain procedures when doctors were unavailable (Marks, *Divided Sisterhood,* 199).

204 Notes to Pages 53–55

21. Department of Health and Welfare, Ciskei Government Service, "Health and Welfare Services," April 17, 1978, 1, Government Publications, Ciskei Health and Welfare Annual Reports, 11, African Studies Documentation Center, University of South Africa Library (hereafter UNISA). See also policy speeches from 1975 on.

22. "New Health Scheme for the Ciskei," *Daily Dispatch*, July 5, 1971; Ciskei Legislative Assembly, 2nd Assembly, 1st Session and Special Session, Debates 1973, 2.1.3/73, 1, 28, Center for Research Libraries, Chicago (hereafter CRL); Ciskei Legislative Assembly, 2nd Assembly, 3rd Session, Verbatim Report, Volume 5, 1975, 2.1.3/75, 2, 200, CRL.

23. "Health and Welfare Services," April 17, 1978, 14–15, UNISA.

24. J. J. Adendorff, "Memorandum on Clinics Preliminary Considerations," October 5, 1971, MS 17 205, Folder 3, Cory Library.

25. Records reveal some frustration and confusion as the system shifted. In 1974 a Mount Coke Hospital report indicated that the hospital and government officials needed to communicate better, especially about staff appointed at clinics, and a year later, the superintendent declared that politicians should stay out of the hospital. "Medical Superintendent's Report, Mount Coke Methodist Hospital, Board Meeting May 17, 1974," MS 17 207, Folder 1, Cory Library. In 1975 the superintendent complained: "We have had over the last week numerous phone calls from Members of Parliament and cabinet ministers regarding minor staff matters at this Hospital. I would like to inform the Board that it is my intention to take a very firm line with staff who have seen it fit to complain to cabinet members or parliamentarians when they do not get their way with the authorities at this Hospital. The elections have come and gone and we were able to keep ourselves aloof of party politics during them and we wish to do the same in the future." "Medical Superintendent's Report to the Mount Coke Hospital Board Meeting Held on the 27th November 1975," MS 17 207, Folder 2, Cory Library. In July of 1971 the St. Matthew's hospital was gearing up to extend its services, send supervisors to clinics, help manage the clinic supplies, and set up health boards but was concerned about not having the medical staff to do it all (St. Matthew's Hospital Board Meeting Minutes, July 29, 1971, AB1354, vol. 3: 1970–1977, HP). Initially, since the Lovedale hospitals still operated under the Cape Provincial Administration at this point, St. Matthew's was assigned to cover the Keiskammahoek, Middledrift, and Alice areas; but the hospital did not have enough full-time doctors to manage this so asked that the Alice region be allocated elsewhere (St. Matthew's Hospital Board Meeting Minutes, March 23, 1972, AB1354, vol. 3: 1970–1977, HP).

26. "Urgent Call for African Hospital," *Daily Dispatch*, April 25, 1967; "Mdantsane to Get Super Hospital Costing R10m," *Daily Dispatch*, July 12, 1967; "Plans Approved for Hospital at Mdantsane," *Daily Dispatch*, May 1, 1969.

27. "Health and Welfare Services," April 17, 1978, 2, UNISA. The plans were reduced to much fewer beds in 1970/71 ("R800 000 lost as hospital plan dropped— plan for Mdantsane," *Daily Dispatch*, February 20, 1971).

28. "Health and Welfare Services," April 17, 1978, 3, UNISA.

29. This hospital was on the edge of the Ciskei, in an urban area that was going to house people relocated from other areas where they were not allowed or those working in East London but forced to live in the Ciskei. Even its location within the township was determined by apartheid tendencies. A letter from the Chief Bantu Affairs Commission of the Eastern Cape to the secretary for Bantu Administration and

Notes to Pages 55–56

Development, Pretoria, in 1967 suggested they choose a site near an entrance to the township so that white hospital staff would not have to drive "a considerable distance through the Township." Letter from Chief Bantu Affairs Commission of the Eastern Cape to the Secretary for Bantu Administration and Development, Pretoria, April 24, 1967, Mdantsane Hospital BAO 7429 P122/1489/2, File 1, National Archives.

30. In 1970 the superintendent wrote that not only did he feel that this was practical but also that the state ought to take responsibility for providing health care. He felt no ethical problems with the change. Recognizing the financial reliance the hospital had on the state, he continued, "The alternative would be to withdraw from the Government scheme and function as a private hospital without any grants. It would be impossible to provide a worthwhile service in this way, as it would mean R180,000 a year increasing by about 10 percent a year." St. Matthew's Hospital Board Meeting Minutes, June 17, 1970, AB1354, vol. 3: 1970–1977, HP.

31. See the discussion of Bethesda Methodist Mission Hospital's response in Hull, *Contingent Citizens*, chap. 3. See also Gelfand, *Christian Doctor and Nurse*, chap. 10.

32. Lovedale Hospital Board, Report for the Year 1971, Pamphlet Box 5, Cory Library.

33. The hospital built new wards in the early 1970s, increasing its specialized services (e.g., physiotherapy and occupational therapy in addition to more surgery) and opening a training school in midwifery in 1973. See "Mount Coke Hospital, Report 1961," Mount Coke Hospital Reports, Newsletters Quarterly Reports, Folder 1, Cory Library. In Adendorff's report to the board in 1972, he described the hospital as "bursting at its seams on all sides" (Mount Coke Hospital Newsletter, August 1972, Mount Coke Hospital Newsletters, Folder 1, Cory Library). With the nurses seemingly "reluctant" to take opportunities to bring in religion in their individual contact with the patients, the hospital added more classes and devotionals. "Mount Coke Hospital, 1970," Mount Coke Hospital Reports, Newsletters Quarterly Reports, Folder 2, Cory Library. Hospital management had found the hospital weak in the area of "individual contact with the patient" although that was "the most effective means of dealing with [the patient's] personal social and spiritual problems."

34. "Mount Coke Mission, The Methodist Church of South Africa, March 1974," Mount Coke Hospital Reports, Newsletters Quarterly Reports, Folder 2, Cory Library; Mount Coke Newsletter, January 1973, Mount Coke Hospital Reports, Newsletters Quarterly Reports, Newsletter Folder 1, Cory Library; "The Roll of Mission Hospitals in the Future," n.d., Methodist Church Mount Coke Hospital Box 3, MS 17 207, Folder 1, Cory Library; St. Matthew's Hospital Board Meeting Minutes, June 17, 1970, AB1354, vol. 3: 1970–1977, HP.

35. Ntsimane, "Amandla Awekho Emuthini, Asenyangeni"; MS 17 211, Transkei and Ciskei Association of Mission Hospitals, Cory Library. Referring to the negotiation process for hospital takeovers in the Transkei, Dr. Ronald Ingle wrote that he sometimes described it as "a three-cornered contest," with one corner holding "those who were concerned to retain the hospitals as institutions for Christian witness," another, "those who saw the absorption of the hospitals into a national and comprehensive health service as appropriate," and the third, "a sometimes perplexed Government" (Ronald Ingle, *An Uneasy Story: The Nationalising of South African Mission Hospitals, 1960–1976, A Personal Account* [Hillcrest, South Africa: The Author, 2010], x).

206 Notes to Pages 56–58

36. Mount Coke and St. Matthew's transferred land to Bantu Trust ownership in order to access more funding. In 1968 the Mount Coke Hospital reported that it received 90 percent of its funds for maintenance costs as a subsidy from the provincial government and fees from the state health department for infectious diseases. "Mount Coke Hospital, 1968 Report," Mount Coke Hospital Reports, Newsletters Quarterly Reports, Folder 1, Cory Library.

37. Radikobo Ntsimane, for example, regarded hospitals who gave in to state take-over as abandoning their communities to homeland governments, as they did not take into account the wishes of the people who actually used the hospital. See Ntsimane, "Amandla Awekho Emuthini, Asenyangeni," chap. 7; Gelfand, *Christian Doctor and Nurse*; and Hull, *Contingent Citizens*.

38. While some white mission hospital staff felt it was time to hand the hospitals over to Africans, others may have had more difficulty giving up their powerful benefactor role. Ntsimane, "Amandla Awekho Emuthini, Asenyangeni." Hospital board reports for the St. Matthew's Mission Hospital reveal that the board only sought "Europeans" for leadership positions in the hospital—even wanted a white person who spoke Xhosa to be the manager of housekeeping instead of entrusting a Xhosa person with it. St. Matthew's Hospital Board Meeting Minutes, December 6, 1960, AB1354, vol. 2: 1956–1969, HP; St. Matthew's Board Meeting Minutes, September 19, 1968, AB1354, vol. 2: 1956–1969, HP; St. Matthew's Hospital Board Meeting Minutes, July 26, 1972, AB1354, vol. 3: 1970–1977, HP. In 1973 the matron said in a board meeting that they could Africanize the laundry, kitchen, and nurses' home supervisor, "but it would take some time to get the right person as the work was very exacting," showing that she did not trust an African could do such work (St. Matthew's Hospital Board Meeting Minutes, October 21, 1974, AB1354, vol. 3: 1970–1977, HP).

39. "Administration Report—Board Meeting 3.6.1976," MS 17 207, Folder 2, Cory Library.

40. "Homeland Hospital Chief Fired on the Spot," n.d., by Rob Hudson, MS 17 211, Folder 5, Cory Library.

41. "Mount Coke Methodist Hospital, Newsletter—September, 1975," Mount Coke Hospital Reports, Newsletters Quarterly Reports, Newsletter Folder 1, Cory Library.

42. Hull also analyzes why nurses had rosy memories of the Christian nature of their work in light of the present day. See Hull, *Contingent Citizens*, chap. 3

43. The Tomlinson Commission of 1955, set up to investigate the viability of an envisioned homeland system, had recommended health care consolidation and the Africanization of hospital personnel in the homelands. "Health and Welfare Services," April 17, 1978, UNISA.

44. Peires, "The Implosion of Transkei and Ciskei"; Cecil Manona, "The Collapse of the 'Tribal Authority' System and the Rise of Civic Associations," in *From Reserve to Region: Apartheid and Social Change in the Keiskammahoek District of (Former) Ciskei, 1950–1990*, edited by Chris de Wet and Michael Whisson (Grahamstown, South Africa: Institute for Social and Economic Research, Rhodes University, 1997), 49–68; Magubane et al., "Resistance and Repression in the Bantustans."

45. Digby, "Bandwagon," 832; Switzer, *Power and Resistance*, 340.

46. Julia Segar, "Health Care at the Village Level: Ciskei and Transkei," in *Political Transition and Economic Development in the Transkei* (East London: Department of Anthropology, Rhodes University, November 1991); Digby, "Bandwagon."

47. See Howard Phillips, "HIV/AIDS in the Context of South Africa's Epidemic History," in *AIDS in South Africa: The Social Expression of a Pandemic*, ed. Kyle D. Kauffman and David L. Lindauer (Basingstoke, UK: Macmillan, 2004), 31–47; John Iliffe, *The African AIDS Epidemic: A History* (Oxford: James Currey, 2006); Rebecca Hodes, "HIV/AIDS in South Africa," *Oxford Research Encyclopedia of African History*, March 2018, http://africanhistory.oxfordre.com/view/10.1093/acrefore/9780190277734 .001.0001/acrefore-9780190277734-e-299.

48. Director-General of the World Health Organization, "Health Implications of Apartheid in South Africa," 5.

49. Packard, *White Plague, Black Labor*, 272–75; Switzer, *Power and Resistance*.

50. Thomas observed in 1970, "A serious problem in this area is that virtually no work is available. In many cases the mother is the sole supporter of her children, but is unable to leave them to go away for work." (St. Matthew's Hospital Board Meeting Minutes, December 7, 1970, AB1354, vol. 3: 1970–1977, HP). Thomas addressed this by starting a home industry scheme for women to engage in sewing and crocheting to earn money. See also Trudi Thomas, *The Children of Apartheid: A Study of the Effects of Migratory Labour on Family Life in the Ciskei* (London: Africa Publications Trust, 1974).

51. South African Institute of Race Relations, *Race Relations Survey 1960–1990*.

52. Switzer, *Power and Resistance*, 340; Digby, "Bandwagon," 849.

53. Clinics, subclinics, and mobile clinics are combined unless otherwise indicated; Mount Coke numbers for 1988 are not clear about how many are static versus subclinics, although the total number appears to have stayed the same.

54. Digby, "Bandwagon," 838.

55. Lulu Msutu Zuma, interview by the author, May 30 and 31, 2012, Jubisa.

56. Victoria Mjikeliso, interview by the author, June 1, 2012, King William's Town.

57. Nobantu Zelpha Baleni, interview by the author, June 6, 2012, Zwelitsha. Also Lumka Someketha, interview by the author, May 29, 2012, King William's Town.

58. "Bisho Needs a Modern Hospital Says Takane," *Daily Dispatch*, June 6, 1985; "New Hospital for Bisho to Cost R15 m," *Daily Dispatch*, October 10, 1985; "Plan to Build General Hospital at Bisho," *Daily Dispatch*, June 12, 1986; "Work Starts on R40m Bisho Hospital Block," *Daily Dispatch*, February 23, 1989; "New Hospital for Bisho," *Daily Dispatch*, June 27, 1989; "Ciskei to Give Up Control of Mount Coke Hospital," *Daily Dispatch*, April 16, 1992.

59. The Ciskei also counted the specialty TB hospital, the Nkqubela Chest Hospital in Mdantsane that had 682 beds, as part of its territory, but it was run by a private company.

60. Saldru Community Health Project, *Health and Health Services in the Ciskei*, 6.

61. Switzer, *Power and Resistance*, 339.

62. Digby, "Bandwagon," 836. See also South African Institute of Race Relations, *Race Relations Survey 1989/90*, 413.

63. "New Health Strategy Planned for Ciskei," *Daily Dispatch*, December 18, 1982. In 1986 a new health policy provided for the coordination of services under an advisory council ("Pieterse Re-Defines National Health Aims," *Daily Dispatch*, July 2, 1986).

64. Victoria Mjikeliso interview, June 1, 2012.

65. Nonzwakazi Gqomfa, interview by the author, October 15, 2013, Lower Gqumashe.

208 Notes to Pages 61–64

66. Alecia Phiwo Dubula interview, May 4, 2012.

67. Segar, "Health Care at the Village Level"; Chris de Wet and Simon Bekker, *Rural Development in South Africa: A Case Study of the Amatola Basin in the Ciskei* (Pietermaritzburg: Shuter and Shooter, 1985). De Wet and Bekker argued that the Komkhulu village that housed the main clinic of the Amathole Basin had an impact on the surrounding community through its health and nutritional education, although malnutrition was still a major problem.

68. "Health for All the Goal," *Daily Dispatch*, December 2, 1983; "Immunization compulsory," *Daily Dispatch*, January 24, 1984; "Measles Jab Campaign Launched," *Daily Dispatch*, August 12, 1986.

69. "Republic of Ciskei, Department of Health, Annual Report, 1988," 29, Government Publications, Ciskei Health and Welfare Annual Reports, UNISA.

70. Digby, "Bandwagon." See also "Qualified Nurses Needed," June 4, 1977, and "More Responsibility for Ciskei Nurses," September 3, 1977, in *Imvo Zabantsundu*.

71. Although available statistics do not give a clear indication of the exact impact this training had on psychiatric health and family planning, reports do indicate an improvement to some degree. The 1988 report noted more psychiatric services and teams in hospitals and an increase in positive attitudes toward contraceptives and condom use. It also noted the increase in cervical cancer screening and education programs. But there are no statistics to evaluate the concrete impact of family planning and psychiatric services.

72. Mashaba, *Rising to the Challenge*, 68; Marks, *Divided Sisterhood*, 199–202.

73. "Only 9 Black State Doctors in Homelands Says MP," *Daily Dispatch*, May 19, 1973. The article "Foreign Staff for Ciskei Hospitals" (*Daily Dispatch*, November 25, 1981) reported that twenty-one doctors were recruited from the Philippines, three from Iran, one from Tanzania, three from India, and seven from the UK. In the 1985 legislature debates, it was acknowledged that the Ciskei was fortunate enough to have recruited para-medical staff and doctors from Israel and West Germany (Ciskei Legislative Assembly, 1st Ass. 4th Session Verbatim Debates, 2.1.4/84, vol. 16, 1985, 499; see also "Britons for Ciskei," *Daily Dispatch*, September 5, 1980, AAS 190, UNISA).

74. Ciskei Commission Manuscript, Memo on Hospitals, 7, MS 16 581, Cory Library.

75. "Republic of Ciskei, Department of Health, Annual Report, 1984," 63 (and 13–14), Government Publications, Ciskei Health and Welfare Annual Reports, UNISA.

76. "Annual Report, 1988," 23–24, UNISA; Digby, "Bandwagon," 842. In 1988 there were 396 VHWs in the Ciskei as a whole who followed up with chronic disorders like TB, psychiatric illness, hypertension, and pediatric malnutrition.

77. In regard to family planning, reportedly, "Village Health Workers are very helpful but need a back up from the professional people." Workers in the S. S. Gida catchment area also at times lacked regular contact with hospital and clinic staff when transportation was hindered but had a big impact in the Hewu district before it had a hospital ("Annual Report, 1988," 18, 103, UNISA).

78. Leslie Anne Hadfield, "Biko, Black Consciousness, and 'the System' EZinyoka: Oral History and Black Consciousness in Practice in a Rural Ciskei Village," *South African Historical Journal* 62, no. 1 (2010): 78–99; Leslie Anne Hadfield, *Liberation and Development: Black Consciousness Community Programs in South Africa* (East Lansing: Michigan State University Press, 2016), chap 3.

Notes to Pages 64–65

79. Lumka Someketha interview, May 29, 2012.

80. Packard, *White Plague, Black Labor*, 251, 272–75. See also de Wet and Bekker, *Rural Development in South Africa*; Phatlane, "Poverty, Health and Disease"; and Diana Wylie's account of state responses to malnutrition in *Starving on a Full Stomach*.

81. "Health and Welfare Services," 17 April, 1978, 14, UNISA.

82. "Programme to Cut Ciskei Malnutrition," *Daily Dispatch*, May 16, 1979.

83. "Malnutrition Ad Shocks Health Secretary," *Daily Dispatch*, September 20, 1979; "Ciskei: Malnutrition Not Great Problem," *Daily Dispatch*, December 15, 1984. The Ciskei Department of Health concluded that these successes came because of the work of school health nurses, mobile immunization teams, clinics, and VHWs. A 1986 survey of rural children reportedly showed a low percentage of malnutrition, with an even better rate in 1987/88. A 1987/88 survey reported that 9.8 percent of children in rural areas had a low weight for their age, claiming that to be a relatively low percentage ("Annual Report, 1988," 33, UNISA). This was compared with 2.9 percent in urban areas in 1986. Cecilia Makiwane Hospital reported a decline in severely malnourished children requiring hospitalization from 428 in 1982 to 121 in 1986. There were 142 cases in 1987 and 137 in 1988, but the numbers reached nowhere near the 428 of five years earlier ("Annual Report, 1988," 76, UNISA). The percentage of children who died of kwashiorkor at the hospital dropped to 8.5 percent in 1988 ("Annual Report, 1988," 85, UNISA). The S. S. Gida Hospital reported that "malnutrition figures stabilized after an early peak to average a figure of 80 per 1000 pediatric admissions which [was] below the 1987 figure." The decline was not as dramatic as that in Mdantsane, but the hospital concluded, "It would seem that the Primary Health Care Services are doing effective work" ("Annual Report, 1988," 99, UNISA).

84. See articles by Peter Davis, "The Face of Starvation," July 19, 1976, "68 per cent Who Suffer," July 20, 1976, and "Malnutrition—Problem on Increase," *Daily Dispatch*, July 21, 1976. See also Ciskei official's remarks in "Resettlement Blamed for Full Hospitals," *Daily Dispatch*, May 24, 1984.

85. Thomas, *The Children of Apartheid*.

86. "Malnutrition—Problem on Increase," *Daily Dispatch*, July 21, 1976.

87. "More Jobs Would End Malnutrition," *Daily Dispatch*, July 18, 1980; "Cholera—Penalty of White Neglect of Blacks," *Daily Dispatch*, March 3, 1982; "Bikitsha: Underdevelopment Is Transkei's Disease," *Daily Dispatch*, April 3, 1986.

88. "Grinding Poverty in Ciskei," *Daily Dispatch*, April 18, 1984. Operation Hunger, a nongovernmental organization, reported in 1984 that it was feeding more than eighty thousand people in the broader region (sixty thousand of whom were children between the ages of three and fifteen) and that relocation settlements were hit the hardest—a reason why Hewlett-Packard and World Vision opened a clinic in Sada in 1986 ("Starvation increases," *Daily Dispatch*, August 24, 1984). In the same article, the Red Cross stated that it usually did not deal with cases of hunger but had been drawn into the Ciskei because of the desperate situation there. In 1985 a study by an Israeli-based education company characterized malnutrition, TB, scabies, and poor drinking water as "acute problems" in rural areas ("Study Finds Acute Health Problems," *Daily Dispatch*, March 19, 1985).

89. For example, in 1986 the Republic promised a loan of R9,000,000 toward the total estimated R15 million cost of building the Hewu Hospital. A large portion of

210 Notes to Pages 65–67

these costs were earmarked for hospital construction (R6,150,000), four clinics to be built (R450,000), one community health center (R1,200,000), upgrading accommodation for nurses (R600,000) and upgrading existing clinics (R600,000). See "Loan Agreement with Regard to Financial and Technical Assistance for 1986," SAB SPM 136 272/1986, National Archives, Pretoria.

90. Pamphlet, "Ciskei . . . the country, the people and its achievements," AAS 190, UNISA.

91. These numbers were compiled from 1980s publications by South African Institute of Race Relations, *Race Relations Survey*.

92. See South African Institute of Race Relations, *Race Relations Survey 1984*, 499–500.

93. South African Institute of Race Relations, *Race Relations Survey 1989/90*, 458–60. Others debated whether the homelands would cost more if they were part of South Africa. Even as the government considered reintegration of the homelands, Pretoria announced it could not meet homeland requests for financial assistance even though allocations for the homelands were 17 percent higher than the year before. A Progressive Federal Party spokesman, Harry Schwarz, posed the question as to whether or not there was any prospect that loans to homelands would ever be repaid and if this "could possibly be regarded as sound budgeting" in the 1987/88 South African parliament debates (South African Institute of Race Relations, *Race Relations Survey 1987/88*, 872). A study published in 1990 by the Development Bank of Southern Africa argued that the development and decentralization policies of the homelands between 1965 and 1985 "had failed to tackle the problems of serious poverty" but rather made the gap between the urban and more rural areas worse (South African Institute of Race Relations, *Race Relations Survey 1989/90*, 465).

94. Les Switzer claimed that although health was a top priority for the Ciskei state, the budget could only fund up to 60 percent of the actual needs. See Switzer, *Power and Resistance*, 340. In 1984 the budget only lasted until September. "Annual Report, 1984," 61–62, UNISA.

95. See South African Institute of Race Relations, *A Survey of Race Relations in South Africa 1983*, 368, for more on KEOSSA. The South African government apparently preferred giving loans because it believed it encouraged self-help.

96. Digby, "Bandwagon," 832.

97. Ciskei Legislative Assembly, 1st Assembly, Special Session and Second Session 1982 Verbatim Report 2.1.4/82, vol. 4, 628–29, CRL. In 1983 a grant from the Johnson & Johnson company allowed the government to pay VHWs R10,000 ("Annual Report, 1983," 36). This continued into 1984 at least. This was particularly helpful for the Hewu district at that time since it had a much more decentralized health services system without a hospital and was experiencing a shortage of staff as well. Johnson & Johnson also donated plastic covers for record keeping in 1986 ("Annual Report, 1986," 120–21, UNISA). In 1984 Operation Hunger helped feed fifteen hundred families biweekly, four hundred preschool children daily, and five thousand school children daily ("Annual Report, 1984," 60, UNISA). The Ford Motor Company donated a mobile mass X-ray unit in 1985 ("Annual Report, 1985," 11, UNISA). And in 1986 Cecilia Makiwane Hospital reported that "as in the previous five years, [it had] received in excess of R 100,000 in cash and goods from independent organizations" and that "much of the work of the

Notes to Pages 67–68

department could not have been accomplished without this massive aid and we are very grateful for it." The report read, "Over the years this has supplied about 5,000 bursaries to destitute children, paid salaries for village health workers, financed courses, maintained an old age complex which now cares for 21 frail old people, provided small 'pensions' and food parcels for hundreds of others, supported day care centres for neglected and malnourished children, as well as other malnourished children and destitute families, provided school meals for children in 22 rural schools as well as seeds, fencing and tanks for their gardens. A play ground for Khayalethemba and a truck which for years made a most successful rural health team possible" ("Annual Report 1986," 123, UNISA). In 1987 the Leprosy Mission in Southern Africa agreed to provide vehicles and staffing to trace and treat leprosy patients ("Annual Report 1987," 22, UNISA).

98. "Republic of Ciskei, Department of Health, Annual Report, 1986," 8, UNISA.

99. "Republic of Ciskei, Department of Health, Welfare, and Pensions, Annual Report, 1983," 4–5, UNISA; South African Institute of Race Relations, *A Survey of Race Relations in South Africa 1983*, 496. That same year, a group of doctors and other medical personnel in the Ciskei came up with a development plan to present to Pretoria to request funds and increase the staff. Whereas mission hospitals received many more applications for nursing positions than they could consider in prior decades, in 1986 the department reported that the difference in salaries between South Africa and Ciskei meant that the Ciskei lost thirty nurses out of just over four thousand total. Thus, for most health practitioners in the Ciskei, salaries were not the reason they stayed or later spoke highly of Ciskei health care. The lack of adequate staff for clinics often appeared in annual reports. Financial constraints even halted the training of VHWs at the S. S. Gida and Mount Coke Hospitals at times ("Annual Report, 1986," 81 and 102, respectively, UNISA). The Ciskei Employment Action Programme (CEAP)—a program funded by South Africa to train people to be self-supporting—helped employ staff in several different categories in 1987; but this continued the reliance on South African funds ("Republic of Ciskei, Department of Health, Annual Report, 1987," 143, UNISA).

100. Ciskei National Assembly 1st Ass. 4th Session Verbatim Debates, 2.1.4/84, vol. 11, 1984, 321–22, CRL.

101. "Annual Report, 1984," 34, UNISA.

102. "Republic of Ciskei, Department of Health, Annual Report, 1985," 9, UNISA.

103. Mission hospitals often had to replace their vehicles because of their use on gravel roads. The St. Matthew's ambulance at times reportedly would not attempt the journey to some places in bad weather (Saldru Community Health Project, *Health and Health Services in the Ciskei*, 28).

104. "Five Cars Wrecked a Day Says Sebe," *Daily Dispatch*, June 14, 1984; "Promote Health Says Minister," *Daily Dispatch*, June 18, 1987; "MPs Attack Health Policy Speech," *Daily Dispatch*, June 7, 1988; "Ckei Govt Vehicles Missing Says Report," *Daily Dispatch*, November 14, 1992. The 1970s reports and debates reveal that Pretoria was reluctant to provide vehicles, and subsequent reports show that a lack of finances stopped the department from making repairs or purchasing new vehicles. The government promised to increase driver training and screening, but the amount of blame placed on drivers and the number of vehicles discovered missing or given to politicians after Sebe's fall also point to possible corruption.

Notes to Pages 68–72

105. "Annual Report, 1985," 46–48, UNISA.

106. See Sasha Polakow-Suransky, *The Unspoken Alliance: Israel's Secret Relationship with Apartheid South Africa* (New York: Pantheon Books, 2010), 57–58.

107. "New Ciskei Hospital: Evidence of Deterioration, *Daily Dispatch*, August 21, 1985; "Prof Says Faults a Potential Health Risk," *Daily Dispatch*, September 12, 1985; South African Institute of Race Relations, *Race Relations Survey 1985*, 300–301; "Ciskei Hospital Unused as Govt Holds Back Cash," July 21, 1986, *Daily Dispatch*.

108. "Ciskei Minister of Health Suspended," *Daily Dispatch*, March 11, 1985; "Beukes Confident He'll Be Cleared," *Daily Dispatch*, March 13, 1985; "Beukes: Bribery and Corruption Findings," *Daily Dispatch*, October 10, 1985.

109. "Annual Report, 1988," 68, 71–72, UNISA).

110. Mashaba, *Rising to the Challenge*, 58–59. Mashaba highlighted prominent cases of Black nurses gaining matron positions in hospitals: Harriet Rita Shezi at a Black hospital in KwaThema Springs in the Transvaal in 1958, three appointed at the Pretoria Non-European Hospital in 1959, and three at Baragwanath in 1960.

111. Marks, *Divided Sisterhood*, 192. Marks described how international and internal pressure led to the 1978 Nursing Act that allowed all registered nurses to vote for a portion of the members of the South African Nursing Council and gave the South African Nurses Association the power to write its own constitution (187–88).

112. The Transkei, as the first homeland to gain independence, made news as it appointed Black superintendents in its hospitals. Dr. Bikithsa was hailed as an example of the Africanization of management positions promised to the homelands when he became the first Black superintendent of the Butterworth Hospital in the Transkei in 1975. Upon the declaration of Transkei's independence in 1976, he was appointed the secretary of health. "Top Medical Post for Bikitsha," *Daily Dispatch*, January 20, 1975; "Bikitsha Appointed Health Secretary," *Daily Dispatch*, July 31, 1976.

113. Lulu Msutu Zuma interview, May 30 and 31, 2012. In a meeting with the author in 2018, she expressed the desire to achieve something for her people in the nursing area—to help nurses transfer their theory to practice.

114. Gamase Doris Sonjica Mtyeku, interview by the author, June 22, 2012, Bhisho.

115. Retired nurses' dialogue with author, November 7, 2018, Ginsberg; "Nurses Go It Alone," *Imvo Zabantsundu*, October 28, 1978.

116. "Goodbye to Baasskap," *Daily Dispatch*, Indaba insert, October 3, 1980, AAS 190, UNISA.

117. "The Ciskeian Nursing Council: Foundation of the Ciskeian Nursing Council (1984)," Booklet produced by the Ciskeian Nursing Council, in possession of Virginia N. Mkosana. Also, retired nurses' dialogue with author, November 7, 2018, Ginsberg.

118. Virginia N. Mkosana, interview by the author, September 23, 2013, Alice.

119. Retired nurses' dialogue with author, November 7, 2018, Ginsberg. Hull also quotes nurses at Bethesda Hospital as finding ways to work around this restriction and providing patients with different addresses at times (Hull, *Contingent Citizens*).

120. Thyra Nomkhitha Mavuso, interview by the author, October 15, 2013, Mavuso Location.

121. Mavis Makubalo, interview by the author, December 3, 2013, Keiskammahoek.

122. Beauty Noziwo Nongauza, interview by the author, October 1, 2013, King William's Town; Beauty Noziwo Nongauza, interview by Lindani Ntenteni and the author,

Notes to Pages 72–79

November 19, 2008, King William's Town. Nongauza was also one who had worked at the Black Consciousness Zanempilo clinic and thus had political leanings against homeland politicians.

123. Mavis Makubalo interview, December 3, 2013.

124. Gamase Mtyeku interview, June 22, 2012.

125. Joan Mavuso, interview by the author, June 22, 2012, Zwelitsha.

Chapter 3. Remembering Clinic Work

1. Thembisa E. Nkonki and Zotshi Mcako, interview by the author, June 15, 2011, Tyutyu Village. Feziwe Leonora Badi (October 7, 2013, Zwelitsha), Thandiwe Millicent Mkwelo (November 27, 2013, Tshatshu Location), and Victoria Mjikeliso (June 1, 2012) also talked about how a nurse had to be independent in the clinics.

2. Nombeko Cecilia Tunyiswa, interview by the author, September 20, 2013, Ann Shaw Location. Nonfundo Rulashe also remarked, "And as a general nurse you did everything!" (Nonfundo R. Rulashe, interview by the author, June 4, 2012, Dimbaza).

3. Penolope Ntshona interview, October 21, 2013.

4. Alecia Phiwo Dubula interview, May 4, 2012.

5. They were prohibited from doing any private nursing and asked to give one month's notice of their resignation (unless they were still in the three-month probationary period, wherein either party could terminate the contract within twenty-four hours). See "Guide to Service Contract Between Employing Body and District Nurse," n.d., Hewu District, Box 78, Cape Town Archives Repository; "Notes on the Establishment of District Nursing Services," n.d., Box 539, Regional Authorities: Clinics, Hospitals, General Folder, Eastern Cape Archives and Records. For a sample contract, see "Contract of Service entered into between: The Middledrift Regional Authority and Nurse Cecilia N. Tunyiswa," Box 535 Regional Authorities: Clinics, Eastern Cape Archives and Records.

6. "Guide to Service Contract Between Employing Body and District Nurse," Cape Town Archives Repository.

7. Report on Visit to Ann Shaw Clinic, Middledrift District, 28.9.1967; Report on Lower Didimana, Hewu, 22.5.68; Report on Burnshill Location, Keiskammahoek, October 3 and 17, 1967, Box 535, Regional Authorities: Clinics, Eastern Cape Archives and Records.

8. Linda Eunice Ngoro, interview by the author, December 5, 2013, Mgxotyeni.

9. Constance Nozipho Thoto, interview by the author, October 18, 2013, Kuntselamanzi.

10. Christina Vuyelwa Magodla, interview by the author, September 19, 2013, Madubela.

11. Zotshi Mcako and Nontsikelelo Biko, interview by the author, December 2, 2008, Ginsberg. Mavis Makubalo remarked that the community would not understand when someone was on leave (Mavis Makubalo interview, December 3, 2013).

12. Evelyn T. N. Magodla, interview by the author, June 7, 2012, King William's Town.

13. Nomali Georgina Gwarabe Bangani, interview by the author, October 9, 2013, Madubela.

14. Nomabali Sara Mbombo, interview by the author, October 4, 2013, King William's Town.

15. Weziwe Tsotsobe, interview by the author, October 2, 2013, King William's Town.

16. Nomathemba Ncukana, interview by the author, October 22, 2013, Ann Shaw Location.

17. Vuyiswa Sodlulashe, interview by the author, September 19, 2013, Madubela.

18. Saldru Community Health Project, *Health and Health Services in the Ciskei*, 21. Well-resourced clinics might have up to four fully qualified nurses. Often, clinics had two fully qualified nurses, with one or two assistant nurses.

19. Nobantu Baleni interview, June 6, 2012.

20. Thembeka Ellen Gantsho, interview by the author, September 19, 2013, Madubela.

21. Celiwe Elizabeth Mbie, interview by the author, October 7, 2013, Bhisho.

22. Mavis Makubalo interview, December 3, 2013.

23. Nomali G. G. Bangani interview, October 9, 2013.

24. Lungelwa Francis Mhlambiso, interview by the author, December 4, 2013, Mqhayiso.

25. Evelyn T. N. Magodla interview, June 7, 2012.

26. Celiwe E. Mbie interview, October 7, 2013.

27. Nomali G. G. Bangani interview, October 9, 2013.

28. Nkonki and Mcako interview, June 15, 2011; Buyiswa Victoria Vakalisa, interview by the author, September 20, 2013, Middledrift; "Nurses: Save Us from Thugs: All-Night Guard Urged," *Daily Dispatch*, Indaba Supplement, November 9, 1973.

29. Eunice Lulama Mkosana, interview by the author, September 25, 2013, Ngcwazi.

30. "Guide to Service Contract Between Employing Body and District Nurse," Cape Town Archives Repository.

31. Pholisa Nombulelo Majiza, interview by the author, October 2, 2013, Burns Hill.

32. Victoria Mjikeliso interview, June 1, 2012.

33. For example, two nurses with five children unsuccessfully appealed to the South African Department of Health for help in housing their children at the Gxulu and Burns Hill clinics in 1968 (Inspection Report on Gxulu Clinic, March 13, 1968, Gxulu file, and Inspection Report on Burnshill clinic, July 22, 1968, Burnshill Location file, both in Box 535, Regional Authorities: Clinics, Eastern Cape Archives and Records).

34. Thyra Nomkhitha Mavuso interview, October 15, 2013; Thandiwe M. Mkwelo interview, November 27, 2013; Nomathemba Ncukana interview, October 22, 2103; and Lungelwa F. Mhlambiso interview, December 4, 2013.

35. Nobantu Baleni interview, June 6, 2012.

36. Celiwe E. Mbie interview, October 7, 2013.

37. Nombeko Cecilia Tunyiswa interview, September 20, 2013.

38. Lumka Someketha interview, May 29, 2012.

39. Nonzwakazi Gqomfa interview, October 15, 2013; Victoria Mjikeliso interview, June 1, 2012.

40. Nomali G. G. Bangani interview, October 9, 2013.

41. Nobantu Baleni interview, June 6, 2012.

42. Nkonki and Mcako interview, June 15, 2011; Constance N. Thoto interview, October 18, 2013. See also Mabel Cetu, "Care of the Child," *Imvo Zabantsundu*, March 9, 1963.

Notes to Pages 87–92

43. Celiwe E. Mbie interview, October 7, 2013.

44. Pholisa N. Majiza interview, October 2, 2013.

45. Celiwe E. Mbie interview, October 7, 2013.

46. Nkonki and Mcako interview, June 15, 2011.

47. Constance N. Thoto interview, October 18, 2013.

48. Lungelwa F. Mhlambiso interview, December 4, 2013.

49. Celiwe E. Mbie interview, October 7, 2013.

50. Hilary K. Mnyanda, interview by the author, September 11, 2013, Bhisho.

51. Thandiwe M. Mkwelo interview, November 27, 2013.

52. Vuyiswa Sodlulashe interview, September 19, 2013.

53. Nobantu Baleni interview, June 6, 2012.

54. Nkonki and Mcako interview, June 15, 2011.

55. Evelyn T. N. Magodla interview, June 7, 2012; Constance Nozipho Thoto interview, October 18, 2013.

56. Saldru Community Health Project, *Health and Health Services in the Ciskei*, 28.

57. Constance N. Thoto interview, October 18, 2013.

58. Vuyiswa Sodlulashe interview, September 19, 2013.

59. Ntshona said she was lonely when she worked as the only nurse at the University of Fort Hare clinic (Penolope Ntshona interview, October 21, 2013).

60. Alecia Phiwo Dubula interview, May 4, 2012.

61. Eunice Lulama Mkosana interview, September 25, 2013.

62. Vuyiswa Sodlulashe interview, September 19, 2013.

63. Pumla Kwatsha, interview by the author, September 17, 2013, King William's Town.

64. Nonfundo R. Rulashe interview, June 4, 2012.

65. Sheila Sonjica, interview by the author, October 14, 2013, Debe Nek; Weziwe Tsotsobe interview, October 2, 2013.

66. Alecia Phiwo Dubula interview, May 4, 2012.

67. Buyiswa V. Vakalisa interview, September 20, 2013.

68. Box 535, Regional Authorities: Clinics, Eastern Cape Archives and Records; MS 17 206, Staff Files for Mount Coke Mission Hospital, Folder 2: 1967–68, Africans, General and Income Tax, Cory Library.

69. South African Institute of Race Relations, *A Survey of Race Relations in South Africa 1973*, 202–5.

70. Barbara Hutmacher, "On Being a Nurse in East London," *Daily Dispatch*, February 21, 1974.

71. South African Institute of Race Relations, *Race Relations Survey 1984*.

72. Roger Southall, "The African Middle Class in South Africa, 1910–1994," *Economic History of Developing Regions* 29, no. 2 (2014): 287–310; Alan Cobley, *Class and Consciousness: The Black Petty Bourgeoisie in South Africa, 1924–1950* (New York: Greenwood, 1990); Owen Crankshaw, *Race, Class and the Changing Division of Labour under Apartheid* (London: Routledge, 1997).

73. Weziwe Tsotsobe interview, October 2, 2013.

74. Of the forty or so who answered this question, ten said it was because of the pay. See also the story of Ntonga struggling to provide for her family on just her salary in chapter 5.

Notes to Pages 92–98

75. Gamase Mtyeku interview, June 22, 2012.

76. Marks, *Divided Sisterhood*, 174.

77. Remedying this has been on the agenda of the King William's Town Retired Nurses' Association.

78. Gamase Mtyeku interview, June 22, 2012.

79. Hadfield, *Liberation and Development*, 106–9.

80. Nonzwakazi Gqomfa interview, October 15, 2013.

81. Nozokolo Hono, interview by the author, October 23, 2013, Middledrift.

82. Vuyiswa Sodlulashe interview, September 19, 2013.

83. Alecia Phiwo Dubula interview, May 4, 2012.

84. Nomali G. G. Bangani interview, October 9, 2013.

85. Lulama "Lulu" Nkani, interview by the author, November 27, 2013, Zwelitsha.

86. Tutors in training hospitals were asked to train in psychiatric nursing in 1986. Nonkululeko Vena, interview by the author, October 11, 2013, Ngqele.

87. Nobantu Baleni interview, June 6, 2012; Buyiswa V. Vakalisa interview, September 20, 2013.

88. Natasha Erlank, "Birth Control in Twentieth Century Africa," presentation at the African Studies Association of the United States, Annual Meeting, November–December 2018, Atlanta, Georgia; "Plea for Control of the Population Explosion," *Daily Dispatch*, November 22, 1968; "Family Planning the Only Way," *Daily Dispatch*, October 15, 1971; "Family Planning Course for 100 Nurses," *Daily Dispatch*, February 16, 1973; "Memorandum: Priorities of the Department of Health and Welfare," September 15, 1978, B-31, D, Ciskei Commission Manuscript MS 16 581, Cory Library; National Research Institute for Nutritional Diseases of the South African Medical Research Council, "An Evaluation of the Nutritional Situation in the Ciskei with Recommendations for Remedial Measures," 18 June 1979, B-36, D, Ciskei Commission Manuscript MS 16 581, Cory Library. Mount Coke established a family planning clinic in 1967 as one of the first clinics in the Ciskei.

89. Susanne M. Klausen, *Race, Maternity and the Politics of Birth Control, 1910–39* (Basingstoke, UK: Palgrave Macmillan, 2004); Amy Kaler, *Running after Pills: Politics, Gender, and Contraception in Colonial Zimbabwe* (Portsmouth, NH: Heinemann, 2003); Catherine Burns, "Controlling Birth, Johannesburg, 1920–60," *South African Historical Journal* 50, no. 1 (2004): 170–98.

90. In fact, Magodla thought the nurses at the hospital did not even want to do family planning but had to because it was a government program. She felt she was chosen to go train in family planning because she was new. She later trained nurses in family planning at Cecilia Makiwane Hospital (Evelyn T. N. Magodla interview, June 7, 2012).

91. Ciskei Legislative Assembly, 2nd Assembly, 3rd Session, Verbatim Report, Volume 5, 1975, 2.1.3/75, 2 of 3, 197, CRL. See also Leslie Xinwa, "The birth control challenge," *Daily Dispatch*, January 5, 1972.

92. Ciskei Legislative Assembly, 2nd Assembly, 5th Session, Verbatim Report, Volume 9, 1977, 2.1.3/77, 3 of 5, CRL; Ciskei Legislative Assembly, 3rd Assembly, 2nd and Special Session, Verbatim Report, Volume 12, 1979/80 2.1.3/80, 1 of 3, CRL. In "Not a Racial Matter at All," *Imvo Zabanstundu*, November 9, 1984, Denis Beckett interviewed M. C. Botha, former minister of Bantu Administration and Development, about a

Notes to Pages 98–103

comment he made encouraging white people to have "apartheid babies." Botha said he was just suggesting that white people have a baby as a gift to the republic, to commemorate its founding, and wasn't trying to call for a change in racial proportions.

93. Klausen, *Race, Maternity and the Politics of Birth Control*, 2.

94. "Malnutrition—Problem on Increase," July 21, 1976, *Daily Dispatch*.

95. Nozokolo Hono interview, October 23, 2013.

96. "A Statement of Policy Objectives: 1979 Department of Health and Welfare," January 22, 1979, B-31, D, Ciskei Commission Manuscript MS 16 581, Cory Library; Sheila Sonjica, "Why Parents Should Tell Children about the Pill," *Daily Dispatch*, Indaba Supplement, September 12, 1980.

97. The 1988 annual Ciskei Department of Health report claimed that people had developed a positive attitude toward family planning, contraceptives were well accepted by the public (especially the injection), there was increased condom use, and that cervical cancer screening was done in all family planning clinics; they had started a small-scale education program and added two male advisors (17); and furthermore, certain high schools had requested aid from family planning nurses because of the incidence of pregnancy and sexually transmitted diseases among their students ("Republic of Ciskei, Department of Health, Annual Report, 1988," 29, Government Publications, Ciskei Health and Welfare Annual Reports, UNISA).

98. De Wet and Bekker, *Rural Development in South Africa*.

99. Nkonki and Mcako interview, June 15, 2011.

100. Nombeko Cecilia Tunyiswa interview, September 20, 2013.

101. Nomali G. G. Bangani interview, October 9, 2013.

102. Feziwe Badi interview, October 7, 2013.

103. Nombeko Hewana, interview by the author, October 8, 2013, Phakamisa Township.

104. Dr. Sino Booi made this comment in a personal conversation on October 30, 2018, in Beacon Bay, East London—maternity cases were "two patients in one," and so she could not just deal with the one patient but had to deal with the effects of what they did to one patient on the other patient and may even have to decide to save one patient over the other.

105. Feziwe Badi interview, October 7, 2013.

106. Nkonki and Mcako interview, June 15, 2011.

107. Thandiwe M. Mkwelo interview, November 27, 2013.

108. Nkonki and Mcako interview, June 15, 2011.

109. Biko and Mcako interview, December 2, 2008.

110. Evelyn T. N. Magodla interview, June 7, 2012.

111. Nkonki and Mcako interview, June 15, 2011.

112. Nombeko Cecilia Tunyiswa interview, September 20, 2013.

113. Thandiwe M. Mkwelo interview, November 27, 2013.

114. Vuyiswa Sodlulashe interview, September 19, 2013.

115. Theresa Nonceba Ntonga, interview by the author, September 26, 2013, Zwelitsha.

116. "She just comes when she is in labor and she doesn't come the first day. She's allowed to go on at home sometimes because there are *matshoko* [a term for old women] there who think they can help her" (Nkonki and Mcako interview, June 15, 2011).

117. Nozokolo Hono interview, October 23, 2013.

118. "Republic of Ciskei, Department of Health, Annual Report, 1985," 97, Government Publications, Ciskei Health and Welfare Annual Reports, UNISA.

119. Celiwe E. Mbie interview, October 7, 2013.

120. Nonfundo R. Rulashe interview, June 4, 2012.

121. Pholisa N. Majiza interview, October 2, 2013.

122. Nobantu Baleni interview, June 6, 2012.

123. Eunice Lulama Mkosana interview, September 25, 2013.

124. Victoria Mjikeliso interview, June 1, 2012.

125. Nkonki and Mcako interview, June 15, 2011.

126. "Ikliniki i-far from isibhedlele. So, wedwa, awuna-advisor ngoku uyenzile [advice ukuthi] i-patient uyitransfere kwihospital." Thembeka E. Gantsho interview, September 19, 2013.

127. Nomabali S. Mbombo interview, October 4, 2013.

128. Nomathemba Ncukana interview, October 22, 2103.

129. Nomathemba Ncukana interview, October 22, 2103.

130. Nosipho Jantjies, interview by the author, September 27, 2013, Ann Shaw Location.

131. Nkonki and Mcako interview, June 15, 2011.

132. Lungelwa F. Mhlambiso interview, December 4, 2013.

133. Linda E. Ngoro interview, December 5, 2013; Qibirha Clinic Maternity Register, 1976–1995, Qibirha Clinic files.

134. Peelton Clinic Maternity Register, 1983–1992, Peelton Clinic files; Tyutyu Clinic Maternity Register, 1983–1992, Tyutyu Clinic files.

135. Lovedale Hospital Board, Report for the Year 1971, Pamphlet Box 5, Cory Library.

136. Retired nurses' dialogue with author, November 7, 2018, Ginsberg.

137. Nkonki and Mcako interview, June 15, 2011.

138. Some were fortunate enough to have worked under older, more experienced nurses who had already worked for years in the clinics. Otherwise, as Celiwe Mbie, remarked, it was "just experience" that trained them for clinic work (Celiwe Elizabeth Mbie interview, October 7, 2013).

139. Nontsikelelo Mfengqe, interview by the author, November 6, 2013, Perksdale; Nomathemba Ncukana interview, October 22, 2103.

140. Nombali Sara Mbombo interview, October 4, 2013.

141. Nozokolo Hono interview, October 23, 2013.

142. Nonzwakazi Gqomfa interview, October 15, 2013.

143. Victoria Mjikeliso interview, June 1, 2012.

144. Constance Nozipho Thoto interview, October 18, 2013.

145. Nomathemba Ncukana interview, October 22, 2103; Ngoro and Majiza also said this in Linda E. Ngoro interview, December 5, 2013; Pholisa N. Majiza interview, October 2, 2013.

146. Theresa Nonceba Ntonga interview, September 26, 2013.

147. Penolope Ntshona interview, October 21, 2013.

148. Mashaba, *Rising to the Challenge*; Egli and Krayer, *"Mothers and Daughters"*; Digby and Sweet, "Nurses as Culture Brokers," 113–29; Horwitz, "'Black Nurses in White,'" 131–46.

Notes to Pages 110–115

149. Pholisa N. Majiza interview, October 2, 2013.

150. Nozokolo Hono interview, October 23, 2013.

151. Pholisa N. Majiza interview, October 2, 2013.

152. Nonzwakazi Gqomfa interview, October 15, 2013.

153. Victoria Mjikeliso interview, June 1, 2012. See also Nomathemba Ncukana interview, October 22, 2013; and Alecia Phiwo Dubula interview, May 4, 2012.

154. Nonfundo R. Rulashe interview, June 4, 2012.

155. Nozokolo Hono interview, October 23, 2013.

Chapter 4. Engaging Xhosa Beliefs and Practices

1. Belsie "Bell" Koliwe Memane, interview by the author, September 26, 2013, Bhisho.

2. Yolisa Ngqokwe, interview by the author, October 4, 2013, King William's Town.

3. Nosipho Jantjies interview, September 27, 2013.

4. Nobantu Baleni interview, June 6, 2012.

5. Ngubane explained that growing up Catholic, in Catholic schools and church, meant that she was herself "raised in a community which presented only part of traditional Zulu culture, thereby leaving gaps in my knowledge and experience." Ngubane, *Body and Mind in Zulu Medicine*, 3.

6. Lumka Someketha interview, May 29, 2012.

7. Program for the Opening Ceremony of Gxulu Clinic at Gxulu Location: Keiskammahoek: September 27, 1967, Gxulu Clinic Folder, Box 535, Eastern Cape Archives and Records.

8. "Care of the Child," *Imvo Zabantsundu*, April 15, 1964; "Yilwa isifo sephepha," *Imvo Zabantsundu*, August 29, 1964.

9. "Mount Coke Hospital 1966 Report," and "Mount Coke Hospital, 1971," Mount Coke Hospital Reports, Folder 2, 1966–1977, Cory Library. In the 1972 August newsletter, Victor Ngowapi, a newly appointed health educator, reflected this approach when he commented on the illogic of people who would not believe in a germ theory because they could not see it, but they would believe in the *impundulu*, which they also did not see. He found that patients who were already ill more readily listened to him. The March 17, 1966, St. Matthew's Board meeting minutes read that they were not doing enough to combat "ignorance which was probably the most important cause of these social diseases. The people needed to be taught nutrition and hygiene and how to limit the size of their families."

10. Digby and Sweet, "Nurses as Culture Brokers." The 1940s saw more respect for cultural relativism in nursing training, but the emphasis on instilling principles of Christian civilization was still underlying training in mission hospitals—and girls and nurses were seen as important to civilizing. Shula Marks pointed out that some nurses had imbibed Western biomedicine pride and a "particular ethos and an entire way of life" in their training, which they held to throughout their careers (Marks, *Divided Sisterhood*).

11. Mashaba, *Rising to the Challenge of Change*, 96.

12. Schuster, "Perspectives in Development"; Hunt, *A Colonial Lexicon*; Digby and Sweet, "Nurses as Culture Brokers"; Digby, *Diversity and Division*.

13. Waltraud Ernst observed that African nurses in mission hospitals "managed to reconcile their role as 'standard bearers of Western medicine' with their allegiance and sympathy for indigenous practices." Waltraud Ernst, ed., *Plural Medicine, Tradition and Modernity, 1800–2000* (New York: Routledge, 2002), 13. Digby also argues that patient pluralism influenced practitioners to be more open to "cross-cultural reshaping" (Digby, *Diversity and Division*, 333).

14. Digby and Sweet, "Nurses as Culture Brokers," 125.

15. Marc Simon Kahn, "The Interface Between Western Mental Health Care and Indigenous Healing in South Africa: Xhosa Psychiatric Nurses' Views on Traditional Healers" (master's thesis, Rhodes University, 1996). Kahn also discusses the various changes or consistencies in Xhosa beliefs due to nursing training (69–70). However, I disagree that the nurses are necessarily in a kind of cultural dissonance.

16. Pholisa N. Majiza interview, October 2, 2013.

17. Alicia Phiwo Dubula interview, May 4, 2012.

18. Nomali Bangani interview, October 9, 2013.

19. Thyra Nomkhitha Mavuso interview, October 15, 2013. She also mentioned a pepper tree and a concoction her sister gave her to help with the effects of a stroke; although she did not remember what it was that her sister gave her.

20. Digby, *Diversity and Division*, 271–72; Nomali Bangani interview, October 9, 2013; Evelyn Magodla interview, June 7, 2012.

21. Feierman, "Struggles for Control."

22. "When a Girl Falls in Love: She Can Sometimes Thank Mr. Wexu," *Daily Dispatch*, Indaba Supplement, November 16, 1973. See also "Witchdoctors Will Hold East London Rally," *Daily Dispatch*, May 12, 1966; "Herbalists: We're Not Quacks," *Daily Dispatch*, Indaba Supplement, January 7, 1977.

23. Tony Dold and Michelle Cocks, *Voices from the Forest: Celebrating Nature and Culture in Xhosaland* (Auckland Park, South Africa: Jacana Media, 2012), 58–61.

24. Nobantu Baleni interview, June 6, 2012.

25. Alan Jeeves, "Public Health and Rural Poverty in South Africa: 'Social Medicine' in the 1940s and 1950s," Seminar Paper (Institute for Advanced Social Research) no. 434 (Johannesburg: University of the Witwatersrand, Institute for Advanced Social Research, 1998).

26. Andile Mayekiso and Munyaradzi Mawere, "Traditional Healers and Medicine in South Africa: A Quest for Legal and Scientific Recognition," in *Between Rhetoric and Reality: The State and Use of Indigenous Knowledge in Post-Colonial Africa*, ed. Munyaradzi Mawere and Samuel Awuah-Nyamekye (Cameroon: Langaa RPCIG, 2015), 109–30.

27. He gained this position by virtue of his Gwali chieftainship. Zilibele Mtumane, "The Poetry of S. M. Burns-Ncamashe" (PhD diss., University of South Africa, 2000).

28. Ciskei Legislative Assembly, 2nd Assembly, 4th Session & 6th Special Session, Verbatim Report, Volume 8, 1976–77, 2.1.3/77, 2 of 4, May 18 and 19, 1976, 435, 445, 451.

29. Ciskei Legislative Assembly, 3rd Assembly, 3rd Session, Verbatim report, Volume 13, 1980, 2.1.3/80, 3 of 3, May 12, 1980, 256. A University of Fort Hare/Rhodes University psychologist also made it into the news with his study: "Witch Doctors Abound in Eastern Cape," *Daily Dispatch*, March 6, 1974.

Notes to Pages 121–122

30. "Can Muti Men Help Doctors?," *Daily Dispatch*, Indaba Supplement, September 19, 1980. He had raised this point in the Ciskei Legislative Assembly the year before when talking about cancer. See Ciskei Legislative Assembly, 3rd Assembly, 2nd and Special Session, Verbatim Report, Volume 12, 1979/80, 2.1.3/80, 1 of 3; 18, May 21–23, 1979, 350–51.

31. "Medicine Men: Maku's Plan," *Daily Dispatch*, February 25, 1981.

32. See Flint's discussion of the licensing of herbalists in Natal and its effects in Flint, *Healing Traditions*.

33. Rüther, "Claims on Africanisation."

34. "Witchdoctors Will Hold East London Rally," May 12, 1966; "Observe Witchcraft Act, Herbalists Told," January 6, 1973; "When a Girl Falls in Love: She Can Sometimes Thank Mr. Wexu," Indaba Supplement, November 16, 1973; "Herbalists: We're Not Quacks," Indaba Supplement, January 7, 1977; "Herbalists in Two-Day Meet," November 3, 1978. See also "Witchdoctors' Secrets May Eventually Aid Modern Medicine Men," by The Chiel, October 1, 1966; "Witchdoctor's Book Calls for Change of Heart in Whites," February 28, 1969; "Protect Plants Used by Witchdoctors—Appeal," June 5, 1971, all in *Daily Dispatch*.

35. "Amagqira kufek'athobel'umbuso—utsho uMnu. Willie," *Imvo Zabantsundu*, June 22, 1963; "Iphumelele iKomfa ebanjwe ngamagqira," *Imvo Zabantsundu*, January 11, 1969.

36. "Herbalists in Two-Day Meet," November 3, 1978; "Observe Witchcraft Act, Herbalists Told," January 6, 1973; "When a Girl Falls in Love: She Can Sometimes Thank Mr. Wexu," Indaba Supplement, November 16, 1973; "Herbalist Is Furious," Indaba Supplement, January 4, 1974, all in *Daily Dispatch*.

37. Some healers saw the establishment of the Ciskei as an opportunity to gain legitimacy and influence. A J. Z. Qethuka, president of the Traditional Healers Organization of the Ciskei (a branch of a larger organization founded in South Africa in 1970), invited Xhosa practitioners to unite with the Ciskei National Independence Party (CNIP) and tried to negotiate for access to forests in the new Ciskei ("Ayamenywa Amagqirha," *Imvo Zabantsundu*, February 8, 1980; "Amagqirha ayabulelwa," *Imvo Zabantsundu*, June 23–27, 1980).

38. Ronald Ingle, medical superintendent at the All Saint's Mission Hospital in the Transkei, held in his archival files a copy of a 1978 journal issue from the Wits Medical School focused on the role of African practitioners in health care along with a newspaper article about a conference on health education in the Transkei that highlighted a call to include herbalists. See *The Leech*, Journal of the University of the Witwatersrand Medical School, 48, no. 2 (1978); "Call to Include Herbalists in Education Plan," *Daily Dispatch*, August 27, 1979.

39. "Republic of Ciskei, Department of Health, Annual Report, 1984," 63 (and 13–14), Government Publications, Ciskei Health and Welfare Annual Reports, 20–22, UNISA. This was part of the efforts of the Ciskeian government to improve its psychiatric health care in general. That same year, in 1984, the department had created a new position in the head office (and proposed a new Mental Health Act, adopted in 1986, that outlined procedures and policies for the care of mentally ill patients). The 1984 report stated that the *amagqirha* had reacted positively to government efforts to enlist their help, but transportation problems prevented effective follow-up in 1985. However,

it is unclear what happened to this initiative. Government reports did not include psychiatric services again until 1988, when the reporting was sparse.

40. As Baranov wrote, biomedicine would enlist the help of African practitioners, not necessarily learning from their approaches but to cooperate with traditional healers "on a limited scale for the benefit of the patient when necessary." Baranov, *The African Transformation*, 22. See also Baranov's discussion of African practitioners brought in to help with the HIV/AIDS epidemic as cultural brokers and translators in chapter 5; "Call to Link Western, Traditional Medicine," *Daily Dispatch*, December 17, 1990; Mayekiso and Mawere, "Between Rhetoric and Reality."

41. Retired nurses' dialogue with author, November 7, 2018, Ginsberg.

42. Kahn, "The Interface." Kahn examines the contours of these various beliefs of Xhosa nurses in the mid-1990s.

43. Gamase Mtyeku interview, June 22, 2012.

44. Nomabali Mbombo interview, October 4, 2013; Feziwe Badi interview, June 6, 2013; Celiwe Mbie interview, October 7, 2013. Vida Mkaza (interview with the author, November 21, 2013, Nkobonkobo) told of TB patients who would come to the South African National Tuberculosis Association (SANTA) Hospital coughing up blood or pieces of their lungs because they had gone to the *amagqirha* and had received medication that was too strong. Bulelwa Ramncwana gave an example of someone who came after two weeks of having stomach pains and resorted to the clinic after Xhosa treatment failed (Bulelwa Ramncwana, interview by the author, December 2, 2013, Peddie). Thandiwe Mkwelo (interview, November 27, 2013) speculated that patients who gave up on *amagqirha* treatment would go to the clinic when they knew their family member was going to die so that they could at least get a death certificate.

45. Celiwe Mbie interview, October 7, 2013; Nonzwakazi Gqomfa interview, October 15, 2013.

46. Segar, "Health Care at the Village Level," 12–13. Ngubane wrote about how the Nyuswa-Zulu considered certain diseases to be European diseases and certain diseases to be African, thus requiring the expertise from their respective medical systems. (Ngubane, *Body and Mind in Zulu Medicine*, 24.)

47. Catherine Burns, "A Long Conversation: The Calling of Katie Makanya," *Agenda* 54 (2002): 134.

48. Thembisa Nkonki and Zotshi Mcako interview, June 15, 2011.

49. Ngubane, *Body and Mind in Zulu Medicine*, 77.

50. Nomali Bangani interview, October 9, 2013.

51. Phiwo Dubula interview, May 4, 2012.

52. Thandiwe Mkwelo interview, November 27, 2013. Mkwelo explained that people would call a swollen limb *umlambo* [river], which indicated to her that the disease was going into the bloodstream and needed antibiotics or it would become septic.

53. Eunice L. Mkosana interview, September 25, 2013.

54. Sheila Sonjica interview, October 14, 2013.

55. Theresa Nonceba Ntonga interview, 26 September 2013. Also Pumla Kwatsha, interview by the author, September 17, 2013, King William's Town; Esther Macaula, interview by the author, September 23, 2013, Madubela. Eunice B. Ntshinga said, "Maybe they knew that at the clinics we always preach, yes" (interview by the author, November 26, 2013, Zwelitsha). While an attitude of scorn characterized earlier times,

Notes to Pages 125–128

Grey Hospital nurse Feziwe Badi acknowledged that some nurses still "snubbed" their patients who clearly used or believed in Xhosa healing in the late twentieth century (Feziwe Badi interview, June 6, 2013).

56. Mavis Makubalo interview, December 3, 2013.

57. Nobantu Baleni interview, June 6, 2012.

58. Nozokolo Hono interview, October 23, 2013.

59. Thyra Nomkhitha Mavuso interview, October 15, 2013.

60. Virginia N. Mkosana interview, September. 23, 2013.

61. Sheila Sonjica interview, October 14, 2013.

62. Nomali Bangani interview, October 9, 2013. For the *Nidorella* plant, see "Fifa Worry about the Use of Muthi," *Sowetan Live*, February 22, 2010, https://www.sowet anlive.co.za/news/2010-02-22-fifa-worry-about-use-of-muthi/.

63. Ntombentsha Anjelina Figlan, interview by the author, December 2, 2013, Peddie.

64. Nobantu Baleni interview, June 6, 2012.

65. Phiwo Dubula interview, May 4, 2012.

66. Ntombentsha Anjelina Figlan interview, December 2, 2013.

67. Celiwe Mbie interview, October 7, 2013.

68. Constance Nozipho Thoto interview, October 18, 2013.

69. Nozokolo Hono interview, October 23, 2013; Lungelwa Mhlambiso interview, December 4, 2013; Nomathemba Ncukana interview, October 22, 2103.

70. Ivy Hermanus, interview by the author, September 18, 2013, Zwelitsha; Lulu Msutu Zuma interview, May 30 and 31, 2012.

71. All Saints' Hospital: District Clinic Course Handbook: Part Three: Health Education, Prepared by Drs. E. R. te Velde, G. W. L. Smeenk, and R. F. Ingle, Produced by Mrs. M. H. Ahlschlager, August 1971, Ronald Ingle personal collection. This handbook compared health education to a bridge. The idea was that if people knew that the nurses recognized their beliefs, they would gain confidence in the nurses who could then introduce new ideas and motivate patients to take new actions. The handbook also stated, "[The health educator] should not aim to destroy all cultural beliefs, but to convince them that certain beliefs have an unfavorable effect upon their health" (2).

72. Julia Segar, "Hard Lives and Evil Winds: Illness Aetiology and the Search for Healing Amongst Ciskeian Villagers," *Social Science and Medicine* 44, no. 10 (1997): 1594; Ngubane, *Body and Mind in Zulu Medicine*, chap. 2; Mthobeli Philip Guma, "Politics of Umoya: Variation in the Interpretation and Management of Diarrheal Illness among Mothers, Professional Nurses, and Indigenous Health Practitioners in Khayelitsha, South Africa" (PhD diss., University of North Carolina, 1998), 185.

73. Segar, "Hard Lives and Evil Winds"; Guma, "Politics of Umoya," 191–200. Guma describes how green colored feces signals to some women that the child has been harmed. See Guma's discussion of the decisions people make regarding where it is necessary to seek care, 157–61, 165; Constance Nozipho Thoto interview, October 18, 2013. Nurses indicated that this sort of belief could also apply to cases of kwashiorkor (retired nurses' dialogue with author, November 7, 2018, Ginsberg).

74. Constance Nozipho Thoto interview, October 18, 2013; Celiwe Mbie interview, October 7, 2013.

75. Phiwo Dubula interview, May 4, 2012.

76. Nombeko Hewana interview, October 8, 2013.

77. Ivy Hermanus interview, September 18, 2013. Yolisa Ngqokwe interview, October 4, 2013.

78. "Yilwa isifo sephepha," *Imvo Zabantsundu*, August 29, 1964.

79. Nobantu Baleni interview, June 6, 2012.

80. Packard, *White Plague, Black Labor*, 277–92.

81. Linda Eunice Ngoro interview, December 5, 2013.

82. Nobantu Baleni interview, June 6, 2012.

83. Nobantu Baleni interview, June 6, 2012.

84. Victoria Mjikeliso interview, June 1, 2012.

85. Digby also found that cross-referrals often happened with certain diseases (like psychosomatic referrals to diviners and TB patients to Western doctors). See Digby, *Diversity and Division*, 354.

86. Marks, *Divided Sisterhood*, 199–202.

87. L. Swartz and C. Lund, "Xhosa-Speaking Schizophrenic Patients' Experiences of Their Condition: Psychosis and Amafufunyana," *South African Journal of Psychology* 28, no. 2 (1998): 63. The *Daily Dispatch* reported committees formed to look at mental health for "non-white" people in 1966.

88. Vera Bührmann, *Living in Two Worlds: Communication Between a White Healer and Her Black Counterparts* (Wilmette, IL: Chiron, 1986). See also Kahn, "The Interface."

89. Ntombentsha Anjelina Figlan interview, December 2, 2013.

90. Ngubane, *Body and Mind in Zulu Medicine*, 144; Julie Parle, "Witchcraft or Madness? The Amandiki of Zululand, 1894–1914," *Journal of Southern African Studies* 29, no. 1 (March 2003): 105–32. See also Julie Parle, *States of Mind: Searching for Mental Health in Natal and Zululand, 1868–1918* (Scottsville, South Africa: University of KwaZulu-Natal Press, 2007).

91. Bührmann, *Living in Two Worlds*, 35; Evelyn Magodla interview, June 7, 2012. When Magodla was first introduced to *amafufunyana* at St. Matthew's Hospital, the other nurses told her the patient would speak in Zulu but said it was just "madness," they really were not possessed. Mabel Cekiso Notshokovu, a traditional healer in Zwelitsha, lamented "the newly fashionable" practice of bewitching people with *amafufunyana*, the magical voices that speak from within an individual, also indicating that people saw it as a new affliction in this time period ("Inkokheli Yamagqirha," *Imvo Zabantsundu*, February 14, 1976).

92. Scholars have noted how Xhosa practitioners identify many different mental disorders and examine the symptoms of epilepsy to make various diagnoses. Hirst, "The Healer's Art," 103; D. J. H. Niehaus et al., "A Culture-Bound Syndrome 'Amafufunyana' and a Culture-Specific Event 'Ukuthwasa': Differentiated by a Family History of Schizophrenia and Other Psychiatric Disorders," *Psychopathology* 37, no. 2 (2004): 59–63; Swartz and Lund, "Xhosa-Speaking Schizophrenic Patients' Experiences of Their Condition: Psychosis and Amafufunyana"; Mpoe Johannah Keikelame and Leslie Swartz, "'A Thing Full of Stories': Traditional Healers' Explanations of Epilepsy and Perspectives on Collaboration with Biomedical Health Care in Cape Town," *Transcult Psychiatry* 52, no. 5 (October 2015): 659–80; Mark Richard Thorpe, "Psycho-Diagnostics in a Xhosa Zionist Church" (master's thesis, Rhodes University, 1982), 40–41.

Notes to Pages 132–136

93. Ngubane, *Body and Mind in Zulu Medicine*, 144–45.

94. A 1984 *Imvo Zabantsundu* article reported that a mentally unstable patient fatally attacked *igqirha* after the *igqirha* realized the patient did not want to take the medicine he asked him to drink and ordered that he be tied with a rope. "Police strongly warned people from keeping at home people who experience mental instability episodes as these people needed to be committed to mental institutions such as the ones in Mzimkhulu and Queenstown" ("Uxhaxhe ngegaba ixhwele ebelimnyanga," *Imvo Zabantsundu*, February 24, 1984). Kahn found that even though nurses could believe that Xhosa practitioners were at times effective, the same nurses did not necessarily believe that Xhosa practitioners had a "positive role" to play in the care of the mentally ill (Kahn, "The Interface," 53). However, 40 percent of his informants also agreed that patients would be better off using both biomedicine and Xhosa medicine, with support for a mutual referral system and statements that Xhosa medical and biomedical treatments did not clash. Yet others said, "Healers should visit hospitals rather than be members of the team" (61–63). Kahn further shows that nurses' distrust of *amagqirha* did not necessarily have to do with the Xhosa system itself, but failures of individual *amagqirha* to finish their training or of a lack of regulation.

95. Nombeko Tunyiswa interview, September 20, 2013.

96. Lumka Someketha interview, May 29, 2012; Thyra Nomkhitha Mavuso interview, October 15, 2013.

97. Thandiwe Violet Mtanga, interview by the author, October 22, 2013, Mgquba Location.

98. Bulelwa Ramncwana interview, December 2, 2013. Evelyn Magodla (interview, June 7, 2012) also talked about the work of missionaries in changing the beliefs of people and persuading people to come to the hospital by giving them food and jobs there.

99. There were a few nurses who talked about faith healing conducted in Christian churches and the refusal of blood transfusions by Seventh-day Adventists as other beliefs that contradicted biomedicine. Thus, it was not just a question of Xhosa beliefs versus biomedicine in the Eastern Cape but also a mixture of beliefs coming from various origins.

100. Nombeko Cecilia Tunyiswa interview, September 20, 2013.

101. Nomabali Mbombo interview, October 4, 2013; Victoria Mjikeliso interview, June 1, 2012.

102. Barbara Mann Wall shows that this corresponded with a wider movement to cooperate more with indigenous healers. She argues that Catholic missions adjusted their relationship with "traditional" healers in the 1970s and 1980s and began sharing knowledge (Wall, *Into Africa*, 120). This was the same time that there was a push for more primary and preventive health care worldwide and greater efforts to work with traditional birth attendants. Baranov also discusses the way that biomedicine sought to work with African practitioners with the HIV/AIDS epidemic. Baranov, *The African Transformation*, chap. 5. See also Rüther, "Claims on Africanisation."

103. Phiwo Dubula interview, May 4, 2012.

104. Lungelwa Mhlambiso interview, December 4, 2013; Linda E. Ngoro interview, December 5, 2013.

105. Nobantu Baleni interview, June 6, 2012.

226 Notes to Pages 136–141

106. Victoria Mjikeliso interview, June 1, 2012.

107. Phiwo Dubula interview, May 4, 2012; Buyiswa V. Vakalisa interview, September 20, 2013; Nonkululeko Vena interview, October 11, 2013.

108. Nomali Bangani interview, October 9, 2013.

109. Vuyiswa Sodlulashe interview, September 19, 2013.

110. Nobantu Baleni interview, June 6, 2012.

111. Constance Nozipho Thoto interview, October 18, 2013; Nomali Bangani interview, October 9, 2013; Victoria Mjikeliso interview, June 1, 2012.

112. Celiwe Mbie interview, October 7, 2013.

113. Digby and Sweet, "Nurses as Culture Brokers," 121. "A simple model of the nurse as the agent of substitution propounded by the missionary societies," they wrote, "thus does not adequately explain her actual role."

114. Phiwo Dubula interview, May 4, 2012.

115. Constance Nozipho Thoto interview, October 18, 2013.

116. Nonfundo Rulashe interview, June 4, 2012.

117. W. D. Hammond-Tooke, *The Bantu-Speaking Peoples of Southern Africa* (London: Routledge & Kegan Paul, 1980), 214. See also Hunt, *A Colonial Lexicon*, 204–5, for similar beliefs in the Belgian Congo.

118. Ngubane, *Body and Mind in Zulu Medicine*, 77–79.

119. See, for example, Guma, "Politics of Umoya," 188–90.

120. Mashaba, *Rising to the Challenge of Change*, 94. Mashaba wrote that in 1963 there were 5,103 black registered midwives, and only 1,582 were single qualified midwives, and that there were thirty-five training hospitals for black midwives run by mission societies in 1964 (101).

121. On infant and maternal mortality, see Michael Gelfand, *Midwifery in Tropical Africa: The Growth of Maternity Services in Rhodesia* (Salisbury: University of Rhodesia, 1978); Hunt, *A Colonial Lexicon*. On maternity care and traditional practices, see Rowley, "Challenges to Effective Maternal Health Care Delivery." On targeting women, see Schuster, "Perspectives in Development"; Holden, "Nursing Sisters in Nigeria, Uganda, Tanganyika"; Pat Holden, "Colonial Sisters: Nurses in Uganda," in *Anthropology and Nursing*, ed. Pat Holden and Jenny Littlewood (New York; London: Routledge, 1991), 71–72; Marks, *Divided Sisterhood*; Hunt, *A Colonial Lexicon*; Digby and Sweet, "Nurses as Culture Brokers"; and Agnes Rennick, "Mission Nurses in Nyasaland: 1890–1916," in *Twentieth Century Malawi: Perspectives on History and Culture*, ed. John McCracken, Timothy J. Lovering, and Fiona Johnson Chalamanda (Stirling, UK: University of Stirling, Center of Commonwealth Studies, 2001), 21–37. On converting people to the clinic and hospital, see Holden, "Colonial Sisters: Nurses in Uganda," 71.

122. Digby, *Diversity and Division*, 263.

123. Mashaba, *Rising to the Challenge of Change*, 7.

124. Retired nurses' dialogue with author, November 7, 2018, Ginsberg.

125. Thyra Nomkhitha Mavuso interview, October 15, 2013.

126. Constance Nozipho Thoto interview, October 18, 2013.

127. Digby, *Diversity and Division*, 393.

128. Belsie Memane interview, September 26, 2013.

129. "Report on Health Education Course for Nurses Sponsored and Arranged by the Transkei and Ciskei Association of Mission Hospitals," held at Tsolo, May 26–30,

Notes to Pages 141–144

1969, Folder 5, MS 17 211, Cory Library. Bosch reportedly spoke frequently in Xhosa and thus likely identified with his Xhosa patients more closely than those who could not speak the language.

130. Nombeko Hewana interview, October 8, 2013.

131. Hilary K. N. Mnyanda interview, September 11, 2013.

132. Lungelwa Mhlambiso interview, December 4, 2013. Also Nosipho Jantjies interview, September 27, 2013, and Nozipho Tom, interview by the author, November 25, 2013, King William's Town.

133. Vuyiswa Sodlulashe interview, September 19, 2013.

134. Thandiwe M. Mkwelo interview, November 27, 2013.

135. Thyra Nomkhitha Mavuso interview, October 15, 2013; Vida Mkaza interview, November 21, 2013; Gamase Mtyeku interview, June 22, 2012.

136. Nosipho Jantjies interview, September 27, 2013.

137. Sandra Rogers, "Since the Women Came': Primary Health Care Nursing in a Nigerian Village" (PhD diss., University of California, San Francisco, 1989); Hunt, *A Colonial Lexicon*; Rowley, "Challenges to Effective Maternal Health Care Delivery"; Digby and Sweet, "Nurses as Culture Brokers."

Chapter 5. Negotiating Marriage and Family Relations

1. Vuyo Mdledle, interview by the author, October 14, 2013, Alice; Nombeko Hewana interview, October 8, 2013; Nombeko Cecilia Tunyiswa interview, September 20, 2013.

2. "Nurses' Pledge of Service," Ciskeian Nursing Association, Democratic Nurses Organization of South Africa (DENOSA), Bhisho Office.

3. Searle merely mentioned, almost in passing, that married female nurses had difficulties in balancing their work with their family responsibilities (Searle, *History of the Development of Nursing in South Africa*, 373–74), and Marks commented that transportation difficulties could affect a nurse's health and cut into time with her children but provided very little evidence or further discussion (Marks, *Divided Sisterhood*, 176). The following are exceptions but deal with later time periods or other countries: Christine Böhmig, *Ghanaian Nurses at a Crossroads: Managing Expectations on a Medical Ward*, African Studies Collection, vol. 23 (Leiden: African Studies Center, 2010); Murray, "The Impact of Divorce on Work Performance of Professional Nurses in Tertiary Hospitals of the Buffalo City Municipality."

4. Senokoanyane, *Their Light, Love and Life*; Buthelezi, *African Nurse Pioneers in KwaZulu/Natal*; Foster, *Lahlekile*. Senokoanyane wrote in the dedication of her book that most people think nurses should be like Florence Nightingale, who serve selflessly, "but they forget that nurses have feelings like everyone else." She pointed out that many chose the profession for economic reasons, which explains why some are unsuited for the work or treat their patients rudely. However, she hardly wrote about her own personal life. Buthelezi acknowledged that a nurse's marriage prospects and family dynamics influenced her professional decisions and performance (18, 316). She discussed the marriage and family life of three of the six nurses she wrote about, delving into her own and her own mother's marriages more, but with the focus on the importance for nurses of marrying an intellectually equal partner and in sharing duties in a marriage (71–75, 238–39, 297–98). She did not analyze further how the nurses' careers

228   Notes to Pages 146–152

intersected with their family lives. Janet Lea Twine similarly addressed the marriage of Bongiwe Bolani in "'I'm Just an Ordinary Nurse': A Life History of Matron Bongiwe Bolani" (bachelor's honors thesis, University of Natal, 1997).

5. For more on these expectations, see E. J. de Jager, "'Traditional' Xhosa Marriage in the Rural Areas of the Ciskei, South Africa," in *Man: Anthropological Essays Presented to O. F. Raum*, ed. E. J. de Jager (Cape Town: C. Struik, 1971), 160–82; Philip Mayer and Iona Mayer, *Townsmen or Tribesmen: Conservatism and the Process of Urbanization in a South African City* (London: Oxford University Press, 1971); Mager, *Gender and the Making of a South African Bantustan*. Women obtained adulthood and womanhood in different stages, tied to her reproductive capacity and status as wife and matriarch (traditionally in many places, women with more than one child gained a higher status, which allowed them to obtain a house and land; mothers-in-law wielded power over daughters-in-law and younger women in families). For more on *lobola*, see Adam Kuper, *Wives for Cattle: Bridewealth and Marriage in Southern Africa* (London: Routledge, 1982).

6. Lulu Msutu Zuma interview, May 30 and 31, 2012.

7. Theresa Nonceba Ntonga interview, September 26, 2013.

8. This description of her wedding resembles Monica Wilson's description of *twala*-initiated marriages in Wilson, "Xhosa Marriage in Historical Perspective," 136.

9. Gladys Noluthando Lucas, interview by the author, November 7, 2013, King William's Town.

10. Marks, *Divided Sisterhood*, 101.

11. See the following for more on gender and marriage changes in the Eastern Cape at the time: Leslie Bank and Linda Qambata, *No Visible Means of Subsistence: Rural Livelihoods, Gender and Social Change in Mooiplaas, Eastern Cape, 1950–1998*, ASC Working Paper 34 (Grahamstown: Institute of Social and Economic Research, Rhodes University, 1999); Mayer and Mayer, *Townsmen or Tribesmen*.

12. "New Role of Black Women Described," April 18, 1972; "Xhosa Woman's Place No Longer in Kitchen," March 13, 1974; "When Women Are Also Breadwinners," October 2, 1984, all in *Daily Dispatch*.

13. "Diary: 'Buzani Kubawo,'" *Imvo Zabantsundu*, March 9, 1963.

14. W. Sangotsha, "Are Our Women Flowers of Homes?," Public Platform, April 13, 1963, and a rebuttal, "An African Women's Position in Our Society," *Imvo Zabantsundu*, April 27, 1963.

15. "Saqonda ubachane eKolweni abafazi," [We realized that he hit the nail in the head with women], September 6, 1969; "Ladies No Longer What They Are Supposed to Be," July 24, 1971; "Amadod'Anengqondo ngaphezu kwabafazi" [Men are more intelligent than women], August 7, 1971; Mabel Mzimba, "Yindoda elikhoboka lomfazi" [It's the man who is a slave of the wife], August 19, 1972; "Esifa Kangaka Nje Amadoda Abulawa Ngabafazi" [High male death rate blamed on women], June 23, 1973; "Men Were Disgruntled," March 2, 1974; "Down with Women's Lib!," April 27, 1974; "You Men—Beware!!," October 26, 1974, all in *Imvo Zabantsundu*.

16. "Sincoma Omazala Nomakoti," September 2, 1972; "Marriage with the Sublime Trade Mark of Eternity," March 10, 1973; "The Future of Our Women in Society," January 18, 1975; Mabel Mzimba, "Ukubaluleka Komfazi kulo ikhaya," January 25,

1975; "Blacks Suffer Oppression from Birth till Death," October 26, 1975, all in *Imvo Zabantsundu*.

17. "Be a Business Woman in Your Own Right, Name and Responsibility," September 23, 1972; "Black Women Put Up a Great Challenge," April 5, 1975; "The Role of the Contemporary Black Woman in Society," January 3, 1976; "The Work of African Women," May 15, 1976; "The African Woman Today—Mrs. P. G. Stamper," October 1, 1977; "Call Me Fez," October 7, 1978 (about the only female legislator in the Ciskei); "Natal Lady Aims for the Bar," October 28, 1978; "Black Women Show Flair for Business and Take the Lead," November 18, 1978; Temba Kente, "Prosecutor Valerie Aims for the Bench," March 31, 1979; "Physiotherapy—All-Female Game in the Ciskei," June 9, 1979, all in *Imvo Zabantsundu*.

18. "Women to Decide What Their Status Must Be," *Imvo Zabantsundu*, February 23, 1971.

19. Mann, *Marrying Well*; Parpart, "'Where Is Your Mother?'"; Sharon Stitcher, "The Middle Class Family in Kenya: Changes in Gender Relations," in *Patriarchy and Class: African Women in the Home and Workforce*, ed. Jane L. Parpart and Sharon Stitcher (Boulder, CO: Westview Press, 1988); Barbara Cooper, *Marriage in Maradi: Gender and Culture in a Hausa Society in Niger, 1900–1989* (Portsmouth, NH: Heinemann, 1997); Allman, Geiger, and Musisi, *Women in African Colonial Histories*; Meghan Healy-Clancy, "The Politics of New African Marriage."

20. See, for example, Thomas and Cole, *Love in Africa*; Mark Hunter, *Love in the Time of AIDS: Inequality, Gender, and Rights in South Africa* (Bloomington: Indiana University Press, 2010); Healy-Clancy, "The Politics of New African Marriage." For other works on love and marriage in African history, see John Mbiti, *Love and Marriage in Africa* (London: Longman, 1973), Nwando Achebe, "Love, Courtship, and Marriage in Africa," in *A Companion to African History*, ed. William H. Worger, Charles Ambler, and Nwando Achebe (Sussex: Wiley Blackwell, 2019), 119–42; Jean-Baptiste and Burrill. "Love, Marriage, and Families in Africa."

21. Thomas and Cole, *Love in Africa*, 13; David Parkin and David Nyamwaya, eds., *Transformations of African Marriage* (Manchester, UK: Manchester University Press, 1987), 13.

22. "Traditional" was often a mix of colonial ideals and African traditions that helped elders maintain authority over youth and women. For two important works on this, see Elizabeth Schmidt, *Peasants, Traders, and Wives: Shona Women in the History of Zimbabwe, 1870–1983* (Portsmouth, NH: Heinemann, 1992); Kristin Mann and Richard Roberts, eds., *Law in Colonial Africa* (Portsmouth, NH: Heinemann, 1991). On the other hand, women, especially in urban areas, engaged in new modernities. See Lynn M. Thomas, "The Modern Girl and Racial Respectability in 1930s South Africa," in the Modern Girl around the World Research Group, *The Modern Girl around the World: Consumption, Modernity, and Globalization* (Durham, NC: Duke University Press, 2008), 96–119.

23. Hunter's work on the changing nature of material exchange linked to intimacy and articles discussing the recent marriage trends of Senegalese women in regard to polygamy are just a few examples. See Hunter, *Love in the Time of AIDS*; Dinah Hannaford and Ellen E. Foley, "Negotiating Love and Marriage in Contemporary Senegal: A Good Man Is Hard to Find," *African Studies Review* 58, no. 2 (September 2015):

230   Notes to Pages 153–154

205–26; Hélène Neveu Kringelbach, "'Marrying Out' for Love: Women's Narratives of Polygyny and Alternative Marriage Choices in Contemporary Senegal," *African Studies Review* 59, no. 1 (April 2016): 155–74.

24. Stitcher, "The Middle Class Family in Kenya"; Parkin and Nyamwaya, *Transformations of African Marriage.* Other authors have pointed to the fact that women continued to bear the burden of childcare even as they took on additional professional or public roles and have highlighted the close links between professional women and kinship networks, particularly when helping with childcare. See Decker, *Mobilizing Zanzibari Women,* 2, 109; Beverly Lindsay, "Issues Confronting Professional African Women: Illustrations from Kenya," in *Comparative Perspectives on Third World Women: The Impact of Race, Sex, and Class,* ed. Beverly Lindsay (New York: Praeger, 1980), 78–95; Harriette McAdoo and Miriam Were, "Extended Family Involvement of Urban Kenyan Professional Women," in *Women in Africa and the African Diaspora,* ed. Rosalyn Terborg-Penn, Sharon Harley, and Andrea Benton Rushing (Washington, DC: Howard University Press, 1989), 133–64; Beatrice Whiting, "The Kenyan Career Woman: Traditional and Modern," in *Women and Success: The Anatomy of Achievement,* ed. Ruth B. Kundsin (New York: William Morrow, 1974), 73. Murray argued that husbands of nurses must accommodate their wife's irregular working hours and must help in managing a home (Murray, "The Impact of Divorce," 2).

25. Van der Vliet found this to be quite common. Virginia van der Vliet, "Traditional Husbands, Modern Wives? Constructing Marriages in a South African Township," in *Tradition and Transition in Southern Africa: Festschrift for Philip and Iona Meyer,* ed. A. D. Spiegel and P. A. McAllister (New Brunswick, NJ: Transaction, 1991), 219–42. For a more contemporary study, see Linda Mary Schwartz, "Grandmothers, Mothers and Daughters: Transformations and Coping Strategies in Xhosa Households in Grahamstown" (master's thesis, Rhodes University, 2006).

26. In Vliet's study, "modern" women whose marriages ended, chose to stay divorced. See Van der Vliet, "Traditional Husbands, Modern Wives?," 235–36. The Mayers wrote that men and women acknowledged that females could gain more independence, but "neither Red nor conservative School men like the idea of an emancipated woman, other than the senior woman who is acting head of a homestead." Mayer and Mayer, *Townsmen or Tribesmen,* 234. Other studies that highlight this dynamic include Healy-Clancy, "The Politics of New African Marriage"; Thomas and Cole, *Love in Africa,* 13, 28, 201; Lynn M. Thomas, *Politics of the Womb: Women, Reproduction, and the State in Kenya* (Berkeley: University of California Press, 2003), chap. 5; Whiting, "The Kenyan Career Woman," 71–75.

27. "Amalungelo abafazi abatshatileyo," *Imvo Zabantsundu,* January 27, 1968.

28. "Women Have Many Rights and Advantages to Enjoy," September 1974; "Husband Has No Right to Know How Much His Wife Earns and Saves," Women's page by Lulama Jijana, December 8, 1973. See also "Men Were Disgruntled," March 2, 1974, all in *Imvo Zabantsundu.*

29. "Charity Kondile Explains: What Breaks Up a Marriage?," November 31, 1970; "Matrimonial Common Sense," January 1, 1972; "No Interference Where Husband and Wife Are Concerned," June 17, 1972; "The End of the Romantic Idealization In Marriage," December 9, 1972; "Husband and Wife Should Work as a Team," January 6, 1973; "Kufuneka Indoda Nomfazi Banyamezelane Bavane," January 27, 1973; "Marriage

with the Sublime Trade Mark of Eternity," March 10, 1973; "Women Complain Husbands Take Them for Granted," February 2, 1974; "Ufuna Ntoni Ngoku Kum? Esitya, enxiba, enendlu" [What does she want from me? She gets food, clothing and she has a house], March 1, 1975; "Happy Marriage," April 24, 1976; "Wives Need Break," March 4, 1978; Ronel Scheffer, "Polygamy Is Out—It's an Insult to Women," March 10, 1979; "Men of Today Exploit and Use Women," July 28–August 1, 1980, all in *Imvo Zabantsundu*.

30. "There Is Companionship and Love in Marriage," *Imvo Zabantsundu*, September 6, 1975.

31. "Makungathwala Nje" [Let's put a stop to abduction of women], *Imvo Zabantsundu*, January 1, 1972.

32. "Uhot'intsuku Wemk'emzini umongikazi," *Imvo Zabantsundu*, November 27, 1976.

33. "The African Woman Today—Mrs. P. G. Stamper," October 1, 1977; Pumla Sangotsha, "Some Tips on Coping with Hubby," June 9, 1973; "Women to Decide What Their Status Must Be," February 23, 1971, all in *Imvo Zabantsundu*.

34. "Lobola—Another Custom Down the Drain?," *Imvo Zabantsundu*, September 1, 1979.

35. Hull deals with this tension as well, although in a different time period and in relation to nurses who migrated overseas (Hull, "International Migration").

36. Hull, "International Migration," 854.

37. Hull, "International Migration," 855; Graeme Reid and Liz Walker, eds., *Men Behaving Differently: South African Men since 1994* (Cape Town: David Philip, 1990); Robert Morrell, *Changing Men in Southern Africa* (Pietermaritzburg, South Africa: University of Natal Press and Zed Press, 2001).

38. Pumla Sangotsha, "Some Tips on Coping with Hubby," *Imvo Zabantsundu*, June 9, 1973.

39. Retired nurses' dialogue with author, November 7, 2018, Ginsberg.

40. On professional women in East Africa, see Whiting, "The Kenyan Career Woman"; McAdoo and Were, "Extended Family Involvement of Urban Kenyan Professional Women"; Thomas, *Politics of the Womb*; Decker, *Mobilizing Zanzibari Women*.

41. "The Working Wife's Marriage Is Always Faced with Some Difficulty," *Imvo Zabantsundu*, March 31, 1973.

42. Nobantu Baleni interview, June 6, 2012. Baleni divorced her husband because he had cheated on her, but she also said that the different levels of education caused friction.

43. Pumla Kwatsha interview, September 17, 2013. This mirrors the emphasis Buthelezi placed on nurses marrying their intellectual and social equals (Buthelezi, *African Nurse Pioneers in KwaZulu/Natal*, 71–75, 238–39, 297–98).

44. Two other studies published in the early twenty-first century found that divorce rates among nurses in Ghana and areas of the former Ciskei were high, citing the difficult working hours, absence from the home or social obligations, and unfaithfulness. See Böhmig, *Ghanaian Nurses at a Crossroads*, 216; Murray, "The Impact of Divorce."

45. Penolope Ntshona interview, October 21, 2013.

46. Pholisa N. Majiza (interview, October 2, 2013) said her husband did not want her to be a nurse at first because people believed nurses wouldn't take care of their

children. Eunice L. Mkosana (interview, September 25, 2013) and Buyiswa V. Vakalisa (interview, September 20, 2013) commented that their husbands feared that they would go around with other men, further indicating that at least some men had this fear, used this to argue against a women's career, or used this to justify their own infidelity. Both Holden and Schuster similarly wrote about how nurses' morality was questioned in Uganda and Zambia as African nurses began to be trained because they were economically independent and living in urban centers. See Holden, "Colonial Sisters: Nurses in Uganda"; Schuster, "Perspectives in Development."

47. At least seven interviewees highlighted the encouragement they received from their parents or other family members to gain training. Other studies have indicated that African women with higher education or professional training tend to have fathers with higher education or fathers who place value on their daughters' education. See, for example, Diane L. Barthel, "The Rise of a Female Professional Elite: The Case of Senegal," *African Studies Review* 18, no. 3 (December 1975): 1–17; Whiting, "The Kenyan Career Woman," 71, 73; Lindsay, "Issues Confronting Professional African Women"; Decker, *Mobilizing Zanzibari Women.*

48. The interviews do not provide very reliable information on the prevalence of this. They were not asked about it directly. It is possible that others also provided economic assistance to their natal families but did not talk about it in the interview.

49. Pumla Sangotsha, "Some Tips on Coping with Hubby," *Imvo Zabantsundu,* June 9, 1973. Sangotsha was not against women obtaining help from their husbands with household duties but argued they would both need to adjust bit by bit and women should not expect to fully adopt Western ideals.

50. Hilary K. Mnyanda interview, September 11, 2013. Mnyanda talked about the difficulties of marrying into a rural family after growing up in the Port Elizabeth area in a family that gave her many opportunities to participate in the family business and learn to drive just like her brother. Indicative of how confined and controlled she felt, she referred to her married name as her "slave name."

51. Southall, "The African Middle Class in South Africa, 1910–1994," 302. Southall provides a good overview of literature on the Black middle class in South African history in this article. He defines the Black middle class as occupying a space between white capital and the Black working class and between "the state and the Black population it ruled," with its status "dictated not only by its resultant standard of living, but by its education, literacy, political authority and, as Maylam implies, its orientation towards material improvement and individual betterment" (290). The professional, semiprofessional, and civil servants of the homelands fit this definition. Other literature on the African middle class defines the group not only according to their income and economic mobility but also according to their aspirations. See Henning Melber, ed., *The Rise of Africa's Middle Class: Myths, Realities, and Critical Engagements* (London: Zed Books, 2016); Roger Southall, *The New Black Middle Class in South Africa* (London: James Currey, 2016). Owen Crankshaw deals more with labor issues in Crankshaw, *Race, Class and the Changing Division of Labour under Apartheid.*

52. Cobley, *Class and Consciousness.*

53. Crankshaw classified nurses as semi-professional partly because their pay was markedly lower than others with more education and managerial opportunities (Crankshaw, *Race, Class and the Changing Division of Labour under Apartheid*, 10). Salaries

Notes to Pages 159–163

varied over the years, and according to a nurse's qualifications, but an African nurse could earn up to R160–200 per month in the late 1960s through the late 1970s (Marks, *Divided Sisterhood*, 264, n. 35; Staff Files, Methodist Church Mount Coke Hospital, MS 17 206, Cory Library.) For a comparison, the estimated average income for African working men in South Africa in 1973 was between R13 and R32 per week (R52–R128 per month), and 61 percent of African female workers earned less than R10 per week (R40 per month) (South African Institute of Race Relations, *A Survey of Race Relations in South Africa 1973*, 202–5).

54. Hilary K. Mnyanda interview, September 11, 2013; Evelyn Magodla interview, June 7, 2012, respectively.

55. "Why, Oh! Why Nurses?," *Imvo Zabantsundu*, August 22, 1964.

56. "Marriages of Convenience," *Imvo Zabantsundu*, May 14, 1977.

57. "Men of Today Exploit and Use Women," *Imvo Zabantsundu*, July 28–August 1, 1980.

58. Hull, "International Migration," 851.

59. Evelyn Magodla interview, June 7, 2012.

60. Lulu Msutu Zuma interview, May 30 and 31, 2012.

61. Maniwe Catherine Mvubu, interview by the author, December 2, 2013, Peddie.

62. Ntombentsha A. Figlan interview, December 2, 2013. This was also mentioned in retired nurses' dialogue with author, November 7, 2018, Ginsberg.

63. "The Working Wife's Marriage is Always Faced With Some Difficulty," *Imvo Zabantsundu*, March 31, 1973.

64. "Umama ophangelayo," *Imvo Zabantsundu*, August 23–29, 1991.

65. "The Working Wife's Marriage Is Always Faced with Some Difficulty," *Imvo Zabantsundu*, March 31, 1973.

66. See also "Sister Dlomo Works Her Way to Top," *Daily Dispatch*, February 20, 1973; "Marg Ndengane to Study Psychiatry at London Institute," *Daily Dispatch*, September 5, 1980.

67. Nomabaso Beatrice Dubula, interview by the author, September 24, 2013, Ann Shaw Location.

68. Ethel Nonkululeko Gwayi, interview by the author, October 16, 2013, Mavuso Location.

69. Lungelwa F. Mhlambiso interview, December 4, 2013.

70. Nomabali S. Mbombo interview, October 4, 2013.

71. Nosipho Jantjies interview, September 27, 2013.

72. Nombeko Hewana interview, October 8, 2013.

73. Pumla Kwatsha interview, September 17, 2013; Theresa N. Ntonga interview, September 26, 2013.

74. For Buthelezi, writing of her own mother who qualified as a nurse in the late 1920s, a teacher made a good spouse for a nurse because they were matched academically, intellectually, and socially, and they were both self-made. She talked about her mother and father sharing household chores. Buthelezi, *African Nurse Pioneers*, 74.

75. Ethel N. Gwayi interview, October 16, 2013.

76. Unmarried women with children could gain senior status as an adult woman. An *inkazana* in Xhosa societies was a woman who had a child outside of marriage, was in her late twenties, and yet did not have marriage opportunities, or had returned from

234 Notes to Pages 163–168

a bad marriage. Her children belonged to her father's lineage where she had an accepted place in the household (Mayer and Mayer, *Townsmen or Tribesmen*, 235–36; Jager, "'Traditional' Xhosa Marriage").

77. Mbie said she finally got a matron at Nompumelelo to understand her situation with her child with health problems, and the matron helped her get a transfer to Mount Coke Hospital in 1992 so she could live near her mother (Celiwe Elizabeth Mbie interview, October 7, 2013).

78. Pumla Kwatsha interview, September 17, 2013.

79. Feziwe Badi interview, October 7, 2013. Also Joan Mavuso interview, June 22, 2012.

80. Guide to Service Contract Between Employing Body and District Nurse, n.d., Box 539, Regional Authorities: Clinics, Hospitals, General Folder, Eastern Cape Archives and Records.

81. Judith Nolde, "South African Women under Apartheid: Employment Rights, with Particular Focus on Domestic Service & Forms of Resistance to Promote Change," *Third World Legal Studies* 10, no. 10 (1991): 203–23.

82. Nomathemba Ncukana (Port Elizabeth, 1969, had to resign and then reapply); Nombeko C. Tunyiswa (1963, Victoria Hospital, had to resign when she got married, no maternity leave); Nobomvu G. Zondani (chased away from Grey when pregnant, 1967–12, and had to beg for her job again).

83. Guide to Service Contract between Employing Body and District Nurse, n.d., Box 539, Regional Authorities: Clinics, Hospitals, General Folder, Eastern Cape Archives and Records.

84. Lumka Someketha (interview, May 29, 2012) also said there was a short amount of time; Celiwe Elizabeth Mbie interview, October 7, 2013.

85. Nonkululeko Vena interview, October 11, 2013.

86. Evelyn Magodla interview, June 7, 2012.

87. Ethel Nonkululeko Gwayi interview, October 16, 2013.

88. Nombeko C. Tunyiswa interview, September 20, 2013.

89. Buyiswa Victoria Vakalisa interview, September 20, 2013.

90. Evelyn Magodla interview, June 7, 2012.

91. Anonymous, interview by the author, December 6, 2013, King William's Town.

92. Nonkululeko Vena interview, October 11, 2013.

93. Nozipho Tom interview, November 25, 2013.

94. Ntombentsha A. Figlan interview, December 2, 2013.

95. Gladys Noluthando Lucas interview, November 7, 2013.

96. Christina Nomqondiso Njamela, interview by the author, June 26, 2012, Zwelitsha.

97. Retired nurses' dialogue with author, November 7, 2018, Ginsberg.

98. Nomabali S. Mbombo interview, October 4, 2013.

99. Nosipho Jantjies interview, September 27, 2013.

100. Nosipho Jantjies interview, September 27, 2013; Pumla Kwatsha interview, September 17, 2013. Hull analyzes the influence of domestic struggles on nurses' decisions to migrate internationally for work in the postapartheid era in Hull, "International Migration." Hull presents evidence on the ways that husbands attempted to

intervene in the career paths of nurses and the social networks that women drew on to provide childcare in their absence. She argues that women's roles as wives and mothers must be considered when assessing their choices and abilities to seek greater status and economic opportunity through international migration.

101. Ciskei Legislative Assembly, 1st Ass. Special Session and Second Session 1982, Verbatim Report, Volume 3, May 26, 1982, CRL.

102. For example, two nurses with five children unsuccessfully appealed to the South African Department of Health for help in housing their children at the Gxulu and Burns Hill clinics in 1968 (Inspection Report on Gxulu Clinic, March 13, 1968, Gxulu File, Inspection Report on Burnshill Clinic, July 22, 1968, Burnshill Location File, both in Box 535, Regional Authorities: Clinics, Eastern Cape Archives and Records).

103. Nontsikilelo Mfengqe interview, November 6, 2013. This sentiment was also voiced in the retired nurses' dialogue with author, November 7, 2018, Ginsberg.

104. St. Matthew's Hospital Board Meeting Minutes, August 31, 1962, AB1354, Minute Books, CPSA Diocese of Grahamstown, St. Matthew's Hospital, Keiskammahoek, vol. 2: 1956–1969, HP.

105. Mount Coke Board Meeting, November 9, 1972, Folder 1, and "Mount Coke Methodist Hospital, Matron's Report to the Mount Coke Hospital Board to be held on Thursday, 27th November 1975," Folder 2, both in Methodist Church Mount Coke Hospital, Box 3, MS 17 207, Cory Library.

106. Ciskei Legislative Assembly, 2nd Ass. 4th Session, Verbatim Report, Volume 8, 1976–77, May 19, 1976, 459, CRL.

107. See comments in "Republic of Ciskei, Department of Health, Annual Report, 1985," 82, and "Republic of Ciskei, Department of Health, Annual Report, 1986," 81, both in Government Publications, Ciskei Health and Welfare Annual Reports, UNISA. The report in 1986 reads that the difference in salaries between Republic of South Africa and Ciskei meant that they lost thirty nurses.

108. "Republic of Ciskei, Department of Health, Annual Report, 1988," 9–10, Government Publications, Ciskei Health and Welfare Annual Reports, UNISA.

109. St. Matthew's Hospital Board Meeting Minutes, March 25, 1969, AB1354, Minute Books, CPSA Diocese of Grahamstown, St. Matthew's Hospital, Keiskammahoek, vol. 2: 1956–1969, HP.

110. Penolope Ntshona interview, October 21, 2013; Buyiswa Victoria Vakalisa interview, September 20, 2013; Patricia Lilly Patiwe Menye, interview by the author, October 8, 2013, Breidbach.

111. Gamase Mtyeku interview, June 22, 2012. Ethel Nonkuuleko Gwayi also hid her marriage and pregnancy at Frere (interview, October 16, 2013).

112. See Rachel Jewkes, Naeemah Abrahams, and Zodumo Mvo, "Why Do Nurses Abuse Patients? Reflections from South African Obstetric Services," *Social Science and Medicine* 47, no. 11 (1998): 1781–95; AFPL d'Oliveira, S. G. Diniz, L. B. Schraiber, "Violence Against Women in Health Care Institutions: An Emerging Problem," *The Lancet* 359 (May 2002): 1681–85. Digby also briefly discusses the perception of nurses as overbearing in *Diversity and Division*, 230–31.

113. Murray, "The Impact of Divorce." Murray later completed a PhD dissertation with recommendations on providing support for divorced nurses.

114. Thoto interview, October 18, 2013.

236 Notes to Pages 171–175

115. Gamase Mtyeku interview, June 22, 2012; Tyileka P. Malo, interview by the author, October 10, 2013, Bhisho; Nomfundo Rulashe interview, June 4, 2012; Weziwe Tsotsobe interview, October 2, 2013.

116. Ethel Nonkululeko Gwayi interview, October 16, 2013; Tyileka P. Malo interview, October 10, 2013. Yolisa Ngqokwe said, "You have to come humble and come as a mother" (interview, October 4, 2013).

117. Pumla Kwatsha interview, September 17, 2013.

118. Nonzwakazi Gqomfa interview, October 15, 2013.

119. Lungelwa F. Mhlambiso interview, December 4, 2013.

Conclusion

1. Peires, "The Implosion of Transkei and Ciskei," 378; Manona, "The Collapse of the 'Tribal Authority' System"; Wotshela, "Insurrection and Locally Negotiated Transition in Stutterheim, Eastern Cape, 1980–1994,"; Southall and De Sas Kropiwnicki, "Containing the Chiefs," 57–59.

2. Southall and De Sas Kropiwnicki, "Containing the Chiefs," 57.

3. Peires, "The Implosion of Transkei and Ciskei," 379.

4. Wotshela, "The Fate of Ciskei."

5. For other leaders' refusal to relinquish their power, see Jason Robinson, "Fragments of the Past: Homeland Politics and the South African Transition, 1990–2014," *Journal of Southern African Studies* 41, no. 5 (2015): 953–67.

6. Colin Stewart White, "The Rule of Brigadier Oupa Gqozo in Ciskei: 4 March 1990 to 22 March 1994" (master's thesis, Rhodes University, 2008), http://letras.comp .filos.unam.mx/wp-content/uploads/2015/03/ColinWhite_TheRuleOfBrigadierOupa GqozoInCiskei.pdf.

7. Stephanie Victor, "The Politics of Remembering and Commemorating Atrocity in South Africa: The Bhisho Massacre and Its Aftermath, 1992–2012," *Journal of Southern African Studies* 41, no. 1 (2015): 83–102.

8. Manona, "The Collapse of the 'Tribal Authority' System"; Southall and De Sas Kropiwnicki, "Containing the Chiefs," 58; Brown Bavusile Maaba, "An Eastern Cape Village in Transition: The Politics of Msobomvu," in *From Apartheid to Democracy: Localities and Liberation*, ed. Christopher Saunders (Cape Town: Department of Historical Studies, University of Cape Town, 2007), 12–48; Wotshela, "Insurrection and Locally Negotiated Transition in Stutterheim, Eastern Cape, 1980–1994"; Wotshela, "The Fate of Ciskei."

9. Celiwe E. Mbie interview, October 7, 2013.

10. "Masa President Sworn In as New Ciskei Health Minister," *Daily Dispatch*, April 20, 1990.

11. "Mdantsane Hospital Crippled by Strike," April 26, 1990; "Government Condemns Union, Warns Strikers," April 27, 1990; "Nurses Arrested as Strike Continues," April 27, 1990; and "Gqozo Warns Union to Stay Out of Ciskei," May 2, 1990, all in *Daily Dispatch*. The strikers demanded a sixty-cent wage increase, reduction of long working hours, increase in night duty allowances, promised casualty pay, reduction of deductions on salaries, and equal privileges and fringe benefits for both married and single staff members. The threat of strikes in hospitals spread across South Africa at this time as the country worked on integrating its previously segregated system and

Notes to Pages 175–178

planned to improve public health care. See also Bafana Mkefa, "Babhokele ucalulo," *Imvo Zabantsundu*, January 11, 1991.

12. "Hospital's Staff Problems Cited," *Daily Dispatch*, May 25, 1991.

13. See the following *Daily Dispatch* articles: "Ciskei Director of Health Suspended," June 25, 1992; "Mdara, Ciskei Fund Row over Relief Aid," November 21, 1992; "SA Asked to Run Ciskei Health Dept," July 19, 1993; "Ciskei Nurses' College Closed after Fees Protest," September 11, 1993.

14. "SA Asked to Run Ciskei Health Dept," *Daily Dispatch*, July 19, 1993.

15. "Health Workers Criticize Services," *Daily Dispatch*, March 3, 1993.

16. "Ciskei Nurses Threaten to Disrupt Services," *Daily Dispatch*, March 18, 1994.

17. Hoosen Coovadia et al., "The Health and Health System of South Africa: Historical Roots of Current Public Health Challenges," *Lancet* 374 (September 5, 2009): 828; "Health Problems Agreed On but Not Solutions," *Daily Dispatch*, August 19, 1991, describing a speech by the ANC's secretary for health, Dr. R. Mgijima, at a conference.

18. Southall and De Sas Kropiwnicki, "Containing the Chiefs," 61. In doing so, they argue, the ANC engaged in a balancing act of incorporating chiefs into a new democratic system.

19. Jenni Horn, "Medical Care in Crisis," *Daily Dispatch*, November 15, 1991; "SA Can't Shake Health Apartheid," *Daily Dispatch*, March 17, 1994.

20. Wotshela, "The Fate of Ciskei"; also Nosipho Jantjies interview, September 27, 2013.

21. "SA, TBVC Health Ministers to Attend Meeting in Ciskei," *Daily Dispatch*, January 24, 1991; "ANC to Discuss Health Policy," *Daily Dispatch*, April 12, 1991. The plan was also to have community input all along the way ("Call for Unitary Health Service," *Daily Dispatch*, April 17, 1991). In 1991 the South African government announced that all primary health care services would be put under local authorities, secondary services such as hospitals under regional governments, and tertiary services under the national system ("Rationalisation Will Not Mean Job Losses—Health Department," *Daily Dispatch*, July 25, 1992).

22. Coovadia et al., "The Health and Health System of South Africa," 828.

23. "Call to Link Western, Traditional Medicine," *Daily Dispatch*, December 17, 1990.

24. Coovadia et al., "The Health and Health System of South Africa," 829.

25. Coovadia et al., "The Health and Health System of South Africa," 829; Hull, *Contingent Citizens*, 119–24.

26. Beauty Noziwo Nongauza interview, October 1, 2013; Nomali G. G. Bangani interview, October 9, 2013.

27. Ntombentsha Anjelina Figlan interview, December 2, 2013.

28. Beauty Noziwo Nongauza interview, October 1, 2013; Nomali G. G. Bangani interview, October 9, 2013; Nomathemba Ncukana interview, October 22, 2103; Lungelwa F. Mhlambiso interview, December 4, 2013; Virginia N. Mkosana interview, September 23, 2013.

29. Evelyn Magodla, though, thought the fact that they had to strike to get better pay meant there was something wrong with the new system (Evelyn T. N. Magodla interview, June 7, 2012).

30. Jewkes, Mvo, and Abrahams, "Why Do Nurses Abuse Patients?"; D'Oliveira, Diniz, and Schraiber, "Violence against Women in Health Care Institutions"; Digby, *Diversity and Division*, 230–31; Coovadia et al., "The Health and Health System of South Africa," 829; Hull, *Contingent Citizens*, 210–11.

31. Nobantu Baleni interview, June 6, 2012.

32. Vuyo Mdledle interview, October 14, 2013.

33. Christina Nomqondiso Njamela interview, 26 June 2012.

34. Lungelwa F. Mhlambiso interview, December 4, 2013.

35. Virginia N. Mkosana interview, September 23, 2013.

36. Linda E. Ngoro interview, December 5, 2013.

37. Retired nurses' dialogue with author, November 7, 2018, Ginsberg.

38. Nonzwakazi Gqomfa interview, October 15, 2013; Nosipho Jantjies interview, September 27, 2013; Yolisa Ngqokwe interview, October 4, 2013.

39. Nomabali S. Mbombo interview, October 4, 2013.

40. Nomathemba Ncukana interview, October 22, 2103.

41. Lulama Nkani interview, November 27, 2013.

42. Dlamini, *Native Nostalgia*, 12.

43. Hull, *Contingent Citizens*, 20.

44. Hull, *Contingent Citizens*, 157–61.

45. Esther Macaula interview, September 23, 2013.

46. Yolisa Ngqokwe interview, October 4, 2013.

47. Victoria Mjikeliso interview, June 1, 2012.

48. Francine/Francis D. Zani, interview by the author, November 19, 2013, Zwelitsha.

49. Francine/Francis D. Zani interview, November 19, 2013; Lydia Liziwe Nohako Tile, interview by the author, September 23, 2013, Brilliant Park Location; Gamase Mtyeku interview, June 22, 2012.

50. Nonfundo R. Rulashe interview, June 4, 2012.

51. Alecia Phiwo Dubula interview, May 4, 2012; Buyiswa V. Vakalisa interview, September 20, 2013.

52. Gamase Mtyeku interview, June 22, 2012.

53. Gamase Mtyeku interview, June 22, 2012; Alecia Phiwo Dubula interview, May 4, 2012; Evelyn T. N. Magodla interview, June 7, 2012.

54. Theresa Nonceba Ntonga interview, September 26, 2013.

55. Hull, *Contingent Citizens*, 172–77.

56. Pholisa Nombulelo Majiza interview, October 2, 2013.

57. Coovadia et al., "The Health and Health System of South Africa"; Robert Marten et al., "An Assessment of Progress Towards Universal Health Coverage in Brazil, Russia, India, China, and South Africa (BRICS)," *Lancet* 384 (April 30, 2014): 2164–71, http://dx.doi.org/10.1016/S0140-6736(14)60075-1.

58. Robinson, "Fragments of the Past," 962; Jonathan Hyslop, "Political Corruption: Before and after Apartheid," *Journal of Southern African Studies* 31, no. 4 (December 2005): 785.

Bibliography

Archival Collections

African Studies Documentation Center, University of South Africa Library (UNISA)
    AAS 151 UNISA—Ciskei Government Accession 1966–1972
    AAS 190 UNISA—Ciskei Collection Accession 1976–1980
    Government Publications—Ciskei Annual Reports
Archives and Records Services, Eastern Cape Department of Sport, Recreation, Arts, and Culture, King William's Town (Eastern Cape Archives and Records)
Center for Research Libraries, Chicago (CRL)
    Daily Dispatch, Microfilmed for Cooperative Africana Microform Project (CAMP)
    Imvo Zabantsundu (CAMP)
    Official Publications of South African States, 1900–1978, Part 2, Ciskei
Cory Library for Historical Research, Rhodes University (Cory Library)
    Lovedale Collection
    Methodist Church of South Africa Archives
Democratic Nursing Organization of South Africa (DENOSA) Library and Bhisho Branch Offices
Historical Papers, William Cullen Library, University of the Witwatersrand (HP)
    CPSA Diocese of Grahamstown
    Jane McLarty Papers
    South African Institute of Race Relations
Killie Campbell Africana Library
National Archives and Records of South Africa
    National Archives Repository, Pretoria (National Archives)
    Cape Town Archives Repository
National Heritage and Cultural Studies Center, University of Fort Hare (NAHECS)
    Periodicals Collection—*Inkqubela*

Newspapers and Periodicals

Daily Dispatch, 1966–90, East London, boxes filed by subject
Imvo Zabantsundu, 1960–95, Amathole Museum

Bibliography

Interviews by the Author

Anonymous, December 6, 2013, King William's Town.
Badi, Feziwe Leonora, October 7, 2013, Zwelitsha.
Baleni, Nobantu Zelpha, June 6, 2012, Zwelitsha.
Bangani, Nomali Georgina Gwarabe, October 9, 2013, Madubela.
Dubula, Alecia Phiwo, May 4, 2012, Bhisho.
Dubula, Nomabaso Beatrice, September 24, 2013, Ann Shaw Location.
Figlan, Ntombentsha Anjelina, December 2, 2013, Peddie.
Gantsho, Thembeka Ellen, September 19, 2013, Madubela.
Gqomfa, Nonzwakazi, October 15, 2013, Lower Gqumashe.
Gwayi, Ethel Nonkululeko, October 16, 2013, Mavuso Location.
Hermanus, Ivy, September 18, 2013, Zwelitsha.
Hewana, Nombeko, October 8, 2013, Phakamisa Township.
Hono, Nozokolo, October 23, 2013, Middledrift.
Hoyana, Eugenia Novela Nixofa, September 24, 2013, Ann Shaw Location.
Jantjies, Nosipho, September 27, 2013, Ann Shaw Location.
Kwatsha, Pumla, September 17, 2013, King William's Town.
Lucas, Gladys Noluthando, November 7, 2013, King William's Town.
Macaula, Esther, September 23, 2013, Madubela.
Magodla, Christina Vuyelwa, September 19, 2013, Madubela.
Magodla, Evelyn T. N., June 7, 2012, King William's Town.
Majiza, Pholisa Nombulelo, October 2, 2013, Burns Hill.
Makubalo, Mavis, December 3, 2013, Keiskammahoek.
Malo, Tyileka Priscilla, October 10, 2013, Bhisho.
Mavuso, Joan, June 22, 2012, Zwelitsha.
Mavuso, Thyra Nomkhitha, October 15, 2013, Mavuso Location.
Mbie, Celiwe Elizabeth, October 7, 2013, Bhisho.
Mbombo, Nomabali Sara, October 4, 2013, King William's Town.
Mcako, Nomazotsho Nyakati, and Nontsikilelo Biko, December 2, 2008, Ginsberg.
Mdledle, Vuyo, October 14, 2013, Alice.
Memane, Belsie "Bell" Koliwe, September 26, 2013, Bhisho.
Menye, Patricia Lilly Patiwe, October 8, 2013, Breidbach.
Mfengqe, Nontsikelelo, November 6, 2013, Perksdale.
Mhlambiso, Lungelwa Francis, December 4, 2013, Mqhayiso (Amathole Basin).
Mjikeliso, Victoria, June 1, 2012, King William's Town.
Mkaza, Vida, November 21, 2013, Nkobonkobo.
Mkosana, Eunice Lulama, September 25, 2013, Ngcwazi.
Mkosana, Virginia N., September 23, 2013, and October 22, 2013, Alice.
Mkwelo, Thandiwe Millicent, November 27, 2013, Tshatshu Location.
Mnyanda, Hilary Kunjuza, September 11, 2013, and September 18, 2013, Bhisho.
Mtanga, Thandiwe Violet, October 22, 2013, Mgquba Location.
Mtyeku, Gamase Doris Sonjica, June 22, 2012, Bhisho.
Mvubu, Maniwe Catherine, December 2, 2013, Peddie.
Ncukana, Nomathemba, October 22, 2013, Ann Shaw Location.
Ngoro, Linda Eunice, December 5, 2013, Mgxotyeni.

Bibliography

Njamela, Christina Nomqondiso, June 26, 2012, Zwelitsha.

Nkani, Lulama "Lulu," November 27, 2013, Zwelitsha.

Nkonki, Thembisa E. (with Zotshi Mcako), June 15, 2011, Tyutyu Village.

Nongauza, Beauty Noziwo, October 1, 2013, King William's Town; interview by Lindani Ntenteni and the author, November 19, 2008, King William's Town.

Ngqokwe, Yolisa, October 4, 2013, King William's Town.

Ntonga, Theresa Nonceba, September 26, 2013, Zwelitsha.

Ntshinga, Eunice Bukeka, November 26, 2013, Zwelitsha.

Ntshona, Penelope, October 21, 2013, Alice.

Ramncwana, Bulelwa, December 2, 2013, Peddie.

Rulashe, Nonfundo R., June 4, 2012, Dimbaza.

Sodlulashe, Vuyiswa, September 19, 2013, Madubela.

Someketha, Lumka, May 29, 2012, King William's Town.

Sonjica, Sheila, October 14, 2013, Debe Nek.

Thoto, Constance Nozipho, October 18, 2013, Kuntselamanzi.

Tile, Lydia Liziwe Nohako, September 23, 2013, Brilliant Park Location.

Tom, Nozipho, November 25, 2013, King William's Town.

Tsotsobe, Weziwe; October 2, 2013, King William's Town.

Tunyiswa, Nombeko Cecilia, September 20, 2013, Ann Shaw Location.

Vakalisa, Buyiswa Victoria, September 20, 2013, Middledrift.

Vena, Nonkululeko, October 11, 2013, Ngqele.

Zani, Francine/Francis D., November 19, 2013, Zwelitsha.

Zondani, Nobomvu Gladys, October 4, 2013, Ginsberg.

Zuma, Lulu Msutu, May 30 and 31, 2012, Jubisa.

Secondary Sources

Achebe, Nwando. *Farmers, Traders, Warriors, and Kings: Female Power and Authority in Northern Igboland, 1900–1960.* Portsmouth, NH: Heinemann, 2005.

———."Love, Courtship, and Marriage in Africa." In *A Companion to African History,* ed. William H. Worger, Charles Ambler, and Nwando Achebe, 119–42. Sussex: Wiley Blackwell, 2019.

Allman, Jean, Susan Geiger, and Nakanyike Musisi, eds. *Women in African Colonial Histories.* Bloomington: Indiana University Press, 2002.

Alpers, Edward. "The Story of Swema: Female Vulnerability in Nineteenth-Century East Africa." In *Women and Slavery in Africa,* edited by Claire Robertson and Martin Klein, 185–219. Madison: University of Wisconsin Press, 1983.

Amadiume, Ifi. *Daughters of the Goddess, Daughters of Imperialism: African Women, Culture, Power, and Democracy.* New York: Zed Books, 2000.

Andersson, Neil, and Shula Marks. "Industrialization, Rural Health, and the 1944 National Health Services Commission in South Africa." In *The Social Basis of Health and Healing in Africa,* edited by Steven Feierman and John M. Janzen, 131–61. Berkeley: University of California Press, 1992.

Bank, Leslie, and Linda Qambata. *No Visible Means of Subsistence: Rural Livelihoods, Gender and Social Change in Mooiplaas, Eastern Cape, 1950–1998.* ASC Working Paper 34. Grahamstown, South Africa: Institute of Social and Economic Research, Rhodes University, 1999.

Bibliography

Baranov, David. *The African Transformation of Western Medicine and the Dynamics of Global Cultural Exchange.* Philadelphia: Temple University Press, 2008.

Barthel, Diane L. "The Rise of a Female Professional Elite: The Case of Senegal." *African Studies Review* 18, no. 3 (December 1975): 1–17.

Beer, Cedric de. *The South African Disease: Apartheid Health and Health Services.* Trenton, NJ: Africa World, 1986.

Beinart, William. "Beyond 'Homelands': Some Ideas about the History of African Rural Areas in South Africa." *South African Historical Journal* 64, no. 1 (March 2012): 5–21.

Berger, Iris. "An African American 'Mother of the Nation': Madie Hall Xuma in South Africa, 1940–1963." *Journal of Southern African Studies* 27, no. 3 (2001): 547–66.

———. *Women in Twentieth-Century Africa.* Cambridge: Cambridge University Press, 2016.

Böhmig, Christine. *Ghanaian Nurses at a Crossroads: Managing Medical Expectations on a Medical Ward.* African Studies Collection 23. Leiden: African Studies Center, 2010.

Bozzoli, Belinda. *Women of Phokeng: Consciousness, Life Strategy, and Migrancy in South Africa, 1900–1983.* Portsmouth, NH: Heinemann, 1991.

Brandt, Allan M., and Martha Gardner. "The Golden Age of Medicine?" In *Medicine in the Twentieth Century,* edited by Roger Cooter and John Pickstone, 21–37. Amsterdam: Harwood Academic, 2000.

Bührmann, Vera. *Living in Two Worlds: Communication Between a White Healer and Her Black Counterparts.* Wilmette, IL: Chiron, 1986.

Burns, Catherine. "Controlling Birth, Johannesburg, 1920–60." *South African Historical Journal* 50, no. 1 (2004): 170–98.

———. "A Long Conversation: The Calling of Katie Makanya." *Agenda* 54 (2002): 133–40.

———. "Louisa Mvemve: A Woman's Advice to the Public on the Cure of Various Diseases." *Kronos* 23 (November 1996): 108–34.

———. "'A Man Is a Clumsy Thing Who Does Not Know How to Handle a Sick Person': Aspects of the History of Masculinity and Race in the Shaping of Male Nursing in South Africa, 1900–1950." *Journal of Southern African Studies,* Special Issue on Masculinities in Southern Africa, 24, no. 4 (December 1998): 695–717.

Burrill, Emily. *States of Marriage: Gender, Justice and Rights in Colonial Mali.* Athens: Ohio University Press, 2015.

Buthelezi, Mazo Sybil T. MaDlamini. *African Nurse Pioneers in KwaZulu/Natal, 1920–2000.* Victoria, BC: Trafford, 2004.

Butler, Jeffrey, Robert I. Rotberg, and John Adams. *The Black Homelands of South Africa: The Political and Economic Development of Bophuthatswana and KwaZulu.* Berkeley: University of California Press, 1977.

Charton, Nancy, ed. *Ciskei: Economics and Politics of Dependence in a South African Homeland.* London: Croom Helm, 1980.

Cobley, Alan. *Class and Consciousness: The Black Petty Bourgeoisie in South Africa, 1924–1950.* New York: Greenwood Press, 1990.

Cohen, David William. "Doing Social History from Pim's Doorway," in *Reliving the Past: The Worlds of Social History,* ed. Olivier Zunz, 191–235. Chapel Hill: University of North Carolina Press, 2014.

Bibliography

Comaroff, Jean, and John Comaroff. "Homemade Hegemony." In *Ethnography and the Historical Imagination: Selected Essays*, edited by Jean Comaroff and John Comaroff. Boulder, CO: Westview, 1992.

———.*Of Revelation and Revolution: Christianity, Colonialism, and Consciousness in South Africa*. Vol. 1. Chicago: University of Chicago Press, 1991.

Cooper, Barbara. *Marriage in Maradi: Gender and Culture in a Hausa Society in Niger, 1900–1989*. Portsmouth, NH: Heinemann, 1997.

Coovadia, Hoosen, Rachel Jewkes, Peter Barron, David Sanders, and Diane McIntyre. "The Health and Health System of South Africa: Historical Roots of Current Public Health Challenges." *Lancet* 374 (September 5, 2009): 817–34.

Crankshaw, Owen. *Race, Class and the Changing Division of Labour under Apartheid*. London: Routledge, 1997.

Decker, Corrie. *Mobilizing Zanzibari Women: The Struggle for Respectability and Self-Reliance in Colonial East Africa*. New York: Palgrave Macmillan, 2014.

Digby, Anne. "'The Bandwagon of Golden Opportunities'? Healthcare in South Africa's Bantustan Periphery." *South African Historical Journal* 64, no. 4 (2012): 827–85.

———."Debating the Gluckman Commission: A Final Rejoinder." *South African Historical Journal* 67, no. 1 (2015): 91–94.

———. *Diversity and Division in Medicine: Health Care in South Africa from the 1800s*. Oxford: Peter Lang, 2006.

———."The Medical History of South Africa: An Overview." *History Compass* 6, no. 5 (2008): 1194–1210.

Digby, Anne, and Howard Phillips. *At the Heart of Healing: Groote Schuur Hospital, 1938–2008*. Auckland Park, South Africa: Jacana Media, 2008.

Digby, Anne, and Helen Sweet. "Nurses as Culture Brokers in Twentieth-Century South Africa." In *Plural Medicine, Tradition and Modernity, 1800–2000*, edited by Waltraud Ernst, 113–29. New York: Routledge, 2002.

Director General, World Health Organization. "Health Implications of Apartheid in South Africa." Notes and Documents/Unit on Apartheid. No. 5/75. United Nations, Department of Political and Security Council Affairs, 1975.

Dlamini, Jacob. *Native Nostalgia*. Auckland Park, South Africa: Jacana Media, 2009.

Dold, Tony, and Michelle Cocks. *Voices from the Forest: Celebrating Nature and Culture in Xhosaland*. Auckland Park, South Africa: Jacana Media, 2012.

Egli, Martina, and Denise Krayer. *"Mothers and Daughters": The Training of African Nurses by Missionary Nurses of the Swiss Mission in South Africa*. Histoire et Héritages—Approche Pluridisciplinaire 4. Lausanne, Switzerland: Le Fait missionnaire, 1997.

Ernst, Waltraud, ed. *Plural Medicine, Tradition and Modernity, 1800–2000*. New York: Routledge, 2002.

Etherington, Norman. "Missionary Doctors and African Healers in Mid-Victorian South Africa." *South African Historical Journal* 19, no. 1 (1987): 77–91.

Etherington, Norman. *Missions and Empire*. Oxford: Oxford University Press, 2005.

Evans, Laura. "Resettlement and the Making of the Ciskei Bantustan, South Africa, c. 1960–1976." *Journal of Southern African Studies* 40, no. 1 (2014): 21–40.

Evans, Laura. "South Africa's Homelands and the Dynamics of 'Decolonization': Reflections on Writing Histories of the Homelands." *South African Historical Journal* 64, no. 1 (2012): 117–37.

Feierman, Steven. "Struggles for Control: The Social Roots of Health and Healing in Modern Africa." *African Studies Review* 28, nos. 2/3 (September 1985): 73–147.

Feierman, Steven, and John M. Janzen, eds. *The Social Basis of Health and Healing in Africa.* Berkeley: University of California Press, 1992.

Flint, Karen E. *Healing Traditions: African Medicine, Cultural Exchange, and Competition in South Africa, 1820–1948.* Athens: Ohio University Press, 2008.

Foster, Doreen Merle. *Lahlekile: A Twentieth Century Chronicle of Nursing in South Africa.* Brentwood, UK: Chipmukapublishing, 2007.

Gasa, Nomboniso, ed. *Women in South African History.* Cape Town: Human Science Research Council Press, 2007.

Gelfand, Michael. *Christian Doctor and Nurse: The History of Medical Missions in South Africa from 1799–1976.* Sandton, South Africa: Aitken Family and Friends, 1984.

———. *Midwifery in Tropical Africa: The Growth of Maternity Services in Rhodesia.* Salisbury: University of Rhodesia, 1978.

Gengenbach, Heidi. "Truth-Telling and the Life Narrrative of African Women: A Reply to Kirk Hoppe." *International Journal of African Historical Studies* 26, no. 3 (1993): 619–27.

Gibbs, Timothy. *Mandela's Kinsmen: Nationalist Elites and Apartheid's First Bantustan.* Melton, Woodbridge, UK: James Currey, 2014.

Gluck, Sherna Berger. "Women's Oral History: Is It So Special?" In *Handbook of Oral History*, edited by Thomas Charlton, Lois E. Myers, and Rebecca Sharpless, 357–83. Lanham, MD: AltaMira, 2006.

Gluck, Sherna Berger, and Daphne Patai, eds. *Women's Words: The Feminist Practice of Oral History.* New York: Routledge, 1991.

Gordon, David. "A Sword of Empire? Medicine and Colonialism at King William's Town, Xhosaland, 1856–91." In *Medicine and Colonial Identity*, edited by Mary P. Sutphen and Bridie Andrews, 41–60. New York: Routledge, 2003.

Groenewald, D. M. "The Administrative System in the Ciskei." In *Ciskei: Economics and Politics of Dependence in a South African Homeland*, edited by Nancy Charton, 82–96. London: Croom Helm, 1980.

Guma, Mthobeli Philip. "Politics of Umoya: Variation in the Interpretation and Management of Diarrheal Illness among Mothers, Professional Nurses, and Indigenous Health Practitioners in Khayelitsha, South Africa." PhD diss., University of North Carolina, 1998.

Gwala, Mafika Pascal, ed. *Black Review 1973.* Durban: Black Community Programmes, 1974.

Hadfield, Leslie Anne. "Biko, Black Consciousness, and 'the System' EZinyoka: Oral History and Black Consciousness in Practice in a Rural Ciskei Village." *South African Historical Journal* 62, no. 1 (2010): 78–99.

———. "Can We Believe the Stories about Biko? Oral Sources, Meaning, and Emotion in South African Struggle History." *History in Africa* 42, no. 1 (2015): 239–63.

———. *Liberation and Development: Black Consciousness Community Programs in South Africa.* East Lansing: Michigan State University Press, 2016.

Bibliography

Hammond-Tooke, W. D. *The Bantu-Speaking Peoples of Southern Africa.* London: Routledge & Kegan Paul, 1980.

———. "The Uniqueness of Nguni Mediumistic Divination in Southern Africa." *Africa* 72, no. 2 (2002): 277–92.

Hannaford, Dinah, and Ellen E. Foley. "Negotiating Love and Marriage in Contemporary Senegal: A Good Man Is Hard to Find." *African Studies Review* 58, no. 2 (September 2015): 205–26.

Hassim, Shireen. *The ANC Women's League: Sex, Gender and Politics.* Ohio Short Histories of Africa. Athens: Ohio University Press, 2014.

———. *Women's Organizations and Democracy in South Africa: Contesting Authority.* Madison: University of Wisconsin Press, 2006.

Healy-Clancy, Meghan. "The Everyday Politics of Being a Student in South Africa: A History." *History Compass* 15, no. 3 (2017): 1–12. https://doi.org/10.1111/hic3.12375.

———. "Introduction: ASR Forum: The Politics of Marriage in South Africa." *African Studies Review* 57, no. 2 (September 2014): 1–5.

———. "The Politics of New African Marriage in Segregationist South Africa." *African Studies Review* 57, no. 2 (September 2014): 7–28.

———. "Women and the Problem of Family in Early African Nationalist History and Historiography." *South African Historical Journal* 64, no. 3 (2012): 450–71.

———. *A World of Their Own: A History of South African Women's Education.* Charlottesville: University of Virginia Press, 2014.

Heyningen, Elizabeth van. "Medical Practice in the Eastern Cape." In *The Cape Doctor in the Nineteenth Century: A Social History*, edited by Harriet Deacon, Howard Phillips, and Elizabeth van Heyningen, 169–94. Amsterdam: Rodopi, 2004.

Higgs, Catharine. "Helping Ourselves: Black Women and Grassroots Activism in Segregated South Africa, 1922–1952." In *Stepping Forward: Black Women in Africa and the Americas*, edited by Catharine Higgs, Barbara A. Moss, and Earline Rae Ferguson, 59–72. Athens: Ohio University Press, 2002.

Hirst, Manton. "Dreams and Medicines: The Perspective of Xhosa Diviners and Novices in the Eastern Cape, South Africa." *Indo-Pacific Journal of Phenomenology* 5, no. 2 (December 2005): 1–22.

———. "The Healer's Art: Cape Nguni Diviners in the Townships of Grahamstown, Eastern Cape, South Africa." *Curare* 16, no. 2 (1990): 97–114.

Hodes, Rebecca. "HIV/AIDS in South Africa." In *Oxford Research Encyclopedia of African History*, March 2018. http://africanhistory.oxfordre.com/view/10.1093/acrefore/9780190277734.001.0001/acrefore-9780190277734-e-299.

Holden, Pat, and Jenny Littlewood, eds. *Anthropology and Nursing.* New York: Routledge, 1991.

Holden, Pat. "Colonial Sisters: Nurses in Uganda." In *Anthropology and Nursing*, edited by Pat Holden and Jenny Littlewood, 67–83. New York: Routledge, 1991.

———. "Nursing Sisters in Nigeria, Uganda, Tanganyika, 1929–1978." Oxford Development Records Project. Oxford: Rhodes House Library, 1984.

Horwitz, Simonne. *Baragwanath Hospital, Soweto: A History of Medical Care, 1941–1990.* Johannesburg: Wits University Press, 2013.

———. "'Black Nurses in White': Exploring Young Women's Entry into the Nursing Profession at Baragwanath Hospital, Soweto, 1948–1980." *Social History of Medicine* 20, no. 1 (2007): 131–46.

Hull, Elizabeth. *Contingent Citizens: Professional Aspiration in a South African Hospital.* New York: Bloomsbury Academic, 2017.

———. "International Migration, 'Domestic Struggles' and Status Aspiration among Nurses in South Africa." *Journal of Southern African Studies* 36, no. 4 (December 2010): 851–67.

———. "The Renewal of Community Health under the KwaZulu 'Homeland' Government." *South African Historical Journal* 64, no. 1 (2012): 22–40.

Hunt, Nancy Rose. *A Colonial Lexicon: Of Birth Ritual, Medicalization, and Mobility in the Congo.* Durham, NC: Duke University Press, 1999.

Hunter, Mark. *Love in the Time of AIDS: Inequality, Gender, and Rights in South Africa.* Bloomington: Indiana University Press, 2010.

Hyslop, Jonathan. "Political Corruption: Before and After Apartheid." *Journal of Southern African Studies* 31, no. 4 (December 2005): 773–89.

Iliffe, John. *The African AIDS Epidemic: A History.* Oxford: James Currey, 2006.

Ingle, Ronald. *An Uneasy Story: The Nationalising of South African Mission Hospitals, 1960–1976: A Personal Account.* Hillcrest, South Africa: The Author, 2010.

Jaffer, Zubeida. *Beauty of the Heart: The Life and Times of Charlotte Mannya Maxeke.* Bloemfontein: SUN, 2016.

Jager, E. J. de. "'Traditional' Xhosa Marriage in the Rural Areas of the Ciskei, South Africa." In *Man: Anthropological Essays Presented to O. F. Raum*, edited by E. J. Jager, 160–82. Cape Town: C. Struik, 1971.

Jean-Baptiste, Rachel, and Emily Burrill. "Love, Marriage, and Families in Africa." In *Holding the World Together: African Women in Changing Perspective*, edited by Nwando Achebe and Claire Robertson, 275–93. Women in Africa and the Diaspora. Madison: University of Wisconsin Press, 2019.

Jeeves, Alan. "Delivering Primary Health Care in Impoverished Urban and Rural Communities: The Institute of Family and Community Health in the 1940s." In *South Africa's 1940s: Worlds of Possibilities*, edited by Saul Dubow and Alan Jeeves, 87–107. Cape Town: Double Storey Books, 2005.

———. "Health, Surveillance and Community: South Africa's Experiment with Medical Reform in the 1940s and 1950s." *South African Historical Journal* 43, no. 1 (November 2000): 244–66.

———. "Public Health and Rural Poverty in South Africa: 'Social Medicine' in the 1940s and 1950s." Seminar Paper (Institute for Advanced Social Research) no. 434. Johannesburg: University of the Witwatersrand, Institute for Advanced Social Research, 1998.

Jensen, Steffen, and Olaf Zenker. "Homelands as Frontiers: Apartheid's Loose Ends—An Introduction." *Journal of Southern African Studies* 41, no. 5 (2015): 937–52.

Jewkes, Rachel, Naeemah Abrahams, and Zodumo Mvo. "Why Do Nurses Abuse Patients? Reflections from South African Obstetric Services." *Social Science and Medicine* 47, no. 11 (1998): 1781–95.

Kahn, Marc Simon. "The Interface Between Western Mental Health Care and Indigenous Healing in South Africa: Xhosa Psychiatric Nurses' Views on Traditional Healers." Master's thesis, Rhodes University, 1996.

Kaler, Amy. *Running after Pills: Politics, Gender, and Contraception in Colonial Zimbabwe.* Portsmouth, NH: Heinemann, 2003.

Bibliography

Kanogo, Tabitha. *African Womanhood in Colonial Kenya: 1900–1950*. Athens: Ohio University Press, 2005.

Keikelame, Mpoe Johannah, and Leslie Swartz. "'A Thing Full of Stories': Traditional Healers' Explanations of Epilepsy and Perspectives on Collaboration with Biomedical Health Care in Cape Town." *Transcult Psychiatry* 52, no. 5 (October 2015): 659–80.

Klausen, Susanne M. *Race, Maternity and the Politics of Birth Control, 1910–39*. Basingstoke, UK: Palgrave Macmillan, 2004.

Kringelbach, Hélène Neveu. "'Marrying Out' for Love: Women's Narratives of Polygyny and Alternative Marriage Choices in Contemporary Senegal." *African Studies Review* 59, no. 1 (April 2016): 155–74.

Kuper, Adam. *Wives for Cattle: Bridewealth and Marriage in Southern Africa*. London: Routledge, 1982.

Lamla, Canasseus Masilo. "Present-Day Diviners (Ama-Gqira) in the Transkei." Master's thesis, University of Fort Hare, 1975.

Liebenberg, Alida M. "Dealing with Relations of Inequality: Married Women in a Transkei Village." In *Culture and the Commonplace: Anthropological Essays in Honour of David Hammond-Tooke*, edited by Patrick McAllister, 349–73. Johannesburg: Witwatersrand University Press, 1997.

Lindsay, Beverly. "Issues Confronting Professional African Women: Illustrations from Kenya." In *Comparative Perspectives on Third World Women: The Impact of Race, Sex, and Class*, edited by Beverly Lindsay, 78–95. New York: Praeger, 1980.

Lissoni, Arianna, and Maria Suriano. "Married to the ANC: Tanzanian Women's Entanglement in South Africa's Liberation Struggle." *Journal of Southern African Studies* 40, no. 1 (2014): 129–50.

Loots, Idalia, and Molly Vermaak. *Pioneers of Professional Nursing in South Africa*. Bloemfontein, South Africa: P. J. de Villiers, 1975.

Loubser, Isabe. "Abuse Suffered by the Amakhoti in the Xhosa Community." PhD diss., University of Stellenbosch, 1999.

Lunde, Martin J. "An Approach to Medical Missions: Dr. Neil Macvicar and the Victoria Hospital, Lovedale, South Africa, circa 1900–1950." PhD diss., University of Edinburgh, 2009.

———. "North Meets South in Medical Missionary Work: Dr Neil Macvicar, African Belief, and Western Reaction." *South African Historical Journal* 61, no. 2 (2009): 336–56.

Lunn, Joe. *Memoirs of the Maelstrom: A Senegalese Oral History of the First World War*. Portsmouth, NH: Heinemann, 1999.

Maaba, Brown Bavusile. "An Eastern Cape Village in Transition: The Politics of Msobomvu." In *From Apartheid to Democracy: Localities and Liberation*, edited by Christopher Saunders, 12–48. Cape Town: Department of Historical Studies, University of Cape Town, 2007.

Magaziner, Daniel. *The Art of Life in South Africa*. Athens: Ohio University Press, 2016.

———. "Pieces of a (Wo)Man: Feminism, Gender, and Adulthood in Black Consciousness, 1968–1977." *Journal of Southern African Studies* 37, no. 1 (2011): 45–61.

Mager, Anne. *Gender and the Making of a South African Bantustan: A Social History of the Ciskei, 1945–1959*. Portsmouth, NH: Heinemann, 1999.

Mager, Anne, and Phiko Jeffrey Velelo. *The House of Tshatshu: Power, Politics and Chiefs North-West of the Great Kei River c 1818–2018.* Cape Town: University of Cape Town Press, 2018.

Maglacas, A. Mangay, and John Simons, eds. *The Potential of the Traditional Birth Attendant.* Geneva: World Health Organization, 1986.

Magubane, Bernard, Lungisile Ntsebeza, Luvuyo Wotshela, Thembela Kepe, Sukude Matoti, Andrew Ainslie, Bernard Mbenga, and Andrew Manson. "Resistance and Repression in the Bantustans." In *The Road to Democracy in South Africa*, vol. 2, edited by South African Democracy and Education Trust (SADET), 749–802. Pretoria: Unisa Press, 2006.

Magubane, Zine. "Attitudes Towards Feminism Among Women in the ANC, 1950–1990: A Theoretical Re-Interpretation." In *The Road to Democracy in South Africa*, vol. 4, *1980–1990*, 975–1034. Pretoria: Unisa Press, 2010.

Mann, Kristin. *Marrying Well: Marriage, Status and Social Change among the Educated Elite in Colonial Lagos.* New York: Cambridge University Press, 1985.

Mann, Kristin, and Richard Roberts, eds. *Law in Colonial Africa.* Portsmouth, NH: Heinemann, 1991.

Manona, Cecil. "The Collapse of the 'Tribal Authority' System and the Rise of Civic Associations." In *From Reserve to Region: Apartheid and Social Change in the Keiskammahoek District of (Former) Ciskei, 1950–1990*, edited by Chris de Wet and Michael Whisson, 49–68. Grahamstown, South Africa: Institute for Social and Economic Research, Rhodes University, 1997.

Marks, Shula. *Divided Sisterhood: Race, Class, and Gender in the South African Nursing Profession.* New York: St. Martin's, 1994.

———. "South Africa's Early Experiment in Social Medicine: Its Pioneers and Politics." *American Journal of Public Health* 87, no. 3 (March 1997): 452–59.

———. "'We Were Men Nursing Men': Male Nursing on the Mines in Twentieth-Century South Africa." In *Deep hiStories: Gender and Colonialism in Southern Africa*, edited by Wendy Woodward, Patricia Hayes, and Gary Minkley, 177–204. Amsterdam: Rodopi, 2002.

Marten, Robert, Diane McIntyre, Claudia Travassos, Sergey Shishkin, Wang Longde, Srinath Reddy, and Jeanette Vega. "An Assessment of Progress Towards Universal Health Coverage in Brazil, Russia, India, China, and South Africa (BRICS)." *Lancet* 384 (April 30, 2014): 2164–71.

Mashaba, Grace. *Rising to the Challenge of Change: A History of Black Nursing in South Africa.* Kenwyn, South Africa: Juta, 1995.

May, Deborah. *You Have Struck a Rock!* DVD. California News Reel, 1981.

Mayekiso, Andile, and Munyaradzi Mawere. "Traditional Healers and Medicine in South Africa: A Quest for Legal and Scientific Recognition." In *Between Rhetoric and Reality: The State and Use of Indigenous Knowledge in Post-Colonial Africa*, edited by Munyaradzi Mawere and Samuel Awuah-Nyamekye, 109–30. Cameroon: Langaa RPCIG, 2015.

Mayer, Philip, and Iona Mayer. *Townsmen or Tribesmen: Conservatism and the Process of Urbanization in a South African City.* 2nd ed. New York: Oxford University Press, 1971.

Mbiti, John. *Love and Marriage in Africa.* London: Longman, 1973.

Bibliography

McAdoo, Harriette, and Miriam Were. "Extended Family Involvement of Urban Kenyan Professional Women." In *Women in Africa and the African Diaspora*, edited by Rosalyn Terborg-Penn, Sharon Harley, and Andrea Benton Rushing, 133–64. Washington, DC: Howard University Press, 1989.

McCord, Margaret. *The Calling of Katie Makanya: A Memoir of South Africa*. New York: John Wiley & Sons, 1995.

Melber, Henning, ed. *The Rise of Africa's Middle Class: Myths, Realities, and Critical Engagements*. London: Zed Books, 2016.

Mhlongo, Thokozani. "Profiling Black South African Nurse Pioneers: Promoting the Black Biography." *Nursing Times Research* 9, no. 65 (2004): 65–72.

Mirza, Sarah, and Margaret Strobel, *Three Swahili Women: Studies in Social and Economic Change*. Bloomington: Indiana University Press, 1989.

Morrell, Robert. *Changing Men in Southern Africa*. Pietermaritzburg, South Africa: University of KwaZulu-Natal Press and Zed Press, 2001.

Mtumane, Zilibele. "The Poetry of S. M. Burns-Ncamashe." PhD diss., University of South Africa, 2000.

Murray, Daphne. "The Impact of Divorce on Work Performance of Professional Nurses in Tertiary Hospitals of the Buffalo City Municipality." Master's thesis, University of Fort Hare, 2012.

Nelson, Nici, ed. *African Women in the Development Process*. London: Frank Cass, 1981.

Ngubane, Harriet. *Body and Mind in Zulu Medicine: An Ethnography of Health and Disease in Nyuswa-Zulu Thought and Practice*. New York: Academic, 1977.

Niehaus, D. J. H., P. Oosthuizen, C. Lochner, R. A. Emsley, E. Jordaan, N. I. Mbanga, and D. J. Stein. "A Culture-Bound Syndrome 'Amafufunyana' and a Culture-Specific Event 'Ukuthwasa': Differentiated by a Family History of Schizophrenia and Other Psychiatric Disorders." *Psychopathology* 37, no. 2 (2004): 59–63.

Noble, Vanessa. "A Medical Education with a Difference: A History of the Training of Black Student Doctors in Social, Preventive and Community-Oriented Primary Health Care at the University of Natal Medical School, 1940s-1960." *South African Historical Journal* 61, no. 3 (September 2009): 550–74.

Nolde, Judith. "South African Women under Apartheid: Employment Rights, with Particular Focus on Domestic Service & Forms of Resistance to Promote Change." *Third World Legal Studies* 10, no. 10 (1991): 203–23.

Ntsimane, Radikobo P. "Amandla Awekho Emuthini, Asenyangeni: A Critical History of the Lutheran Medical Missions in Southern Africa with Special Emphases on Four Mission Hospitals, 1930s-1978." PhD diss., University of KwaZulu-Natal, 2010.

Oliveira, A. F. P. L. d', S. G. Diniz, and L. B. Schraiber. "Violence Against Women in Health Care Institutions: An Emerging Problem." *The Lancet* 359 (May 2002): 1681–85.

Oppong, Christine. "Nursing Mothers: Aspects of the Conjugal and Maternal Roles of Nurses in Accra." Canadian African Studies Association Meeting, Toronto, 1975.

Osborn, Emily. *Our New Husbands Are Here: Households, Gender, and Politics in a West African State from the Slave Trade to Colonial Rule*. Athens: Ohio University Press, 2011.

Packard, Randall M. "Review: A History of Nursing." *Journal of African History* 37, no. 2 (1996): 324–26.

———. *White Plague, Black Labor: Tuberculosis and the Political Economy of Health and Disease in South Africa.* Berkeley: University of California Press, 1989.

Parkin, David, and David Nyamwaya. *Transformations of African Marriage.* Manchester: Manchester University Press, 1987.

Parle, Julie. *States of Mind: Searching for Mental Health in Natal and Zululand, 1868–1918.* Scottsville, South Africa: University of KwaZulu-Natal Press, 2007.

———. "Witchcraft or Madness? The Amandiki of Zululand, 1894–1914." *Journal of Southern African Studies* 29, no. 1 (March 2003): 105–32.

Parle, Julie, and Vanessa Noble. "New Directions and Challenges in Histories of Health, Healing and Medicine in South Africa." *Medical History* 58, no. 2 (April 2014): 147–65.

Parpart, Jane L. "'Where Is Your Mother?': Gender, Urban Marriage, and Colonial Discourse on the Zambian Copperbelt, 1924–1945." *International Journal of African Historical Studies* 27, no. 2 (1994): 241–71.

Peires, Jeff. *The Dead Will Arise: Nongqawuse and the Great Xhosa Cattle-Killing Movement of 1856–7.* Bloomington: Indiana University Press, 1989.

———. "Ethnicity and Pseudo-Ethnicity in the Ciskei." In *Segregation and Apartheid in Twentieth-Century South Africa*, edited by William Beinart and Saul Dubow, 256–84. London: Routledge, 1995.

———. *The House of Phalo: A History of the Xhosa People in the Days of Their Independence.* Johannesburg: Jonathan Ball, 2003.

———. "The Implosion of Transkei and Ciskei." *African Affairs* 91, no. 364 (1992): 365–87.

Phatlane, Stephens Ntsoakae. "Poverty, Health and Disease in the Era of High Apartheid: South Africa, 1948–1976." PhD diss., University of South Africa, 2009.

Phillips, Howard. "The Grassy Park Health Centre: A Peri-Urban Pholela?" In *South Africa's 1940s: Worlds of Possibilities*, edited by Saul Dubow and Alan Jeeves, 108–28. Cape Town: Double Storey Books, 2005.

———. "HIV/AIDS in the Context of South Africa's Epidemic History." In *AIDS in South Africa: The Social Expression of a Pandemic*, edited by Kyle D. Kauffman and David L. Lindauer, 31–47. Basingstoke, UK: Macmillan, 2004.

Polakow-Suransky, Sasha. *The Unspoken Alliance: Israel's Secret Relationship with Apartheid South Africa.* New York: Pantheon Books, 2010.

Potgieter, Eugéne. *Professional Nursing Education, 1860–1991.* Pretoria: Academica, 1992.

Prince, Ruth J., and Rebecca Marsland, eds. *Making and Unmaking Public Health in Africa: Ethnographic and Historical Perspectives.* Cambridge Center of African Studies Series. Athens: Ohio University Press, 2014.

Rankin, John. *Healing the African Body: British Medicine in West Africa, 1800–1860.* Columbia: University of Missouri Press, 2015.

Reh, Mechthild, and Gudrun Ludwar-Ene, eds. *Gender and Identity in Africa.* Munster: Lit, 1995.

Reid, Graeme, and Liz Walker, eds. *Men Behaving Differently: South African Men since 1994.* Cape Town: David Philip, 1990.

Bibliography

Rennick, Agnes. "Mission Nurses in Nyasaland: 1890–1916." In *Twentieth Century Malawi: Perspectives on History and Culture*, edited by John McCracken, Timothy J. Lovering, and Fiona Johnson Chalamanda, 21–37. Stirling, UK: University of Stirling, Center of Commonwealth Studies, 2001.

Roberts, Jonathan. "Western Medicine in Africa to 1900, Part 1: North, West and Central Africa." *History Compass* 15, no. e12400 (2017): 1–8. https://doi.org/10.1111/hic3.12400.

———. "Western Medicine in Africa, Part 2: Ethiopia, East and Southern Africa to 1900." *History Compass* 15, no. e12393 (2017): 1–8. https://doi.org/10.1111/hic3.12393.

Robinson, Jason. "Fragments of the Past: Homeland Politics and the South African Transition, 1990–2014." *Journal of Southern African Studies* 41, no. 5 (2015): 953–67.

Robinson, Pearl T. "Fatimata Traore, Nurse-Midwife: Combining a Successful Family Planning Program with Community Development." *Sage* 7, no. 1 (1990): 55–56.

Rogers, Sandra. "'Since the Women Came': Primary Health Care Nursing in a Nigerian Village." PhD diss., University of California, San Francisco, 1989.

Rowley, Chishamiso. "Challenges to Effective Maternal Health Care Delivery: The Case of Traditional and Certified Nurse Midwives in Zimbabwe." *Journal of Asian and African Studies* 35, no. 2 (2000): 251–64.

Rüther, Kirsten. "Claims on Africanisation: Healers' Exercises in Professionalisation." *Journal for the Study of Religion* 15, no. 2 (2002): 39–63.

Saldru Community Health Project. *Health and Health Services in the Ciskei*. Saldru Working Papers, no. 54. Cape Town: Saldru, 1983.

Schmidt, Elizabeth. *Peasants, Traders, and Wives: Shona Women in the History of Zimbabwe, 1870–1983*. Portsmouth, NH: Heinemann, 1992.

Schuster, Isa. "Perspectives in Development: The Problem of Nurses and Nursing in Zambia." In *African Women in the Development Process*, edited by Nici Nelson, 77–97. London: Frank Cass, 1981.

Schwartz, Linda Mary. "Grandmothers, Mothers and Daughters : Transformations and Coping Strategies in Xhosa Households in Grahamstown." Master's thesis, Rhodes University, 2006.

Searle, Charlotte. *The History of the Development of Nursing in South Africa, 1652–1960*. Cape Town: Struik, 1965.

———. *Towards Excellence: The Centenary of State Registration for Nurses and Midwives in South Africa, 1891–1991*. Durban: Butterworths, 1991.

Segar, Julia. "Hard Lives and Evil Winds: Illness Aetiology and the Search for Healing Amongst Ciskeian Villagers." *Social Science and Medicine* 44, no. 10 (1997): 1585–1600.

———. "Health Care at the Village Level: Ciskei and Transkei." In *Political Transition and Economic Development in the Transkei*. East London: Department of Anthropology, Rhodes University, November 1991.

Senokoanyane, Ntsoaki. *Their Light, Love and Life: A Black Nurse's Story*. Cape Town: Kwela Books, 1995.

Shapiro, Karin A. "Doctors or Medical Aids—The Debate over the Training of Black Medical Personnel for the Rural Black Population in South Africa in the 1920s and 1930s." *Journal of Southern African Studies* 13, no. 2 (January 1987): 234–55.

Sheldon, Kathleen. *African Women: Early History to the 21st Century.* Bloomington: Indiana University Press, 2017.

Smith, Andrew. *A Contribution to South African Materia Medica.* 3rd ed. Grahamstown, South Africa: Cory Library, 2011.

Soga, John Henderson. *The Ama-Xhosa: Life and Customs.* Lovedale, South Africa: Lovedale, 1932.

South African Institute of Race Relations. *Race Relations Survey.* Johannesburg: South African Institute of Race Relations, 1984–95. Published annually.

———. *A Survey of Race Relations in South Africa.* Johannesburg: South African Institute of Race Relations, 1952–83. Published annually.

Southall, Roger. "The African Middle Class in South Africa, 1910–1994." *Economic History of Developing Regions* 29, no. 2 (2014): 287–310.

———. *The New Black Middle Class in South Africa.* London: James Currey, 2016.

Southall, Roger, and Zosa De Sas Kropiwnicki. "Containing the Chiefs: The ANC and Traditional Leaders in the Eastern Cape, South Africa." *Canadian Journal of African Studies* 37, no. 1 (2003): 48–82.

Stephens, Rhiannon. *A History of African Motherhood: The Case of Uganda, 700–1900.* New York: Cambridge University Press, 2013.

Stitcher, Sharon. "The Middle Class Family in Kenya: Changes in Gender Relations." In *Patriarchy and Class: African Women in the Home and Workforce,* edited by Jane L. Parpart and Sharon Stitcher. Boulder, CO: Westview Press, 1988.

Swartz, L., and C. Lund. "Xhosa-Speaking Schizophrenic Patients' Experiences of Their Condition: Psychosis and Amafufunyana." *South African Journal of Psychology* 28, no. 2 (1998): 62–70.

Sweet, Helen. "Mission Nursing in the South African Context: The Spread of Knowledge During the Colonial and Apartheid Periods." In *Transnational and Historical Perspectives on Global Health, Welfare and Humanitarianism,* edited by Michael Marten, Ellen Fleischmann, Sonya Grypma, and Inger Marie Okkenhaug, 137–55. Kristiansand, Norway: Portal Books, 2013.

Switzer, Les. *Media and Dependency in South Africa.* Africa Series 47. Athens: Ohio University Monographs in International Studies, 1985.

———. *Power and Resistance in an African Society: The Ciskei Xhosa and the Making of South Africa.* Madison: University of Wisconsin Press, 1993.

Thomas, Lynn M. *Politics of the Womb: Women, Reproduction, and the State in Kenya.* Berkeley: University of California Press, 2003.

———. "The Modern Girl and Racial Respectability in 1930s South Africa." In *The Modern Girl Around the World: Consumption, Modernity, and Globalization.* The Modern Girl Around the World Research Group, 96–119. Durham, NC: Duke University Press, 2008.

Thomas, Lynn M., and Jennifer Cole, eds. *Love in Africa.* Chicago: University of Chicago Press, 2009.

Thomas, Trudi. *The Children of Apartheid: A Study of the Effects of Migratory Labour on Family Life in the Ciskei.* London: Africa Publications Trust, 1974.

Thorpe, Mark Richard. "Psycho-Diagnostics in a Xhosa Zionist Church." Master's thesis, Rhodes University, 1982.

Bibliography

Tollman, Steve, and Derek Yach. "Public Health Initiatives in South Africa in the 1940s and 1950s: Lessons for a Post-Apartheid Era." *American Journal of Public Health* 83, no. 7 (July 1993): 1043–50.

Twine, Janet Lea. "'I'm Just an Ordinary Nurse': A Life History of Matron Bongiwe Bolani." Bachelor's honors thesis, University of Natal, 1997.

Van Allen, Judith, and Kathleen Sheldon. "ASR Forum on Women and Gender in Africa: Part 2." *African Studies Review* 59, no. 1 (2016): 123–25.

Vaughan, Megan. *Curing Their Ills: Colonial Power and African Illness.* Stanford, CA: Stanford University Press, 1991.

Victor, Stephanie. "The Politics of Remembering and Commemorating Atrocity in South Africa: The Bhisho Massacre and Its Aftermath, 1992–2012." *Journal of Southern African Studies* 41, no. 1 (2015): 83–102.

Vliet, Virginia van der. "Traditional Husbands, Modern Wives? Constructing Marriages in a South African Township." In *Tradition and Transition in Southern Africa: Festschrift for Philip and Iona Meyer,* edited by P. A. McAllister and Andrew Spiegel, 219–42. New Brunswick, NJ: Transaction, 1991.

Walker, Cherryl. "Conceptualising Motherhood in Twentieth Century South Africa." *Journal of Southern African Studies* 21, no. 3 (September 1995): 417–37.

Walker, Cherryl, ed. *Women and Gender in Southern Africa to 1945.* Cape Town: David Philip and James Currey, 1990.

———. *Women and Resistance in South Africa.* New York: Monthly Review Press, 1991.

Walker, Liz. "'They Heal in the Spirit of the Mother': Gender, Race and Professionalisation of South African Women." *African Studies* 62, no. 1 (2003): 99–123.

Wall, Barbra Mann. *Into Africa: A Transnational History of Catholic Medical Missions and Social Change.* New Brunswick, NJ: Rutgers University Press, 2015.

Wells, Julia C. *We Now Demand! The History of Women's Resistance to Pass Laws in South Africa.* Johannesburg: Wits University Press, 1993.

Wet, Chris de, and Simon Bekker. *Rural Development in South Africa: A Case Study of the Amatola Basin in the Ciskei.* Pietermaritzburg, South Africa: Shuter and Shooter, 1985.

White, Colin Stewart. "The Rule of Brigadier Oupa Gqozo in Ciskei: 4 March 1990 to 22 March 1994." Master's thesis, Rhodes University, 2008.

Whiting, Beatrice. "The Kenyan Career Woman: Traditional and Modern." In *Women and Success: The Anatomy of Achievement,* edited by Ruth B. Kundsin, 71–75. New York: William Morrow, 1974.

Wilson, Monica. "Xhosa Marriage in Historical Perspective." In *Essays on African Marriage in Southern Africa,* edited by Eileen Jensen Krige and John Comaroff, 133–47. Cape Town: Juta, 1981.

Wotshela, Luvuyo. "The Fate of Ciskei and Adjacent Border Towns: Political Transition in a Democratic South Africa, 1985–1995." In *Road to Democracy in South Africa,* vol. 4, part 3, 1855–99. Ibadan, Nigeria: Pan-African University Press, 2019.

———. "Homeland Consolidation, Resettlement and Local Politics in the Border and the Ciskei Region of the Eastern Cape, South Africa, 1960–1996." PhD diss., Oxford University, 2001.

———. "Insurrection and Locally Negotiated Transition in Stutterheim, Eastern Cape, 1980–1994." In *From Apartheid to Democracy: Localities and Liberation,* edited by Christopher Saunders, 49–68. Cape Town: Department of Historical Studies, University of Cape Town, 2007.

———. "Territorial Manipulation in Apartheid South Africa: Resettlement, Tribal Politics, and the Making of the Northern Ciskei, 1975–1990." *Journal of Southern African Studies* 30, no. 2 (June 2004): 317–37.

Wright, Marcia. *Strategies of Slaves & Women: Life-Stories from East/Central Africa.* New York: Lilian Barber Press, 1993.

Wylie, Diana. *Starving on a Full Stomach: Hunger and the Triumph of Cultural Racism in Modern South Africa.* Charlottesville: University Press of Virginia, 2001.

Zondi, Welcome Siphamandla. "Medical Missions and African Demand in KwaZulu-Natal, 1836–1918." PhD diss., University of Cambridge, 2000.

Index

accommodation (nurses'), 40, 64, 67, 77, 81–84, 86, 93, 165

Adendorff, J. J., 55, 56

African National Congress (ANC), 5, 10, 17, 173–74, 176

AIDS, 9, 58, 87, 97, 135, 137, 176, 177

amafufunyana, 120, 131–32

amagqirha (sing. *igqirha*), 23, 25–27, 30, 33–34, 44–46, 104, 112–15, 122–24, 134–35, 140; and advertisements, 118–19; cooperation with, 119–22, 124, 127–31, 133, 135–36, 138; nurses' use of, 113–17

amaxhwele (sing. *ixhwele*), 25–26, 27, 113–14, 116–17, 120–21

ambulances, 18, 40, 88, 102, 104, 105, 106, 107, 177

Ann Shaw clinic, 80, 81, 90, 102

antenatal, 54, 78, 87, 93, 102–4, 140

apartheid, 4–6, 8–11, 38, 46–48, 50, 53, 55–58, 60, 63, 66, 72, 99, 147, 176, 182

Baragwanath Hospital, 7, 47, 108, 164, 168

Beukes, Hennie C., 67–68

Bhisho, 10, 54, 60, 68, 95, 105, 106

Bhisho Hospital, 60, 86, 97, 149, 175

Bhisho Massacre, 174–75

Bikitsha, Charles, 65, 212n112

biomedicine: history of, 7, 11–13, 21–23, 28–30, 33–35. See also *amagqirha*:

cooperation with; *amagqirha*: nurses' use of; doctors (biomedical); health education; mission hospitals; training

birth. *See* maternity cases

birth attendants, 13, 22, 103, 138–40

Burns-Ncamashe, Chief Sipho Mangindi, 120, 131

Cecilia Makiwane Hospital, 55, 59–60, 62, 69, 70, 72, 98, 108, 133, 162, 175

childbirth. *See* maternity cases

childcare (by nurses), 14, 144–45, 148–49, 153, 163–67, 169–70

Ciskei: Department of Health, 8, 14, 55–57, 62, 97–98, 120, 175–76; finances, 65–68; history, 7, 8, 17, 30; nurses' views of, 69–73; politics, 8, 10, 14, 49, 51–54, 57, 60, 63–64, 68, 173–75, 204n25

Ciskeian Nursing Council, 15, 49, 70–71, 125

Colani, Mina, 35–36

commitment (of nurses), 4, 36, 73, 75, 107–11, 117, 144, 148, 178, 181, 182–83

community relations, 7, 34, 53, 75–76, 95–97, 108–10, 113, 121–22, 126–27, 136–38, 141

comprehensive health care, 4, 7–8, 49, 50, 53, 54, 60–62, 70, 75, 95, 118–20

Index

Daily Dispatch, 15, 91, 98, 121
democracy, 178–80
diabetes, 54, 75, 93, 94, 123
diarrhea, 63, 94–96, 127–29, 176. *See also* gastroenteritis
district nursing, 36, 38–41, 47, 49–51, 127, 139, 177
divorce, 92, 148, 155–56, 158, 159, 170–71
doctors (biomedical), 29, 34–35, 40–41, 43, 61, 115; relations with nurses, 7, 47, 74, 100, 128, 133, 141, 147; relations with Xhosa practitioners, 21, 32–33, 44, 46, 120; shortages, 5, 7, 9, 41, 51, 53–54, 56, 63, 67–68, 74. *See also amagqirha*

family. *See* childcare; divorce; in-laws; marriage; motherhood
family planning, 61–62, 65, 75, 79, 97–99, 104, 108, 164, 177
Fitzgerald, John Patrick, 30–33
Frere Hospital, 42, 55, 70, 92, 148, 170, 199n120, 201n1
funding, of health care, 17, 32, 38–40, 51, 56, 62, 175, 177, 178, 183. *See also* Ciskei: finances

gastroenteritis, 38, 54, 58, 63, 64, 75, 93–96, 122, 127–29, 176, 143
gender, 7, 32, 36–37, 109–10, 112–13, 138–42
Gluckman Report (and Commission), 40, 53
Grey Hospital, 7, 31–33, 41, 87, 100, 105, 164
Grey, Sir George, 30, 33
Gxulu clinic, 51, 79, 81, 85–86, 88, 114

health education, 4, 49, 54, 63, 68, 75, 86, 94, 95, 99, 127–31, 133, 135–38
Hewu Hospital, 60, 68
hierarchy in nursing, 46, 70, 76, 90–91, 178–80
HIV, 9, 58, 87, 97, 135, 137, 176, 177
homelands, 57, 65, 92, 159, 185n4; and health care, 3, 4, 6–9, 11, 49–50, 53, 55–59, 62, 70, 120, 136, 176–77; and history, 6, 8–11, 17, 182–83; and politics, 6, 8, 50, 52, 56, 66–67, 69, 174
hypertension, 54, 75, 93, 94, 104

igqirha. See *amagqirha*
immunizations, 29, 34, 39, 50, 54, 60–63, 67, 78, 87, 93, 96, 97, 136, 137, 177
impundulu, 24, 28, 114, 120, 129
Imvo Zabantsundu, 15, 117–19, 121, 152, 154–55, 159, 161
indigenous medicine and healers, 21, 44, 135
infant mortality rate, 5, 7, 9, 58–59
in-laws, 145, 146, 151, 153–55, 157, 158, 166
intambo, 117, 120
Israel, 67–68
ixhwele. See *amaxhwele*

job satisfaction (of nurses), 58, 61, 70, 90, 91, 95–97, 99, 100, 106–7, 110–11, 136, 172

King Edward VIII Hospital, 108, 199
King William's Town, 7, 8, 10, 14–18, 30, 31, 34, 40, 41, 52, 64, 87, 150
kwashiorkor, 58, 64, 95

Livingstone Hospital, 108, 150
lobola, 146, 150, 155. *See also* marriage: Xhosa
Lovedale mission, 14, 20, 32, 35, 40; hospitals, 10, 14, 20, 35, 39, 40, 55, 80, 108, 204n25; and strikes, 47–48. *See also* Victoria Hospital; Macvicar Hospital
Lucas, Thando, 149–51, 153, 155, 158, 162, 163, 166, 170

Macvicar, Neil, 35, 44
Macvicar Hospital, 39, 47
Makiwane, Cecilia, 8, 20, 35–36
malnutrition, 38, 53, 54, 58, 63–65, 67, 75, 94–95, 98, 99, 176, 182
marasmus, 58, 64, 95

Index

marital tensions, 19, 145, 155–61, 170, 183

marriage: changes in, 5, 14, 145–46, 151–55, 160; companionate, 145, 153–54, 160, 161, 166; Xhosa, 146, 150, 153–55. *See also* childcare; divorce; in-laws; marital tensions

masculinity, 152, 154, 156, 160

maternity cases, 36, 38, 54, 75, 80, 84, 99–108, 138–40, 165, 171, 182

maternity leave, 64, 76, 144, 163–65, 170

McCord's Zulu Hospital, 108, 139, 196n76

measles, 58, 62, 63, 94, 176

midwifery, 36, 39, 41, 42, 62, 63, 70, 108, 115, 131, 139, 151, 162. *See also* district nursing; maternity cases

mission hospitals, 30, 34–35, 38, 39–44, 47, 49, 55–57, 60, 114–15, 139, 181–82

mobile clinics, 11, 54, 55, 59–62, 67, 68, 77, 97, 137, 177

motherhood, 14, 110, 147, 148–49, 151, 153, 163–67, 171

Mount Coke Hospital, 14–15, 37–39, 42, 43, 44–45, 60, 103, 129, 150, 163, 169; and clinics, 38, 40–42, 51, 55, 59, 64, 88–89, 100, 101, 133; and mission, 14, 37, 43–44, 56, 115. *See also* Bhisho Hospital

Nginza, Dora, 36, 152

Nompumelelo Hospital, 55, 56, 59–60, 63, 87, 104, 126

Ntonga, Theresa Nonceba, 103, 109, 124, 148–49, 151, 159–60, 162, 167, 181

nurse's uniform, 43, 76–77, 111

nurses, relationship with colleagues, 89–91. *See also* hierarchy in nursing

nurses' quarters, 43, 76, 81, 84, 144, 150, 157, 165, 167. *See also* accommodation (nurses')

oral history, 15–18, 74–75, 93–94, 156

patient pluralism, 11, 115, 122–24, 140

pay. *See* rural clinics: and pay

pellagra, 58, 64, 95

politics, and health care, 4, 37–40, 46–48, 63–64. *See also* Ciskei: politics; homelands: and politics

primary health care, 5, 53, 54, 61, 93, 135, 176, 177, 182

psychiatric nursing, 62, 63, 75, 79, 97–98, 108, 120, 122, 127, 131–35, 143

Qibirha clinic, 77, 78, 107, 130

Rabula clinic, 51, 61–62, 88, 102, 123, 140

racism/racial discrimination, 5, 10, 46, 69–70, 72. *See also* apartheid

Ramphele, Mamphela, 65, 98

rural clinics: buildings, 40, 42, 81–88; case load, 38, 41, 51, 53, 54, 58, 64, 74–75, 79–81, 93–105, 178; distribution of, 16, 55–56, 59, 63–64, 87–88, 113–14, 122–23; equipment, 86–88; establishment of, 40, 50–51, 59; and management, 51, 54–56, 69–72, 76–77, 177–78; and pay, 89, 91–93, 159–60; security, 81; staffing, 41, 54, 69, 73, 79–80, 168–69; and working contracts, 55, 75–78, 91–92. *See also* community relations; district nursing

salaries. *See* rural clinics: and pay

school health services, 54, 60–62, 99

Sebe, Lennox L., 10, 52, 55, 57, 68, 173–74

sexually transmitted infections, 38, 54, 93, 98, 123. *See also* family planning

South African Department of Health, 8, 9, 39–40, 50–51, 53, 76, 82

S. S. Gida Hospital, 59–62, 68, 72, 74, 77, 80, 81, 128. *See also* St. Matthew's Hospital

St. Matthew's Hospital, 14, 36–38, 42–44, 54, 58, 60, 68, 78, 95, 98, 166, 169–70; and clinics, 51, 55, 61, 74, 80, 81, 87, 88, 126, 128, 135; and mission, 37, 43, 56. *See also* S. S. Gida Hospital

strikes, 47–48, 174–76, 178

258 Index

Thomas, Trudi, 58, 64, 95
Thornhill, 52, 60
training, 41–45, 55, 62–63, 91, 108, 127, 181–82; and family life, 144–45, 150, 162, 164
transition from apartheid, 93, 175–78
Transkei, 6, 8, 10, 50, 52, 57, 93, 147; and health care, 55, 56, 59, 65, 69, 115, 141, 156, 176, 177
transportation, 60, 67–68, 73, 75, 81, 84, 88–89, 91, 102, 104, 122, 162
tuberculosis (TB), 38, 39, 53, 58, 60–62, 64, 68, 75, 93–94, 96, 97, 120, 176; and Xhosa beliefs and practices, 24, 120, 123; and health education and cooperation, 122, 125–27, 129–31, 133, 137. See also *impundulu*
typhoid, 38, 58, 94

umhlonyane, 25, 125
University of Fort Hare, 47–48, 62

vaccination. *See* immunization
Victoria Hospital, 8, 14, 20–21, 35–39, 41, 47, 72, 164, 165; and clinics, 59, 77, 86, 126, 128, 137, 140; and mission character, 43; and strikes, 47–48. *See also* Lovedale: hospitals

village health workers (VHWs), 13, 61–63, 67, 68, 94, 126, 136–37, 177–78

well-baby clinic, 54, 61, 78, 93, 96, 140
witchcraft, 26, 31, 33–34, 37, 116–17, 119, 121, 131, 133
witches, 23, 24, 26, 30, 31, 33, 46, 114, 121
women's economic power, 13, 91–92, 149, 151–55, 158–60
women's liberation, 152, 154–55
World Health Organization (WHO), 53, 58, 62

Xhosa Cattle Killing, 25, 31
Xhosa medicine: history of, 12, 17, 21–30. See also *amagqirha*; *amaxhwele*; doctors (biomedical): relations with Xhosa practitioners; patient pluralism; Xhosa medicines
Xhosa medicines, 27–28, 114, 116, 118–19, 122–26, 128–29, 132, 140, 166
Xuma, Alfred Bitini, 23, 24, 46

Zanempilo Community Health Center, 64, 65, 95
Zuma, Lulu Msutu, 10, 59, 69, 145–51, 153, 155–56, 158, 161, 164

Women in Africa and the Diaspora

Holding the World Together: African Women in Changing Perspective
Edited by Nwando Achebe and Claire Robertson

Engaging Modernity: Muslim Women and the Politics of Agency in Postcolonial Niger
Ousseina D. Alidou

Muslim Women in Postcolonial Kenya: Leadership, Representation, and Social Change
Ousseina D. Alidou

Silenced Resistance: Women, Dictatorships, and Genderwashing in Western Sahara and Equatorial Guinea
Joanna Allan

I Am Evelyn Amony: Reclaiming My Life from the Lord's Resistance Army
Evelyn Amony; edited and with an introduction by Erin Baines

Rising Anthills: African and African American Writing on Female Genital Excision, 1960–2000
Elisabeth Bekers

African Women Writing Resistance: An Anthology of Contemporary Voices
Edited by Jennifer Browdy de Hernandez, Pauline Dongala, Omotayo Jolaosho, and Anne Serafin

Genocide Lives in Us: Women, Memory, and Silence in Rwanda
Jennie E. Burnet

Tired of Weeping: Mother Love, Child Death, and Poverty in Guinea-Bissau
Jónína Einarsdóttir

Embodying Honor: Fertility, Foreignness, and Regeneration in Eastern Sudan
Amal Hassan Fadlalla

A Bold Profession: African Nurses in Rural Apartheid South Africa
LESLIE ANNE HADFIELD

Women's Organizations and Democracy in South Africa: Contesting Authority
SHIREEN HASSIM

Slave Trade and Abolition: Gender, Commerce,
and Economic Transition in Luanda
VANESSA S. OLIVEIRA

Gossip, Markets, and Gender: How Dialogue Constructs Moral Value
in Post-Socialist Kilimanjaro
TUULIKKI PIETILÄ

Claiming Civic Virtue: Gendered Network Memory in the
Mara Region, Tanzania
JAN BENDER SHETLER

Gendering Ethnicity in African Women's Lives
Edited by JAN BENDER SHETLER

Surviving the Slaughter: The Ordeal of a Rwandan Refugee in Zaire
MARIE BÉATRICE UMUTESI; translated by JULIA EMERSON